INTERNATIONAL HEALTH CARE MANAGEMENT

ADVANCES IN HEALTH CARE MANAGEMENT

Series Editors: John D. Blair, Myron D. Fottler and Grant T. Savage

ADVANCES IN HEALTH CARE MANAGEMENT   VOLUME 5

INTERNATIONAL HEALTH CARE MANAGEMENT

EDITED BY

GRANT T. SAVAGE
University of Alabama, AL, USA

JON A. CHILINGERIAN
Brandeis University, MA, USA

MICHAEL POWELL
Griffith University, Brisbane, Australia

ASSISTANT EDITOR

QIAN XIAO
University of Alabama, AL, USA

2005

ELSEVIER
JAI

Amsterdam – Boston – Heidelberg – London – New York – Oxford
Paris – San Diego – San Francisco – Singapore – Sydney – Tokyo

ELSEVIER B.V.
Radarweg 29
P.O. Box 211
1000 AE Amsterdam,
The Netherlands

ELSEVIER Inc.
525 B Street, Suite 1900
San Diego
CA 92101-4495
USA

ELSEVIER Ltd
The Boulevard, Langford
Lane, Kidlington
Oxford OX5 1GB
UK

ELSEVIER Ltd
84 Theobalds Road
London
WC1X 8RR
UK

First edition 2005

British Library Cataloguing in Publication Data
A catalogue record is available from the British Library.

ISBN: 0-7623-1228-9
ISSN: 1474-8231 (Series)

∞ The paper used in this publication meets the requirements of ANSI/NISO Z39.48-1992 (Permanence of Paper).
Printed in The Netherlands.

CONTENTS

v

LIST OF CONTRIBUTORS

Douglas Adam	Graduate School of Management, University of Western Australia, Australia
Volker Amelung	Hannover Medical School, Germany
Jonathan Broomberg	Praxis Capital, Houghton, South Africa
Jon A. Chilingerian	Heller School of Social Policy and Management, Brandeis University, USA
Rosina Cianelli	School of Nursing, Pontificia Universidad Católica de Chile, Chile
Michael A. Counte	School of Public Health, Saint Louis University, USA
Lilian M. Ferrer	School of Nursing, Pontificia Universidad Católica de Chile, Chile
Blair D. Gifford	School of Business, University of Colorado, Denver, USA
Michele Issel	School of Public Health, University of Illinois at Chicago, USA
Katharina Janus	Hannover Medical School, Germany
John R. Kimberly	Wharton School, University of Pennsylvania, USA
Angelina Kouroubali	Institute of Computer Science, Foundation for Research and Technology-Hellas, Crete, Greece
Shuen-Zen Liu	College of Management, National Taiwan University, Taiwan, Republic of China

Tim Mazzarol   Graduate School of Management,
                        University of Western Australia,
                        Australia

Anne Mills   Health Economics and Financing
                        Programme, London School of Hygiene
                        & Tropical Medicine, UK

Etienne Minvielle   INSERM and CNRS, Paris, France

Stelios C.   University of Crete-Heraklion and
Orphanoudakis   Foundation for Research and
                        Technology-Hellas, Crete,
                        Greece

Petri Parvinen   Executive School of Business, Helsinki
                        University of Technology, Finland

Michael Powell   Griffith Business School, Griffith
                        University, Australia

James C. Romeis   School of Public Health, Saint Louis
                        University, USA

Grant T. Savage   Culverhouse College of Commerce &
                        Business Administration, University of
                        Alabama, USA

Geoffrey N. Soutar   Graduate School of Management,
                        University of Western Australia,
                        Australia

Manolis Tsiknakis   Institute of Computer Science,
                        Foundation for Research and
                        Technology-Hellas, Crete, Greece

Pirkko Vartiainen   Department of Public Management,
                        University of Vaasa, Finland

Dimitris Vourvahakis   Foundation for Research and
                        Technology-Hellas, Crete, Greece

Rachel Collins Wilson   College of Business Administration,
                        University of Nebraska at Omaha,
                        USA

David Wood	ChinaCare Group, Beijing, People's Republic of China
Qian Xiao	Culverhouse College of Commerce & Business Administration, University of Alabama, USA

REVIEW BOARD MEMBERS

REVIEWERS

Sarita Bhalotra	Heller School of Social Policy and Management, Brandeis University, USA
Thomas D'Aunno	Health Care Management Initiative, INSEAD, France
Jullet Davis	Culverhouse College of Commerce & Business Administration, University of Alabama, USA
Michael Doonan	Heller School of Social Policy and Management, Brandeis University, USA
Myron D. Fottler	College of Health and Public Affairs, University of Central Florida, USA
Stephen Fournier	Royal Institute of Technology (KTH), Sweden
Leonard Friedman	College of Health and Human Sciences, Oregon State University, USA
Deborah Garnick	Schneider Institute for Health Policy, Brandeis University, USA
Tia Gilmartin	Health Care Management Initiative, INSEAD, France
Michele Kacmar	Culverhouse College of Commerce & Business Administration, University of Alabama, USA
Louis D. Marino	Culverhouse College of Commerce & Business Administration, University of Alabama, USA
Ann Scheck McAlearney	School of Public Health, Ohio State University, USA
Reuben R. McDaniel	College of Business and Administration, University of Texas at Austin, USA

Melissa Morley	Heller School of Social Policy and Management, Brandeis University, USA
Stephen O'Connor	School of Health Related Professions, University of Alabama at Birmingham, USA
Donald S. Shepard	Schneider Institute for Health Policy, Brandeis University, USA
Richard Shewchuk	School of Health Related Professions, University of Alabama at Birmingham, USA
Sharon Topping	College of Business Administration, University of Southern Mississippi, USA
Eric Williams	Culverhouse College of Commerce & Business Administration, University of Alabama, USA
Jacqueline Zinn	Fox School of Business and Management, Temple University, USA

PREFACE: A FRAMEWORK FOR THE DEVELOPING FIELD OF INTERNATIONAL HEALTH CARE MANAGEMENT

WHAT CAN WE LEARN FROM AN INTERNATIONAL PERSPECTIVE ON HEALTH CARE MANAGEMENT?

We hope this research volume will change the way scholars and managers think about health care management in two fundamental ways. First, we want to challenge the superficial separations between national and international health care management. To dissolve these distinctions, the "not-invented-here" or "who cares about a Belgian, Indian, or Thai medical center," or "that won't work in our policy system" attitudes must change. Second, we want scholars and managers to learn how to transfer innovative ideas and management practices across cultures and around policy barriers. Cultural, language, and policy differences present formidable barriers, but we believe lessons about managing human resources, informatics, quality, services, and strategies in health care organizations can be transferred.

International health care management is a multidisciplinary field that examines how health care organizations can become more effective from a global perspective. There are good reasons why health care management should become international in scope. Increasingly, Asian, African, and South American philosophy and management approaches are forcing European and North American companies to learn and adapt their strategies, production and quality control systems, human resource practices, and managerial ideas. Business managers in service, manufacturing, and other sectors have discovered that they are not only competing with the best in the world, but they can learn from the best in the world. In other words, if managerial ideas learned from global experiences can be transferred in the business world, the same should hold true for health care organizations.

Moreover, we believe programs educating health care managers should include this international learning perspective. Globalization in health care delivery is an infant enterprise. However, if current trends continue, the future will see more and more health care delivery becoming and remaining international. Many nations may believe they have a high-performing and well-managed health care systems. However, information becomes evidence only by showing data in relation to other data, and international comparisons are necessary. Only the measurement and reporting of health care organization performance, comprehensive case studies of management practices and organizational behaviors, and other international comparisons can substantiate the claims of the superiority of one or another country's health system. Moreover, international comparisons of health care organizations can uncover strategic and operational performance differences that remain hidden in analyses of organizations and "best practices" within a single country.

A FRAMEWORK FOR UNDERSTANDING INTERNATIONAL HEALTH CARE MANAGEMENT

We have selected papers from around the world that attempt to make sense of the complex environments and organizations that provide health services and that draw lessons for health care management, both from a theoretical and a practical perspective. Authors from Australia, Chile, Finland, France, Germany, Greece, South Africa, Taiwan, the United Kingdom, and the United States of America are included in this volume. They explore the delivery and organization of care in health systems from Africa, Asia, Australia, Europe, North America, and South America, encompassing over 20 countries in their comparisons. The papers included in this volume were only accepted following a rigorous peer-review process. Each paper, whether solicited or responding to our open call, went through a double-blind review and revision process. The result is a select collection of outstanding papers.

When we initially envisioned this research volume, we issued a broad call for papers that would address the following issues:

- Globalization and the development of international health care markets
- Innovative management practices in the coordination of care
- Identification and evaluation of clinical best practices
- Innovations in care programs or delivery systems
- Emerging new consumer segments and service strategies
- Focused factories and/or the privatization of health care delivery
- Innovative organizational designs, management practices, and governance structures

- Managing of quality health care
- Changing roles of health professionals
- Impact of information or innovative technologies on performance.

We were delighted to receive contributions that addressed many of these issues, but then faced the dilemma of determining how best to organize such a diverse set of papers! Fig. 1 represents our attempt to frame the contributions of this research volume into three sections: patients and providers, policy, and performance. Patients and providers of health care services are key stakeholders in any health system; hence, the issues that face these stakeholders often are universal. Nonetheless, each nation has particular population needs, wants, and demands that influence patient behaviors. In turn, providers struggle to address patient needs, wants, and demands using various strategies, structures, and behaviors.

Health policy traditionally has focused on the issues of access, quality, and cost. From an international management perspective, health care policies create the institutional rules and incentives for health care organizations and their patients. Understanding how organizational and individual actions are constrained and enabled by health policy decisions is important to both providers and patients, respectively. Lastly, every nation is

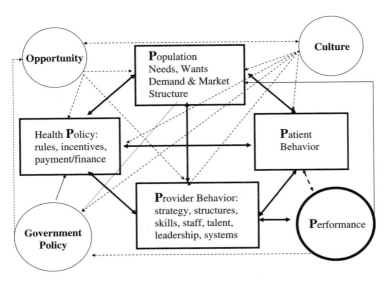

Fig. 1.   Framework for the Volume.

concerned about the performance and management of its health care organizations. Questions of organizational efficiency and effectiveness are the focus of many debates among health care policy makers, managers, and scholars. These debates encompass concerns ranging from health care quality to the use of information technology to human resource management.

OVERVIEW OF THE VOLUME

This fifth volume of *Advances in Health Care Management* consists of 12 papers, one of which serves as an introduction, with the other papers arranged into three sections based on the framework shown in Fig. 1. The first section on patients and providers focuses on such issues as how socio-cultural forces affect health care experiences; how hospital providers function differently under various governance structures; how global strategies affect providers and patients; and why and how provider organizations should consider integrating within a health delivery system. The second section on policy and management addresses such dilemmas as whether some health care issues are impossible to solve through traditional policy reforms; how international refugees' should receive health care; and whether policy reform lessons from other countries can be adapted and applied to transform another country's health system. The third and final section on performance and management addresses issues such as whether the quality of care can be managed at the hospital level; how human resource management can be benchmarked within and across health care organizations; how health care informatics can improve the continuity of care; and whether different ways of accessing care within health systems can be systemically compared and improved.

As an introduction, Jon A. Chilingerian and Grant T. Savage address why international health care management is emerging as an important field of study among scholars and a significant concern to health care managers. Their discussion of international health care management examines seven issues: global business blindness; global challenges and opportunities; meta-national knowledge management; best practice sharing; lessons lost in translation; learning from worst cases; and learning from an international perspective.

Patients and Providers

How do socio-cultural forces affect health care experiences? Lilian M. Ferrer, Michele Issel, and Rosina Cianelli, use patient narratives to reveal organizational and managerial issues related to providing ethical and quality HIV/AIDS health care in Chile. The purpose of their study is to understand, from the perspective of FONASA (National Health Fund) users, key problems with FONASA and to identify the strategies that HIV/AIDS advocacy groups and activists use to make those problems known. They begin by providing background information on the HIV/AIDS epidemic in Chile and its neighboring countries, with particular attention to the Chilean health system. Ferrer, Issel, and Cianelli use patient and activists' narratives to develop a conceptual model of the forces for change that includes stakeholders, strategies, and targets of change. Importantly, this model advances the notion of organizational environmental dynamism. The need for managing organizational culture and change, with consideration of equity, access, and quality of basic health care, are consistent with the renewed emphasis by the Pan American Health Organization and World Health Organization (2003) on health system responsiveness. The construct of environmental dynamism has international applicability, particularly to governmental health systems that are influenced by strong socio-cultural forces.

What can hospital providers learn by making significant comparisons between different governance structures? Anne Mills and Jonathan Broomberg compare management differences in structures, styles, and incentives among three different groups of South African hospitals: public hospitals; contractor hospitals publicly funded but privately managed; and private hospitals owned and run by private companies. These comparisons illuminate how these differences in management structure, style, and incentives affected hospital functioning, including cost per patient and various quality indicators. They found that individual hospitals rank consistently by group, with contractor hospitals the lowest cost, then public, and then private. Although public hospitals in South Africa are, in general, better equipped and staffed, they have worse standards of maintenance and cleanliness than contractor hospitals. Nursing quality is systematically better in the contractor hospitals. Mills and Broomberg conclude that there is potential for governments in transitional economies to profit from the management expertise in the private sector by contracting out service management. In addition, they discuss improving public hospital management by delegating substantial management authority to the hospital level, making changes to the structure and functioning of management teams at both hospital and head office level, and paying attention to the incentives facing hospital and head office managers.

How should health care organizations think about global strategy? Blair D. Gifford and David Wood focus on the primary strategies that would be used to enter an international market for the American health care firms deciding to globalize their product or service lines. The paper examines the differing market entry and early development strategies into the Chinese hospital market by two American-based hospital development companies. These firms' market entry strategies range from "greenfield" operations, where the hospital does little to change its corporate and managerial style from what it uses domestically, to a localization strategy, where the firm is quite sensitive to fitting into the Chinese culture and being accepted by the Chinese government. Gifford and Wood conclude that what is learned from the experiences of enterprising American hospital firms in China may well portend the future for international developments by many other Western-based health organizations. Their contribution also highlights the potential for developing and testing strategic theories of international health care management.

Many countries are thinking about integrated delivery systems – but how much effort is needed to develop an integrated health system? Examining recent experiences in the San Francisco Bay area, Katharina Janus and Volker Amelung end this section with an investigation of why integrated health care delivery (IHCD) offers appropriate care, but fails to provide efficient health care. They draw extensively upon transaction cost economics to explore a new understanding of IHCD, which focuses on actual integration through virtual integration instead of aggregation of health care entities. With the emergence of information technology and the trend toward maintaining looser but coordinated relationships, virtual integration combines various care services provided by separate – but seamlessly organized – entities that offer services under contract to each other. Janus and Amelung conclude with a discussion of the implications of virtual IHCD for the German health system, highlighting lessons that may be valuable for other health systems that rely extensively on social health insurance.

Policy and Management

Are some health care issues impossible to solve through reforms? This section on policy opens with Pirkko Vartiainen's exploration of the wickedness of health care management issues through an analysis of Finnish and Swedish health care reforms. The concept of a wicked issue can be described as a policy problem that is difficult to identify and solve through linear thinking and singular policy reforms. The reason for choosing the concept of wicked issues as the framework for this study is the hypothesis that most serious health care management problems are wicked problems. As

Vartiainen examines how health care management deals with system-wide problems, he focuses on solutions and new styles of managing that have been introduced to solve these problems in Finland and Sweden, illustrating how the concept of wicked health care issues helps to explain and understand the social complexity involved in health care policy and management.

How should international refugees' health issues be handled? Rachel Collins Wilson focuses on the health care policy and systemic financial ramifications of refugee and asylum-seeker influx in seven countries: Iran, the United Kingdom, Serbia and Montenegro, Germany, Guinea, the United States, and the Gaza Strip/West Bank region. Her article identifies each country's issues, policies, and strategies regarding refugee health, and presents the short-term tactics and long-term strategies undertaken to care for the refugees. She examines the refugee problems and the international efforts that are in place to aid countries around the world in their assistance to refugees, focusing on the multilateral, bilateral, and nongovernmental organizations outside the host countries. To evaluate the refugee health care practice of countries used as focal examples in the paper, she employs a model of a sound health care management system. Wilson concludes by discussing the major issues – including resource development, coordination activity, and outcome measurement – and recommends a set of strategies for moving toward effective policies for refugee care.

What works and what does not work in health care? James C. Romeis, Shuen-Zen Liu, and Michael A. Counte close the policy section with a review and reflection on a decade of comparative health system research. They focus on Taiwan's changing policies for its delivery system and the selected adaptations of health care management by providers, as well as patients. Following a general description of the changes in Taiwan's health policy, they provide research findings from two previously published studies as an indication of methods and outcomes of comparative health services research. Romeis, Liu, and Counte call attention to such horizon issues as managing financing and implementing quality mechanisms, and draw an interesting conclusion: when socio-cultural forces are taken into consideration with appropriate cultural adjustments, a policy reform that has never worked in one country could work in another country.

Performance Management

Can quality of care be managed at the hospital level? Etienne Minvielle and John R. Kimberly examine this question by describing and analyzing the current reforms in the French system of "assurance maladie," or its health insurance system. Their work is particularly significant since the "iron triangle" in health care – the relationship among, and concern about, cost, quality, and access – has stimulated manifold initiatives around the globe for the measurement and management of hospital performance and quality. The measurement and management of quality play a vital role in the French reforms, thus providing a particularly timely example for policy makers, researchers, and managers in health care to consider. The COMPAQH Project, featuring in the current French reforms, is designed to identify a set of Quality Indicators (QI) that could be generalized to all French hospitals. Minvielle and Kimberly demonstrate that many lessons about culture and health care management can be learned from the French experience.

If management is about getting work done through people, it is an understatement to say that people are the most important asset in health care services. Tim Mazzarol, Geoffrey N. Soutar, and Douglas Adam outline the design and development of a diagnostic tool for use in health care organizations to assist in benchmarking the management of human resources. To begin with, a five-part HRM framework for the effective management of people with measurable performance indicators was identified: work organization, leadership, availability for work, utilization of people, and performance development. Using a cross-section of metropolitan and regional health services, the study used focus groups and large-scale survey research to capture data on the way in which employees perceived their work roles, work loads, satisfaction with their work life, and their views of clients, peers, front line supervisors, and senior management. The diagnostic tool developed in the present study provides a potentially useful way to measure employee perceptions and attitudes that can supplement existing HR performance indicators.

What is the role of informatics in the performance management of health care organizations and systems? Manolis Tsiknakis, Angelina Kouroubali, Dimitris Vourvahakis, and Stelios C. Orphanoudakis try to answer this question by focusing on the common problems facing all industrialized countries: chronic illnesses and the continuous aging of the population. They conclude that health care delivery organizations should be redesigned around relationships and exchanges of information to address patient needs within local and regional communities. They analyze the impact of HYGEIAnet, an integrated regional health information network in Crete, on health care performance. The fundamental objective of HYGEIAnet is to enable information sharing and medical collaboration among all stakeholders of the regional health economy and assist in the re-organization of the health care system based on innovative technological solutions and e-health services. Novel e-health services were deployed such as prehospital emergency services; home tele-management of patients; e-health services, and an integrated e-health record. Tsiknakis and his colleagues demonstrate that advanced IT strategies can provide significant economic and quality of care benefits if they are well executed and managed.

How should people access health services? Petri Parvinen and Grant T. Savage examine seven industrialized countries and provide an overview of some institutional characteristics of their health systems. They compare the different modes of financing national health systems with how each system structures access to primary and specialist care. Parvinen and Savage define and categorize health care access systems, identify the components of a health care access system, explore the notion of a strategic fit between health care financing systems and access system configurations; and propose that the health care access system is a key determinant of process-level cost efficiency. By systematically examining the experiences in seven health systems, Parvinen and Savage develop three propositions: (1) the attributes of the health care access system are correlated with health care spending and costs; (2) the fit between the health care access and financing systems affects system- and process-level efficiency in health care; and (3) health care access systems differ in their patient and process-level efficiency.

CONCLUSION

Clearly, learning from the best in the world, borrowing best practices, sharing expertise, or even globalization of health care are not new ideas, but challenge our assumptions, our cultural biases, and our theories about health care management. We believe that if scholars and managers can draw on the lessons from health care management from other nations and systems, they will better achieve the goals of improving quality, providing services efficiently, and implementing innovative care practices.

Jon A. Chilingerian, Guest Editor
Grant T. Savage, Series Editor
Michael Powell, Guest Editor
Qian Xiao, Assistant Editor

INTRODUCTION

THE EMERGING FIELD OF INTERNATIONAL HEALTH CARE MANAGEMENT: AN INTRODUCTION

Jon A. Chilingerian and Grant T. Savage

ABSTRACT

To underscore the significance of international health care management, we focus on three themes: the problem of global blindness; global health care challenges and opportunities; and learning from international health care management. The problem of global blindness highlights how health care managers' inattentional blindness to competitors' operational performance and market strategies lead to avoidable and expensive failures. To address global challenges and opportunities, health care organizations are employing two different strategies: (1) building and marketing a world-class health care facility internationally, and (2) organizing and integrating multinational health care operations. The first strategy exploits the medical-tourism market. The second strategy requires either multinational health care networks or transnational health care organizations. One of the lessons to be learned from international health care management is that an organization can create a meta-national competitive advantage. Another lesson is that by examining best practices from around the world, health care organizations can obtain new insights and

International Health Care Management
Advances in Health Care Management, Volume 5, 3–28
ISSN: 1474-8231/doi:10.1016/S1474-8231(05)05001-9

3

become more innovative within their home markets. A corollary and third lesson is that while health care organizations can learn a great deal from examining international best clinical practices, sometimes the most important management lessons are lost in clinical translations. The fourth and last lesson is that worst cases – serious international management failures – offer perhaps the most valuable insights into the role of culture, complexity, and leadership for health care organizations.

INTRODUCTION

Health is a worldwide pursuit. If health policy provides the beacon for health aspirations and action, it is the medical care system that directly touches the lives of people and affects the economy of every nation. Medical care systems are complex networks of providers and patients, impressive technologies, and communities of clinical practices that benefit people by increasing their longevity and their quality of life. The health system in every country faces two basic questions: (1) how much money should be allocated to health, and (2) how can a nation be sure that their medical care system is well managed, achieving ready access and high quality at a reasonable – or politically acceptable – cost?

The sources of financing the medical care system are largely determined by a nation's health policy decisions. In addition to paying something out-of-pocket, every health care system relies primarily on one of the three sources of health financing: (1) taxes (e.g., Australia, Italy, and the United Kingdom), (2) social security funds (e.g., France, the Netherlands, and Japan), or (3) private health insurance (e.g., Switzerland and the United States). Although health is a universal pursuit, the health policy issues in underdeveloped, transitional, welfare state, socialist, and free enterprise countries are different (Roemer, 1977; Raffel, 1997). The challenge of promoting access in developing nations is very different from that of controlling health care costs. Whether to reduce health disparities or to deal with capacity problems and bottlenecks, policymakers typically try to improve the availability of health services.

The rapid increase in health care expenditures has led to a variety of policy experiments in every industrialized country, including balancing public and private coverage, mixing for-profit and not-for-profit providers, and experimenting with market forces and various degrees of regulation.

These experiments include highly centralized payment and management structures, formularies for pharmaceuticals, price controls, and provider payment systems, and a variety of managed care ideas such as global budgets, capitation payments to providers, and/or restricted patient access to selected clinics, hospitals, and specialty care (Raffel, 1997). While successful at improving the availability of care, virtually every nation's policy attempts to remedy rising costs have failed. Health care costs, and hospital costs in particular, continue to rise in every country (Preker & Harding, 2003). This state of affairs suggests that policy reforms can only address certain aspects of the iron triangle of access, cost, and quality. Comparative studies of international health care management, illuminate not only why many health reforms fall short, but also delineate innovative ways to improve the quality and the efficiency of health care delivery.

This chapter is divided into four sections. The first section lays out the case for studying international care management. The second section addresses the problem of global blindness, highlighting how health care managers' inattentional blindness to competitors' operational performance and market strategies lead to avoidable and expensive failures. The third section explores global health care challenges and opportunities. To address global challenges and opportunities, health care organizations are employing two different strategies: (1) building and marketing a world-class health care facility internationally, and (2) organizing and integrating multinational health care operations. The first strategy exploits the medical-tourism market. The second strategy requires either multi-national health care networks or transnational health care organizations. The fourth and final section discusses how we can learn from international health care management. One of the lessons to be learned from international health care management is that an organization can create a meta-national competitive advantage. Another lesson is that by examining best practices from around the world, health care organizations can obtain new insights and become more innovative within their home markets. A corollary and third lesson is that while health care organizations can learn a great deal from examining international best clinical practices, sometimes the most important management lessons are lost in clinical translations. The fourth and last lesson is that sometimes managers and clinicians can learn more from the worst mistakes than from best practices (Walshe & Shortell, 2004). The worst cases – serious international management failures – offer perhaps the most valuable insights into the role of culture, complexity, and leadership for health care organizations.

THE CASE FOR INTERNATIONAL HEALTH CARE MANAGEMENT

The desire to improve health care can be seen in the unrelenting increase in the quantity of health products and services available to patients. Yet, even with these increases, health care seems to offer fewer perceived benefits to patients in relation to their perceived sacrifices (see Anderson, Reinhardt, Hussey, & Petrosyan, 2003; Bristol Royal Infirmary Inquiry, 2001; New-house, 2002). Hence, one of our core arguments is that for a medical care system to perform, management matters.

A recent five-country comparison of outcomes concluded that while every country performed better than the rest in a few areas, every country could improve their outcomes in other areas (Hussey et al., 2004). As one econ-omist has proclaimed, "Despite the lack of a summary measure of its ef-ficiency, many seem convinced that the industry's performance falls short" (Newhouse, 2002, p. 14).

Figures 1 and 2 tell an interesting story about the United States. In 2000, although the United States spent more per capita than any other country, the World Health Organization (WHO, 2000) ranked its performance 37th overall. The United States continues to provide the most money for health spending; however, citizens of Italy, France, and Japan pay much lower prices for the same health care services and outperform the United States.

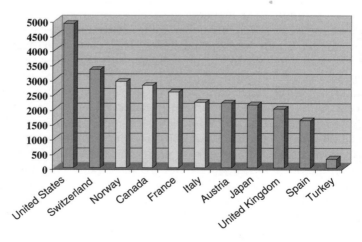

Fig. 1. Per Capita Expenditure on Healthcare (Purchasing Power Parity Interna-tional Dollars). OECD Data, 2002.

- 1 — France
- 2 — Italy
- 3 — San Marino
- 4 — Andorra
- 5 — Malta
- 6 — Singapore
- 7 — Spain
- 8 — Oman
- 9 — Austria
- 10 — Japan

- 11 — Norway
- 18 — United Kingdom
- 20 — Switzerland
- 22 — Columbia

- 30 — Canada
- 36 — Costa Rica
- 37 — United States of America
- 38 — Slovenia

Fig. 2. WHO National Ranking of Overall Health System Performance. The World Health Report 2000.

For example, while breast cancer survival rates in the United States are higher than in other countries, asthma mortality rates are increasing, and transplant survival rates are lower than in other countries (Hussey et al., 2004). Moreover, the number of physicians per 1000 population, primary care visits per capita, acute beds per capita, hospital admissions per capita, and hospital days per capita were below the median of most other developed countries (Anderson et al., 2003).

Are the quality and productive efficiency of some national health care systems really lower than that of many other industrialized nations? Does health care management account for these performance differences? A recent international poll of 538 hospital executives from Australia, Canada, New Zealand, United Kingdom, and the United States revealed that all executives perceived inadequate funding, reimbursement, and staffing shortages as major problems (Blendon et al., 2004). Moreover, the executives from every country (except the United States) reported that their facilities were a major problem.

In January 2005, a group of 30 international health care leaders were discussing the kinds of strategic decisions they were currently making with the senior author. Their list of strategic decisions included the following:

- outsourcing of diagnostic services;
- nurse staffing;
- creating regional alliances with some health care organizations versus competing with others;
- integrating the continuum of services under one structure;
- coordination of primary and acute care;
- rationalizing and closing down specialty services in a hospital system; and
- achieving 2–5% reductions in financial targets.

Although the payment and financing systems and rules and regulations that this group of executives faced were vastly different, everyone agreed that the major health care management issues were similar and familiar to everyone. Everyone shared an interest in measuring, reporting, and improving their performance, and making information on management practices available to each other. These executives believed there was an advantage in learning how these management problems were being solved around the world.

THE CHALLENGE OF GLOBAL BLINDNESS

To survive in a world economy, businesses have had to learn some hard lessons about benchmarking their performance against their global competitors. Pride and success can lead to global blindness – a lack of attention to competitors' sales, markets, and production approaches. Although many businesses have learned some hard lessons about international management from their competitors, often these business failures have developed gradually, not exponentially. Typically, long before these failures appeared on the financial statements, the problems were embedded in the culture of these organizations.

The story of the discovery and marketing of the anti-ulcerant, cimetidine, is a case in point. In 1972, Dr. James Black, a scientist working at a British lab for the pharmaceutical company SmithKline, discovered a new class of anti-ulcerants called H2-antagonists.[1] By 1976, SmithKline had launched the new drug called Tagamet (cimetidine), which by 1981 accounted for $780 million of SmithKline's sales.

In 1986, SmithKline's competitor in the United Kingdom, Glaxo Holdings plc, despite being priced 20–75% higher, overtook Tagamet in global sales with an essentially similar drug called Zantac. Zantac became the first drug to earn one billion dollars in global pharmaceutical sales, despite the fact that the FDA noted that Zantac offered little or no contribution over Tagamet. In 1989, as Dr. James Black was awarded a Nobel Prize in Medicine for cimetidine, Zantac dominated 42% of the worldwide market, beating Tagamet's sales in Italy, the United Kingdom, the United States, France, and Japan. How could SmithKline, with first mover advantage, patent protection, and a Nobel Prize, have lost the battle for global sales?

In the early 1980s, the United States was 37% of the worldwide market. Tagamet easily captured 90% of sales in the United States. As Angelmar and Pinson (1992) observed: "News from Europe slowly made its way to the SmithKline organization in the US...the news tended to emphasize

Tagamet's continued sales progression in Europe, and its good showing in the UK" (p. 9). Strategic thinking must make sense out of temporal patterns such as changes in sales as they unfold. According to one psychologist, human beings appear to have difficulty seeing and interpreting developments over time (Dörner, 1989). Between 1982 and 1989, Glaxo was steadily eroding SmithKline's market share; however, its managers appeared to hardly notice until it was too late.

When Glaxo first heard about Dr. Black's discovery, it decided to improve on Tagamet. By 1978, Glaxo had begun clinical trials in 20 countries, and by 1981 it had launched Zantac. Since its research revealed that physicians saw Zantac as a similar drug with no added medical benefit, they simplified the dosage regiment to once-a-day and although the marketing division wanted to price it 10% below Tagamet's daily treatment cost, the CEO insisted on charging a 75% higher price. Based on published studies, Glaxo positioned the drug as having superior effectiveness with the tag line: "faster, simpler, and safer." Lastly, Glaxo had a much stronger international sales force than SmithKline, having created co-marketing alliances with companies in Japan, Germany, and France.

There are two explanations for Zantac's success. First, Glaxo managed this product better than SmithKline managed Tagamet. Second, the early commercial success of Tagamet led to "inattentional blindness" (Simons & Chabris, 1999) within SmithKline. The lesson of inattentional blindness is that it is necessary to pay attention to competitive responses in retrospect. However, proud organizations court psychological denial and cynical reactions to threatening information; unless someone influential draws attention to the threatening information, the patterns will neither be seen nor understood.

Although there is a great deal to learn from studying health care management around the world, global blindness is a challenge to be overcome. As we will discuss in some depth, domestic borders are not an insurmountable barrier to health care delivery. Some health care organizations are thinking globally, deciding on the countries in which they want to operate, and whether they will partner, license, or even franchise their medical care knowledge. In the next section, we discuss some global health trends.

GLOBAL HEALTH CARE: NEW CHALLENGES AND OPPORTUNITIES

A global strategy is one in which a health care organization targets patients across national borders and employs some type of integrated health care management (see Porter, 1990). Comparative advantage, when applied to health care, refers to significant differences in one nation's cost, quality, or access such that health activities or services could be offered elsewhere in the world. Porter (1987, p. 45) argues that "the global competitor can locate activities wherever comparative advantage lies, decoupling comparative advantage from the firm's home base or country of ownership."

A good example of relocating a primary clinical activity is using radiologists located in Australia, India, Israel, and Lebanon to read patient X-rays, CAT scans, and MRIs performed in the United States (Pollack, 2003). For many small hospitals with low demand, paying $50 per investigation saves on the salary of a full-time radiologist, or paying a physician to work on a third shift from midnight to daylight. A medical director summarizes this advantage: "We used to do maybe three or four a night after midnight, and now we do in the range of 60 CAT scans after hours" (Tanner, 2004, p. 2).

Doz and his co-workers (2001) have identified a three-phase evolution of global strategies. Phase one is to build on the innovations and the financial success of a high-performing domestic organization. During phase two, organizations leverage their domestic success on a global scale, first by offering low-cost services to nearby culturally homogeneous markets to maximize revenue and minimize costs. Gradually they expand and move production to countries with lower factors costs as their products mature. The third, and final phase, is to expand into more markets by balancing local responsiveness with global integration, generating both economies of scale and scope, where being local accommodates cultural and customer desires.

The belief that health care is a local is being swept away by an emerging international market (Burns, D'Aunno, & Kimberly, 2004). The digital age has begun to link patients, providers, and payers previously unknown to each other (Lerer & Piper, 2003). If any document on the internet is an average of 19 clicks away from any other document (Barbasi, 2003), there is a potential for collaboration and communication, global learning via alliances, shared services, and shared medical talent pools. If global organizations organize their services for world markets, how international is health care?

Two Global Health Care Delivery Strategies

There are two global health care delivery strategies: (1) build a world-class health care facility domestically and market it to international patients; or

(2) organize multinational health care operations with varying degrees of integration. If we measure a global health care organization by geographic distributions of sales (i.e., patient care delivered outside the country), some health care organizations would qualify as more internationally developed. Although most hospitals that promote international patients have less than 10% of their patients from foreign countries, there are some interesting exceptions. One example is Shouldice Hospital in Canada, where only 56% of the patients are Canadian; most of the rest are from nearby, English-speaking United States (42%), while the remaining 2% come from Europe (Urquhart & O'Dell, 2004). Another example is Bumrungrad Hospital in Bangkok, with five-star hotel services and accreditation from the Joint Commission for International Accreditation; it treated 300,000 international patients from 154 countries in 2002, accounting for 37% of its patient revenues (Intel Corporation, 2004).

Moreover, global medical-tourism business is beginning to blossom. For many years, patients from the Middle East, Latin American and Asia have come to the United States, Canada, Germany, France, and Belgium for health care. Medical centers in the United States, such as Johns Hopkins Medical Services Corporation (Johns Hopkins Hospital, Baltimore, MD), The Cleveland Clinic Foundation (Cleveland, OH), The Methodist Hospitals (Houston, TX), and the Mayo Clinic (Rochester, MN) market their services to attract foreign patients. However, in 2002, the United States reported a drop in international patient revenues from Saudi Arabia and the United Arab Emirates between $750 million and $1.25 billion (Landers, 2002). Patients are not only going to the United States, Canada, and Western Europe, but are also going to Thailand, Malaysia, and India for their health care. One of the leading providers of health care in developing countries is the Apollo Hospital Group of India.

Understanding the Demand for International Health Services

Why would people from England, Canada, and other parts of the world go to Thailand, Singapore, or India for health care? Apollo's service concept is to offer low cost and immediate access for people who want to avoid lengthy waits and high cost alternatives. One patient from Canada facing a lengthy one-year wait for a hip replacement went to Apollo and paid a total of $4,500 for the entire procedure versus an average price of $15,000 or more in Western Europe or the United States (Solomon, 2004).

Lengthy waits can be psychologically and physically damaging to older patients. For example, a study conducted in Scotland of older people needing hip and knee replacements found that patients were waiting as long as 30 months and non-urgent cases waited as long as 78 months (Roy & Hunter, 1996). These patients experienced great pain, mobility restrictions, an inability to go out or climb stairs, and one-fourth had been forced to retire. A Canadian study of patients waiting for hip and knee replacements found that some patients had been waiting up to three years (Williams et al., 1997). Another study of cataract patients from Canada, Denmark and Spain were asked if they would be willing to pay out of pocket to shorten their wait times (Anderson, Modrow, & Tan, 1997). Approximately 38% of the Canadians, 17% of the Danes, and 29% of the Spanish were willing to pay $500 for a shorter wait.

In July 2002, the British Medical Association conducted a survey of 2,000 adults in the United Kingdom. These citizens, entitled to free care from the National Health Service (NHS), were asked how far they would be willing to travel if they faced a lengthy wait for health care services. More than 40% were willing to travel outside the United Kingdom; 15% would travel anywhere in Europe; and 26% would travel anywhere in the world (Beecham, 2002). For citizens within the European Union, the right to travel abroad to receive health care stems from a 1988 ruling by the European Court of Justice. The now famous Kohl and Dekker cases established that health care resources should be treated as any other part of the European Union economy with regard to the free movement of goods and services. Patients can seek treatment across borders unless the same treatment can be provided conveniently within their own country.

Three Successful Approaches to Global Organization

Doz, Santos, and Williamson (2001) argue that there are three basic approaches to global organization, based on the degree of standardization versus customization. This model can be adapted to health care organizations. In Fig. 3, each quadrant is a response to the integration-adaptation dilemma. The strategy represented in the bottom left quadrant would only require a health care organization to buy or build a health facility in another country. This strategy would not draw on the health care organization's domestic advantages through sharing services or transferring clinical or non-clinical knowledge. If the hospital or facility was successful, the international organization would hold it; if it was not, the international

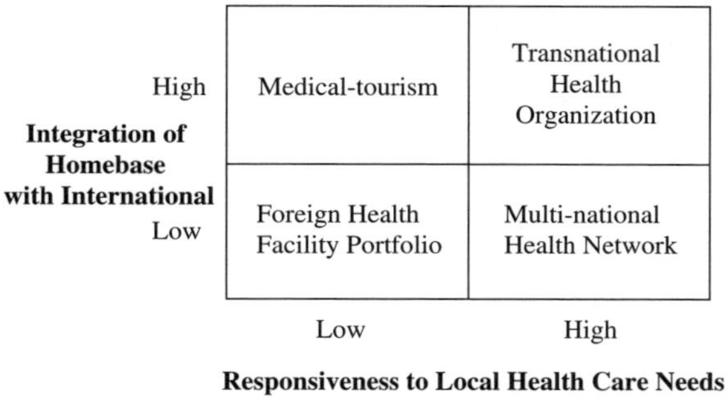

High	Medical-tourism	Transnational Health Organization
Low	Foreign Health Facility Portfolio	Multi-national Health Network

Integration of Homebase with International

Low	High

Responsiveness to Local Health Care Needs

Fig. 3. Multinational Strategy: Standardization versus Adaptation. Source: Adapted from Doz et al. (2003).

organization would divest it. However, several hospital chains that have tried this low-intensity international strategy have not been successful (Burns, D'Aunno, & Kimberly, 2004).

The upper left quadrant emphasizes scale efficiency with a high degree of coordination. This may be where most health care organizations are today that engage in international services. For example, most U.S. academic medical centers have an international one-stop shopping office with airport pick-up, appointment coordination, diagnostic, surgical, and medical services. Other health care organizations draw on added benefits to attract foreign patients. For instance, Phuket International Hospital (2005) advertises that it provides "high quality and cost efficient hospital services, coupled with the warmth and caring nature that only true Thai hospitality can provide."

The multi-national network form in the bottom right quadrant emphasizes a high degree of local adaptation. A leading example is United Healthcare's partnership with BUPA International, which offers expatriates a strong network of facilities worldwide. Multi-lingual help is available 24 hours a day, along with air ambulance services and medical advice from English-speaking physicians.

The transnational form in the upper right quadrant emphasizes both domestic integration and a high degree of local adaptation. Galbraith argues that international development occurs when an organization "creates more assets and employees outside the home country, thereby enlarging the role that its subsidiaries can play in contributing and leading in the creation of the firm's advantages" (1998, p. 104). By this measure there are just a few examples of global health care organizations that have begun to uncover the value of a transnational approach. Two will be discussed: Apollo Hospital of India and Sweden's Capio.

Apollo Hospital

In 1983, Dr. Prathap C. Reddy, founder and chair of the Apollo Hospital Group, launched its first private 150-bed hospital in Chennai, India. The website for Apollo now states: "Our mission is to bring health care of international standards within the reach of every individual...we are now in a position to offer our services to people throughout the world" (http://www.apollohospitalgroup.com/mission.htm). This mission statement has become a credible threat to domestic health care delivery in Asia, where Apollo has become one of Asia's largest private health care providers.

Apollo offers health services in India and abroad, through a network of 36 hospitals, 46 clinics, 135 pharmacies, and 35 telemedicine centers, as well as managed care plans. Apollo has defined a global strategy to make India the preferred global healthcare destination, targeting the Middle East, South East Asia, CIS countries, and parts of Africa, Pakistan, Bangladesh, Nepal, and Myanmar. It has telemedicine centers in Kazakistan, Sudan, and Ethiopia, and it is providing managed care in Mauritius, Ghana, Nigeria, Kuwait, Malaysia, and Nepal.

Capio

Most recent health care acquisitions in Europe have taken place within single domestic markets such as Germany or France. Between 1997 and 2001, Capio, founded in Sweden in 1994, acquired hospitals throughout Europe, including 17 hospitals in Sweden, 12 in Norway, 3 in the United Kingdom, 12 in Spain, and 1 in Switzerland, and 1 in Denmark. Today Capio has become Europe's leading independent provider of hospital services, specialty hospitals, and diagnostic clinics.

Capio's global strategy blends European standardization (large-scale efficient hospitals and clinics) with local labor/local services. By applying a rigorous business model based on putting people first, standardized care processes, benchmarking best practices, performance aimed at the "right quality" at the lowest price, redesign of clinical jobs, medical, operational, and financial scorecards, and management of patient and employee satisfaction, Capio has been both efficient and profitable (see http://www.capio.com/BusinessInformation/).

LEARNING FROM INTERNATIONAL HEALTH CARE MANAGEMENT

Meta-National Knowledge Management in Health Care

Doz, Santos, and Williamson (2001) have identified a new competitive capability they call meta-national advantage. A meta-national organization has an ability to acquire knowledge scattered worldwide and a capacity to create innovative services and systems. By transcending home country boundaries, these multi-cultural organizations not only respect cultural and geographic differences, they turn diversity into success. Today the opportunity to learn from around the world has never been greater. Health care managers and policymakers have an opportunity to find, mobilize, and transfer medical knowledge, clinical knowledge and expertise, and management practices from the best in the world. Moreover, medical innovations have always been scattered around the world. Three examples of the diffusion of medical knowledge follow.

Organ Transplants
Transplantation is a highly effective therapy, but until the 1980s the idea of transplanting organs was considered a dream. During World War II, Dr. Peter Medawar observed skin grafts on soldiers in England, and began breakthrough research on foreign tissue rejection. During 1954, the first kidney transplant took place with identical twins in Boston, and Dr. Christian Barnard at Groote Schuur Hospital in Cape Town, South Africa, performed the first heart transplant in 1967. However, few organ transplants were performed until the 1980s when a new immunosuppressant drug called, cyclosporine, was approved for use. Although cyclosporine was discovered in 1970 from a Norwegian soil fungus by Jean F. Borel at Sandoz laboratories in Switzerland, it took many years to be put it into practice (Chilingerian & Vanderkerckhove, 2005, in press).

Kangaroo Mother Care
Neo-natal intensive care is very expensive, and often is unavailable in developing countries. In 1978, Bogota, Columbia, did not have enough neonatal intensive care beds, and their infant mortality rate for low-birth weight ($<2500\,g$) or premature infants (<37 weeks gestation) was a gruesome 70%. Two Columbian neonatologists, Dr. Edgar Rey and Dr. Hector Martinez, developed an inexpensive alternative, where mothers of

premature newborns were instructed to hold their babies 24 hours a day, keeping them under their clothes. The innovation, coined "Kangaroo Mother Care" reduced mortality rates, and led to much shorter hospitals stays (Charpak, Ruiz-Pelaez, Figueroa, & Charpak, 1997). This efficient innovation has slowly diffused around the world, and only recently reaching the health care systems in Africa, Asia, and North America.

Buprenorphine Treatment
Buprenorphine, a medication developed in 1969 in England for the treatment of pain, was reported in 1978 by researchers in the United States to be effective as a substitution medication by blocking the euphoria produced by opiates. In 1996, the French National Health System approved the use of buprenorphine to treat patients with opiate dependencies. French physicians quickly adopted this drug, and today over half of all opiate addicts in France are taking this drug permanently. Studies suggest that mortality rates from drug overdoses have been substantially reduced, and many former addicts have returned to more normal lives. Although France has found this drug to be effective, physicians in the United States were prohibited from utilizing buprenorphine until 2002; consequently, there has been limited awareness and adoption of this drug in the United States (Vastag, 2003).

In all three examples, new technologies and medical knowledge needed to provide state-of-the-art health care was not found in one country, but dispersed around the world. Knowledge diffuses gradually as papers are published; workshops, medical congresses, and health care conferences attended; and people slowly digest new ways of thinking and behaving. However, as Doz, Santos, and Williamson (2001) argue, innovative and efficient organizations must be more proactive by "accessing, mobilizing, and leveraging pockets of knowledge drawn from around the world" (p. 3). To become a meta-national health care organization, managers and clinicians have to learn how to transcend national and regional borders in order to tap into the massive human, intellectual, and social capital situated around the world.

Limits to Learning and Transfer

On the one hand, the opportunity to access and exchange skills, expertise, technology, and new information at a distance has never been easier. New alliances and collaborations are possible through the internet, electronic workshops and symposiums, and telemedicine. Consequently, the costs associated with time-space have been reduced, so innovative health care management practices could be adapted to any local health care setting. On the other, sharing medical care knowledge and expertise worldwide is limited. Clinicians and managers may not want to share knowledge and expertise, or they may not be capable of cultivating and harvesting widely dispersed information.

This latter perspective comes from the work of Herbert Simon (1981) on bounded rationality and the work of John Seely Brown. Brown and Duguid (2000) argue that people bound by occupational roles develop identities and social networks. For example, each year 1,400 patients who had hernia surgery attend a reunion in Toronto. Hernia patients throughout the world (or physiotherapists, nurses, or transplant surgeons) could be linked into a global village of hernia survivors via the internet. This is the difference between face-to-face communities with dense connections and global networks bounded – and separated – by culture and language (Brown & Duguid, 2000).

Clinicians who work closely together in face-to-face groups develop similar ideas about practices, especially around the quality of care. Their beliefs about best practices often are an artifact of age or educational biases rather than evidence-based. Consequently, best practice information rarely travels efficiently through a network of practice; sometimes it cannot be transferred.

Creating Global Advantage

Medical specialities such as emergency services, oncology, transplantation, hypertension, and clinical activities, including admission, investigation, therapy, recovery, etc. are the sources of advantage in health care delivery. An organization enacts an operating strategy when it performs clinical activities better than other organizations. Strategic positioning occurs when health care organizations offer different medical services and perform clinical activities in novel or unique ways.

Globalization takes place if there is some distinct advantage in integrating medical specialties and/or clinical activities worldwide (Porter, 1990). The creation of service value, shown in Fig. 4, identifies the primary clinical activities that create value for patients: admission, investigation, therapy, recovery, and follow-up. There are also four secondary activities: organizing the care processes, managing human resources, developing and maintaining clinical information, and supporting the primary clinical activities.

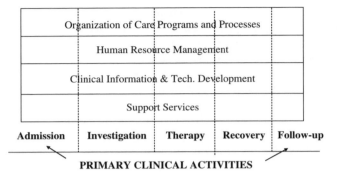

Fig. 4.   Primary Clinical and Non-Clinical Activities.

A health care organization that wants an international presence has to think about the coordination across all these activities. This might include managing medical devices and suppliers, creating clinical standards, branding the name, or transferring skills and sharing activities. Should health care strategies become more global? If so, how should health care organizations execute these nine primary and secondary activities? How can they become positioned to be perceived as providing better services in each locality?

Sharing Best Practices

There are many examples of international knowledge sharing. In 2004, Apollo Hospital of India announced a new collaboration with the Boltzmann Institute for Applied Radiation Research in Vienna. They will exchange researchers and physicians, exchange knowledge and innovative practices in medical physics and radiation oncology via the internet, and develop state-of-the-art treatment guidelines and exchange.

Clinical practice allows each provider, whether a nurse, a physician, or a therapist, to evolve somewhat independently of the organization. A care process binds people to a routine or a "one best way;" however, collaboration and improvisation can also lead to new ideas and innovations. As Brown and Duguid (2002) argue, there needs to be a balance between practices and processes. By looking at international examples of best practices, health care organizations and systems can obtain new insights.

For example, a recent study of 11 leading causes of acute hospital admissions and utilization in England's NHS when compared with data from

Kaiser Permanente of California found that Kaiser provided more efficient care (Ham, York, Sutch, & Shaw, 2003). Although admission rates in Kaiser were higher for heart failure, acute myocardial infarction, knee replacements, and kidney infections, the NHS had four to five times the admission rates for bronchitis, angina, or asthma. For 11 acute admissions, NHS bed use was three and a half times the Kaiser rate.

The NHS could learn several lessons from Kaiser's approach to integrated care. The design of Kaiser as a multi-specialty group allowed generalist and specialist physicians to work as a team, allowing patients to move from hospitals to skilled nursing facilities. Since physicians at Kaiser have more efficient access to diagnostic services, patients are quickly diagnosed and offered treatments. Patients with heart failure or asthma are "actively" managed with evidence-based guidelines. Kaiser's discharge specialists avoid patients waiting for discharge. Finally, patients are highly involved in their own care. Orthopedic patients are taught how to dress, exercise, and take their medicine.

The competence and performance of clinicians and provider organizations can have a normal distribution (Gawande, 2004). Figure 5 shows a hypothetical distribution of physicians, some of whom have poorer outcomes on average. The Aravind Eye Hospital of India and Shouldice

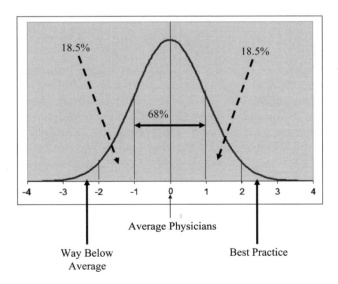

Fig. 5. A Normal Distribution of Physicians.

Hospital in Toronto, Canada, are interesting examples of providers who get better outcomes by focusing on a small set of procedures. Aravind concentrates on blindness and Shouldice on simple inguinal hernias. They are not only efficient but offer high-quality care.

A study published in *American Family Physician* in 1999 found evidence for the bell curve when specialty hospitals doing hernia surgeries were compared with general hospitals. The investigators found that complications rates were between 0.3 and 13% and recurrences were 0.1–2% in specialty hospitals versus complication rates of 6–28% and recurrences rates of 2–14% for general hospitals (Bax, Sheppard, & Crass, 1999).

International Lessons Lost in Translation

Although general hospitals can learn a great deal from international examples of clinical best practices, the management lessons are often lost in the clinical translation. A recent example of this occurred in 2002, when the *British Journal of Surgery* reported on a randomized trial of two surgical approaches: the recent Lichtenstein mesh technique versus the Shouldice technique developed in 1940. Although there was no significant differences in postoperative complications, pain, and recovery, the researchers concluded that the Lichtenstein repair was easier to learn, took less time (the Shouldice technique took 7 min longer to perform), and there was a slight difference in recurrence rates (Nordin, Bartelmess, Jansson, Svensson, & Edlund, 2002).

For the randomized trial, five surgeons were taught both techniques in a typical surgical training program, and surgery was performed under general anesthesia in an ambulatory setting. The clinical objective was a quick repair, less time in the operating room, and same day outpatient discharge. From a health care management perspective the clinical trial not only missed what the Shouldice technique is about; the study completely missed the key service lessons.

Communities of Practice Make a Difference

The Shouldice hernia repair almost never uses general anesthesia; in well over 95% of the cases operations are performed under local infiltration and a light sedative (Glassow, 1986). The avoidance of general anesthesia significantly reduces the risk of harm to patients. Moreover, Shouldice surgeons are carefully selected and trained over 4 months before they are allowed to operate. Whereas a general surgeon may perform 50 hernia repairs a year, each Shouldice surgeon performs over 600 per year. Additionally, the surgery is not done on an outpatient basis; each patient stays for a minimum of 3 days.

Shouldice is not just a hernia repair technique; it is a well-designed service proposition that has clinical value for a specific group of patients (Urguhart & O'Dell, 2004). The care process includes a stay in a pleasant and relaxed environment, continuity of relationships, low prices, and high quality. The primary clinical activities of admission, investigation, therapy, recovery, and follow-up (see Fig. 4) are performed in very unique ways. Patients are carefully screened and not admitted if they have a cold, or are obese. Obese patients are instructed to begin a special diet, and are admitted only when their health will facilitate excellent outcomes.

Once selected for Shouldice, patients are educated to become partners and co-producers in every aspect of the care process, which builds both trust and self-confidence. For example, they walk into the operating room, they are awake and can talk with the surgeons during the surgery, and they are invited to get off the operating table and walk (with the help of the surgeon) to the post-operative room because early ambulation is part of the recovery process.

The physician patient interaction differs from most surgical encounters; when patients are admitted, the first person they see is their surgeon who confirms their diagnosis, explains the procedure, and informs them about what to expect. All patients go into a semi-private room with the understanding that they have been matched up with a surgical buddy who will share the experience and help to ease any fears.

Recovery is completely programed to include wake-up, medication, breakfast, exercise classes, rest periods, lunch in the dining room, more exercise, dinner, and more activity. To encourage mobility and interaction there are no televisions or telephones in the rooms. Meals must be eaten in a dining room, and patients must take themselves to the toilets. The facility has stairs with low risers, putting greens, exercise cycles, walking paths, and other activities aimed at a speedy recovery. Once discharged, patients are invited to annual reunions and membership in the Shouldice patient network.

Every patient, physician, nurse, and employee at Shouldice is a member of a "community of practice" (Brown & Duguid, 2002). Patients, providers, and staff are fully engaged, understand their roles and responsibilities, and share an attitude and an outlook. Through mutual interaction, learning and understanding, they are committed to the mission and goals of the clinical care process and adopt a Shouldice identity. The nurses know that their job is not to perform menial tasks, but to educate patients, help them to exercise, and relieve physicians of simple non-clinical tasks. These are powerful lessons in the repositioning of the primary clinical activities and the role of management in the formulation of care practices into a care process.

From Communities of Practice to Focused Health Care Strategies

From a patient perspective, quality is not a simple concept, but best understood in terms of five underlying dimensions shown in Fig. 6 (Chilingerian, 2004). If we analyze the Shouldice case in terms of these five dimensions, we find a complex configuration of quality outcomes, as delineated in Table 1.[2] Our discussion of the Shouldice case, however, begs the question: Why does a focused strategy work in health care? Gittell (2004) argues that an effective focus strategy is also associated with both effective coordination and positive relationships among participants: "The bottom line of this theory is that relationships of shared goals, shared knowledge, and mutual respect, enable participants to coordinate more effectively the work processes in which they are engaged" (p. 687).

In addition to shared goals and knowledge, and mutual respect, the other elements of relational coordination include frequent, timely, accurate, and problem-solving communication. A high order of leadership is required to develop the competencies of relational coordination: the enabling condi-

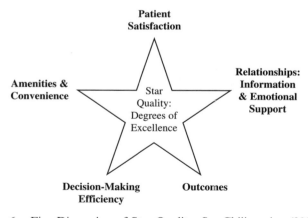

Fig. 6.   Five Dimension of Star Quality. See Chilingerian (2004).

Table 1. An Analysis of the Shouldice Experience using the Five
Dimensions of Star Quality.

Dimensions of Star Quality	Results
Outcomes	Low recurrence rates of less than 1% over 50 years
	Complications are less than 0.5%
	On average patients go back to work in 8 days
Patient satisfaction	98% are extremely satisfied with the care, and 2% "merely" satisfied
	Excellent pain management
	100% willing to recommend Shouldice
Decision-making efficiency	High degree of coordination of patient care across operating units
	Average cost per case at Shouldice is $1,342 less than the average local community hospital
	Quick diagnosis to treatment
	45 min surgery
	Optimal involvement of the patient in the care process
Amenities and convenience	Short waits once admitted
	Excellent dining services and food
Relationships: information and emotional support	High degree of trust and confidence
	Nurses and physicians spend time answering questions
	Annual reunions/long-term relationship

tions, the coaching, and the team skills. Reporting on a study of joint replacement patients in nine hospitals, Gittell (2004) found that providers who focused on one type of care program for a targeted patient population had higher levels of relational coordination. She hypothesized that part of the effect of clinical focus on quality and efficiency may be due to relational coordination.

Learning but not Transferring Best Practices

Are international lessons transferable? For many years, nearly every week, physicians and managers visit Shouldice to learn. Curiously, whatever new knowledge and new ideas they acquire seems to stay inside their heads because there are very few examples of Shouldice Hernia Hospitals. Failure to transfer best practices is not a new discovery, but it is one of the "wicked" problems in health care management. It is not about the difficulty of international transfer due to culture and language, because there are no examples of hospitals like Shouldice in Canada, let alone Toronto. In the words of Brown and Duguid: "Best practices can have as much trouble traveling across town as they do across continents" (2004, p. 123).

Learning Lessons from Worst Cases

There is another reason why health care organizations should pay attention to small side effects and repercussions, as well as trends and events abroad: we can learn how to avoid failures before they happen at home. Managers in organizations invite failure in predictable ways. By enlarging the pool of information about clinical practices, we can learn how to avoid some of the worst mistakes.

The retired American General Norman Schwartzkopf once came to a leadership class and told the students that he had learned more from bad than from good management. Do managers actually learn by making mistakes, or from being successful? We do know that if managers can avoid confronting the consequences of mistakes for an extended period, they can create an illusion of good management. The most gruesome example of this took place at the Bristol Royal Infirmary, a hospital in England.

The hospital received special funding to become a Supra Regional Service center for pediatric cardiac surgical care. However, the Bristol hospital experienced pediatric mortality rates as high as 32% when the national average was 11%. This program received funding over a 14-year period, despite significantly higher mortality and morbidity rates, as well as poor physician performance, than warranted based on national comparisons. According to the Bristol Royal Infirmary Investigation (2001, p. 4):

> Bristol had a significantly higher mortality rate for open-heart surgery on children under 1 than that of other centres in England. Between 1988 and 1994 the mortality rate at Bristol was roughly double that elsewhere in five out of seven years.

What went wrong at Bristol? The Bristol Royal Infirmary Investigation did not find bad people, willful harm, or lack of caring clinicians. What the investigators did find was bad health care management. Health care managers relied on weak control structures, provided no mechanisms for managing performance, and developed a culture that did not cherish safety, quality, accountability, or collaborative teamwork. Pediatric cardiac surgery became a community of normal accidents and poor practices, with disrespect for patients. Although the hospital was awash with data, the organizational culture was entrapped in mediocrity (Weick & Sutcliffe, 2003).

While the story about Bristol hospital illuminates a major health care failure, it is not about a sudden catastrophe, or about a lack of resources or clinical expertise. Most people deal with problems on an ad hoc basis, and they typically do not think about problems that do not have immediacy. Over many years, few individuals accumulate enough experience to deal with all the problems they might encounter. When novel situations arise, most people rely on routine methods successfully used in the past. Consequently, international cases like the Bristol Royal Infirmary offer new insights for any health care manager, especially, in terms of the role of culture, complexity, and leadership.

Noel Tichy (2002) argues that the essence of modern leadership is challenging basic business assumptions and developing a teachable point of view: "a cohesive set of ideas and concepts that a person is able to articulate clearly to others" (p. 74). Breaking inattentional blindness requires one to see emerging situations as new, and not in terms of old, established routines and practices that merely need to be activated (Dörner, 1996). If nothing else, health care managers need to develop teachable points of views from local, national, and international examples of medical errors and other avoidable failures.

CLOSING REMARKS

International health care management is a newly emerging field with much unexplored territory. However, throughout the world, the managers of health care organizations face similar issues. Health care organizations appear to be among the most complex organizations to manage; however, the apparent complexity of health organizations may be merely a reflection of the complexity of the environment in which health care takes place. Hence, we believe it is advantageous to learn from comparative, international health care management research.

Health care executives face a number of challenges, but global blindness is perhaps the most serious one for them to overcome. If they can overcome this inattentional blindness, a global strategy can enhance the comparative advantage of a health care organization, especially in the context of an emerging international market. Indeed, health care organizations can create a global advantage both by acquiring new technologies and medical knowledge dispersed worldwide and by performing clinical activities in novel or unique ways.

While health care organizations can obtain new insights from international examples of best practices, the management lessons are often lost in the clinical translation. Failure to transfer best practices is not a new discovery, but it is one of the "wicked" problems in health care management. Lastly, health care organizations may gain their greatest insights by learning lessons from the worst cases of failure in international health care management.

There are arguments against seeking knowledge from the world's best practices. National pride, autonomy, language, and culture are all barriers to adopting ideas. But as Don Berwick (2004, p. 4) said succinctly: "If the world has something to teach us, why would we not learn?" We believe that if managers and scholars can draw on the lessons from international health organizations, they can advance the field of health care management in ways that will have the most far reaching and profound impact.

NOTES

1. This section is based on lectures by Reinhard Angelmar of INSEAD, and the case by Reinhard Angelmar and Christian Pinson, *Zantac (A)* European Case Programme (1992).

2. These data have been accumulated over a 55-year period, with annual follow-ups of over 280,000 patients (Urquhart & O'Dell, 2004).

REFERENCES

Anderson, G. F., Reinhardt, U. E., Hussey, P. S., & Petrosyan, V. (2003). It's the prices, stupid: Why the United States is so different from other countries. *Health Affairs, 22*(3), 89–105.

Angelmar, R., & Pinson, C. (1992). *Zantac (A)*. (European Case Program) Fontainebleau, France: INSEAD.

Barbasi, A-L. (2003). *Linked: How everything is connected to everything else and what it means for business, science, and everyday life.* New York: Penguin Books.

Bax, T., Sheppard, B. C., & Crass, R. A. (1999). Surgical options in the management of groin hernias. *American Family Physician, 59*(4), 893–906.

Beecham, L. (2002). British patients willing to travel abroad for treatment. *British Medical Journal, 325*, 10.

Berwick, D. M. (2004). *Escape fire: The designs for the future of health care.* San Francisco: Jossey-Bass.

Blendon, R. J., Schoen, C., DesRoches, C. M., Osborn, R., Zapert, K., & Raleigh, E. (2004). Confronting competing demands to improve quality: A five-country hospital survey. *Health Affairs, 23*(3), 119–135.

Bristol Royal Infirmary Inquiry. (2001). *Learning from Bristol: The report of the Public Inquiry into children's heart surgery at the Bristol Royal Infirmary 1984–1995* (No. CM 5207(1)). London: The Stationery Office.

Burns, L. R., D'Aunno, T., & Kimberly, J. (2004). Globalization in healthcare. In: H. Gatignon & J. Kimberly (Eds), *The INSEAD-Wharton alliance on globalizing: Strategies for building successful global businesses* (pp. 395–421). Cambridge: Cambridge University Press.

Charpak, N., Ruiz-Pelaez, J. G., Figueroa de, C. Z., & Charpak, Y. (1997). Kangaroo mother versus traditional care for newborn infants <2000 grams: A randomized, controlled trial. *Pediatrics, 100*(4), 682–688.

Chilingerian, J. A. (2004). Who has star quality? In: R. E. Herzlinger (Ed.), *Consumer-driven health care: Implications for providers, payers, and policy-makers* (pp. 443–453). San Francisco: Jossey-Bass.

Chilingerian, J. A., & Vandekerckhove, P. (2005). Managing a transplant decision at University Medical Center Leuven: (A). Fontainebleau: INSEAD (in press).

Dörner, D. (1989). *The logic of failure: Recognizing and avoiding error in complex situations.* Reading, Massachusetts: Perseus Book.

Dörner, D. (1996). *The logic of failure: recognizing and avoiding error in complex situations.* New York: Metropolitan Books.

Doz, Y., Santos, J., & Williamson, P. (2001). *From global to metanational.* Boston: Harvard Business School Press.

Gawande, A. (2004). The bell curve. *The New Yorker, 80,* 82–91.

Gittell, J. H. (2004). Achieving focus in hospital care: The role of relational coordination. In: R. E. Herzlinger (Ed.), *Consumer-driven health care: Implications for providers, payers, and policy-makers* (pp. 627–634). San Francisco: Jossey-Bass.

Glassow, F. (1986). The shouldice hospital technique. *International Surgery, 71*(3), 148–153.

Ham, C., York, N., Sutch, S., & Shaw, R. (2003). Hospital bed utilisation in the NHS, Kaiser Permanente, and the US Medicare programme: Analysis of routine data. *British Medical Journal, 327*(7426), 1257.

Hussey, P., Anderson, G., Osborn, O., Feek, C., McLaughlin, V., & Millar, J. (2004). How does the quality of care compare in five countries? *Health Affairs, 23*(3), 89–99.

Intel Corporation. (2004). *Bumrungrad hospital transforms healthcare delivery with integrated information system on Intel architecture.* Retrieved March 24, 2005, from http://www.intel.com/business/casestudies/bumrungrad.pdf

Landers, S. J. (2002). *Heightened security keeping international patients away: U.S. hospitals with substantial international programs see a decline in revenue; doctors see a boost in telemedicine consults.* Retrieved March 20, 2005, from http://www.amaassn.org/amednews/2002/09/16/hlsc0916.htm

Lerer, L., & Piper, M. (2003). *Digital strategies in the pharmaceutical industry.* New York: Palgrave Macmillan.

Newhouse, J. (2002). Why is there a quality chasm? *Health Affairs, 21*(4), 13–25.

Nordin, P., Bartelmess, P., Jansson, C., Svensson, C., & Edlund, G. (2002). Randomized trial of Lichtenstein versus Shouldice hernia repair in general surgical practice. *British Journal of Surgery, 89*(1), 45–49.

Phuket International Hospital. (2005). Retrieved March 20, 2005, from http://www.phuket-interhospital.co.th/index.htm

Pollack, A. (2003). Who's reading your x-ray? *New York Times,* p. 3.1.

Porter, M. (1987). Changing patterns of international competition. In: D. J. Teece (Ed.), *The competitive challenge.* Cambridge: Ballinger Publishing Company.

Porter, M. (1990). *The competitive advantage of nations.* New York: The Free Press.

Preker, A., & Harding, A. (2003). The economics of hospital reform: From hierarchical to market-based incentives. *World Hospitals and Health Services, 39*(3), 3–10, 42, 44.

Raffel, M. W. (Ed.) (1997). *Health care and reform in industrialized countries.* University Park: Pennsylvania State University Press.

Roemer, M. (1977). *Comparative national policies on health care.* New York: Marcel Dekker.

Roy, C. W., & Hunter, J. (1996). What happens to patients awaiting arthritis surgery? *Disability and Rehabilitation, 18*(2), 101–105.

Simon, H. (1981). *The sciences of the artificial* (2nd ed.). Cambridge: MIT Press.

Simons, D. J., & Chabris, C. F. (1999). Gorillas in our midst: Sustained inattentional blindness for dynamic events. *Perception, 28,* 1059–1074.

Solomon, J. (2004). Traveling cure: India's new coup in outsourcing: Inpatient care; Facing expense, long waits at home, Westerners fly in; A hospital empire grows; Mr. Salo has "real doubts". *Wall Street Journal,* p. A.1.

Tanner, L. (2004). CT scans, MRIs sent overseas for outsourcing. *Beaumont Enterprise,* p. D.9.

Tichy, N. M. (2002). *The cycle of leadership: How great leaders teach their companies to win.* New York: Harper.

Urquhart, D. J. B., & O'Dell, A. (2004). A model of focused health care delivery. In: R. E. Herzlinger (Ed.), *Consumer-driven health care: Implications for providers, payers, and policy-makers* (pp. 627–634). San Francisco: Jossey-Bass.

Vastag, B. (2003). In-office opiate treatment "not a panacea": Physicians slow to embrace therapeutic option. *Journal of the American Medical Association, 290*(6), 731–735.

Walshe, K., & Shortell, S. (2004). When things go wrong: How health care organizations deal with major failures. *Health Affairs, 23*(3), 103–111.

Weick, K. E., & Sutcliffe, K. M. (2003). Hospitals as cultures of entrapment. *California Management Review, 45*(2), 73–84.

WHO. (2000). *The World health report 2000: Health systems: Improving performance.* Geneva: World Health Organization.

Williams, J. I., Llewellyn Thomas, H., Arshinoff, R., Young, N., & Naylor, C. D. (1997). The burden of waiting for hip and knee replacements in Ontario. *Journal of Evaluation in Clinical Practice, 3*(1), 59–68.

PATIENTS AND PROVIDERS

STORIES FROM SANTIAGO: HIV/AIDS AND NEEDED HEALTH SYSTEMS CHANGE

Lilian M. Ferrer, Michele Issel and Rosina Cianelli

ABSTRACT

The incipient HIV/AIDS epidemic in Chile poses challenges for respon-siveness of the Chilean national health care system, Fondo Nacional de Salud (FONASA) (National Health Funds), especially given the soci-ocultural forces for inertia in FONASA. Thus, the issue is what is the nature of the forces for change. A grounded theory approach was applied to interview data from two qualitative studies, one with HIV/AIDS ad-vocates and activists as interviewees and the other with Chilean low-income women. The stories of their experiences with and perceptions of FONASA revealed major issues facing FONASA, including quality of care and ethics. Ways in which these issues are being addressed by the activists result in constructed environmental dynamism. A conceptual model of the forces for change was developed including actors, strategies, and targets of change that constitutes organizational environmental dy-namism. The construct of environmental dynamism has international ap-plicability, particularly to governmental health systems, which are influenced by strong sociocultural forces.

International Health Care Management
Advances in Health Care Management, Volume 5, 31–72
Copyright © 2005 by Elsevier Ltd.
All rights of reproduction in any form reserved
ISSN: 1474-8231/doi:10.1016/S1474-8231(05)05002-0

The presence of HIV/AIDS has resulted in a high mortality rate internationally (Levy & Kates, 2000) and poses challenges for health care system responsiveness in many nations, including Chile. UNAIDS (2004a) described Chile as a country with an incipient epidemic, meaning that the prevalence of HIV/AIDS is precariously close to a full epidemic. The fact that HIV/AIDS is a looming epidemic has created, among some groups, a sense of urgency that the Chilean health service delivery be responsive to the clients' HIV/AIDS related needs by addressing the pending epidemic, partly because the culture of Chile, like that of many developing nations, stresses stability and supports a strong power differential within the society. *Fondo Nacional de Salud* (FONASA) (National Health Fund) also receives no financial incentives or rewards for providing long-term or costly care to clients living with HIV/AIDS. As a governmental entity, the Chilean national health system, FONASA, is cumbersome and slow to change. Reinforcing the slow pace of change is the professional culture of health care providers to maintain the professional status quo.

Potentially countering the forces for stability are three overarching forces for change. One is a growing public awareness that the nascent HIV/AIDS epidemic in Chile is poised to grow (Dayton & Merson, 2000). However, this is not necessarily accompanied by the awareness that HIV/AIDS prevention programs and care will put demands on FONASA that will require organization's structural and cultural changes. Another force is the recent, and novel in Chile, AIDS related Law mandating a specific level of care be provided to individuals living with HIV/AIDS and HIV/AIDS prevention. The law essentially requires that providers under the control of the Ministry of Health change their practice. Achieving change of this magnitude will require a change in the nature of the health system in which the providers work. A third force for systems change is the adoption and importation by HIV/AIDS activists of international norms regarding social justice, ethical health care, and equality in access to health care for all persons.

HIV/AIDS activists, who have the determination to make their needs known, are themselves stakeholders for FONASA. They are also, most likely, the voice of the marginalized homosexual men and persons living with HIV/AIDS. Thus, a role of activists is to stimulate organizational changes in the FONASA system, changes needed to adequately address health problems of disadvantaged groups. Having an understanding of the strategies the activists use to create change contributes to development of a global model of organization and environment interaction, particularly in nations that have strong sociocultural barriers to the delivery of equitable health care. Therefore, the purpose of this study was to understand, from the perspective of FONASA users, key problems with FONASA and to identify the strategies that HIV/AIDS advocacy groups and activists use to make those problems known.

Our focus on the role of activists is consistent with the views of Frooman (1999) and Rowley (1997) regarding how stakeholders can influence and change organizations. In this case, HIV/AIDS advocates are the stakeholders and the organization is FONASA. Clients of FONASA provide stories and descriptions of their experiences with FONASA, revealing organizational and managerial issues related to providing ethical and quality HIV/AIDS health care. Their stories reveal several issues needing to be addressed in order to implement HIV/AIDS prevention, early diagnosis, and treatment in Chile. Based on the data, we propose a model for how HIV/AIDS related advocacy groups are contributing to actualizing changes through their actions within the organizational environment of FONASA. The need for management of organizational culture and change, consideration of equity, access, and quality of basic health care are consistent with the renewed emphasis by PAHO and WHO (2003) on health care responsiveness.

We begin by providing background information on the HIV/AIDS epidemic in Chile and its neighboring countries, with particular attention to the Chilean health system. This is followed by a description of the process by which qualitative data from HIV/AIDS advocates, clients, and low-income women at high risk for exposure to HIV/AIDS were used to generate a grounded theory that delineates key strategies being used to create changes to FONASA. After presenting key findings from the interviews, we discuss the theoretical and practice implications of our analysis for international health services development.

THE CHILEAN SITUATION

HIV/AIDS in Latin America

Latin America is a region disproportionately affected by HIV/AIDS. Approximately 1.6 million people were living with HIV in Latin America by the end of 2003, or 0.6% of the adult population. Of those, approximately 84,000 died from HIV/AIDS-related illnesses and 200,000 were newly infected (UNAIDS, 2004a). Each day, 567 people are newly infected with HIV in Latin America and the Caribbean area (Patz, Mazin, & Zacarias, 1999). Countries in the southern portion of Latin America (Argentina, Bolivia, Chile, and Peru) have an incipient HIV/AIDS epidemic, with infection rates between 0.1% and 0.7% among adults (UNAIDS, 2004a). These contiguous countries share cultural norms, religious beliefs, gender roles, and languages, all of which contribute to a similar pattern for the HIV/AIDS epidemic in these countries.

Overall, many public policies in Argentina, Bolivia, Chile, and Peru have not been clear, followed, or useful in building egalitarian societies (Varas & Toro-Alfonso, 2001). The Latino cultures of these countries are described as a conglomerate of communities that share inequalities in different spectrums of life (ARC, 1998; Peragallo, 1996). Latinos are at higher risk for acquiring HIV/AIDS, not only because of these inequities, but also because of traditional cultural norms, gender roles of *marianismo* and *machismo*, limited governmental responses to the epidemic, and lack of public awareness that HIV/AIDS affects persons regardless of sexual orientation, ethnicity, and socioeconomic status. An overview of the HIV/AIDS situation in these countries provides a context for understanding the response of the Chilean health care system. Basic HIV/AIDS epidemic data are summarized in Table 1.

Bolivia

HIV infection data are gathered from sites in four cities. In Bolivia, 333 AIDS cases were reported through 2001. There were 4,800 adults (age 15–49), including 1,300 women (age 15–49), living with HIV or AIDS at the end of 2003 (UNAIDS, 2004c). Heterosexual contact was the most common mode of transmission (51%), followed by men who had sex with men (41%), intravenous drug use (3%), perinatal transmission (3%), and blood transfusion (2%) (UNAIDS, 2004c). Among those who have been tested, results revealed very low HIV seroprevalence levels. Registered sex workers are required to have quarterly sexually transmitted infection exams and semiannual HIV tests in order to retain their health certificates. Thus, reliable data are available. In 2001, HIV prevalence among registered sex workers was 0.0%, with one site reporting a prevalence rate of 0.46% (UNAIDS, 2004a).

Argentina

In Argentina, at the end of 2003, UNAIDS (2004b) estimated that 120,000 adults were living with HIV or AIDS, of whom 24,000 were women aged 15–49. During 2003, 1,500 adults and children died from AIDS. The

Table 1.   Latest HIV/AIDS-Related Information of Chile and Neighboring Countries.

	Chile[a,b]	Bolivia[a,c]	Argentina[a,d,e]	Peru[a,f]
Population (UN, 2002)	15,211,000	8,329,000	37,032,000	27,567,000
National HIV/AIDS incidence rate for 2001	4.6/100,000	NA	4.71/100,000	NA
Estimated number of people living with HIV/AIDS (UNAIDS 2004a, b, c, d)				
Adults (15–49)	24,000	4,800	120,000	80,000
Women (15–49)	8,000	1,300	24,000	27,000
Modes of transmission				
Sexual (%)	93.5	92.0	63.9	82.0
Homo/bisexual (%)	69.0	41.0	17.6	42.0
Heterosexual (%)	31.0	51.0	46.3	40.0
Blood (including intravenous drug users and transfusions) (%)	5.0	5.0	19.6	NA
Perinatal transmission (%)	1.5	3.0	5.2	NA

NA, not available.
[a]UNAIDS (2004a).
[b]CONASIDA (2001).
[c]UNAIDS (2004c).
[d]UNAIDS (2004b).
[e]Ministerio de salud de la nación (2003).
[f]UNAIDS (2004d).

Argentinean Ministry of Health reported that in 2002 the HIV/AIDS incidence rate was 47.1 per 100,000, with a sex distribution of 2.6 men every woman. Of all HIV/AIDS cases reported since 1982, 87.5% are in large urban areas. For the year 2002, sexual contact was recorded as the most common mode of transmission (63.9%), mainly through heterosexual contact (46.3%), followed by intravenous drug use (19.1%), and perinatal transmission (5.2%) (Ministerio de salud de la nación, 2003). HIV infection reports are collected semiannually from sentinel sites across the country. Only data from pregnant women and blood donors are sent by all jurisdictions. Between 1998 and 2001, the prevalence of HIV among pregnant women decreased from 0.75% to 0.46%. The blood donor prevalence rate declined from 0.23% to 0.13% and HIV prevalence among sex workers from four jurisdictions declined from 6% to 2.3%. However, the prevalence of HIV among prison inmates increased during the same time period from 17.9% to 23.1%. In the provinces of Buenos Aires and Cordoba, the prevalence among intravenous drug users increased slightly from 18.3% to 19.4% (UNAIDS, 2004b), but the national cumulative distribution for intravenous drug users is 36.3%.

Perú

Reports on HIV infection are obtained from 24 geographic departments across Perú. At the end of 2003, Perú had 80,000 adults living with HIV or AIDS, of whom 27,000 were women, and a total of 4,200 persons died of AIDS during the year 2003 (UNAIDS, 2004d). HIV prevalence among intravenous drug users increased from 1% to 28% between 1986 and 1990. HIV prevalence increased among sex workers from 2% to 19% between 1986 and 1990. A single-site study conducted in 1995 found that 7% of patients at the sexually transmitted disease clinics tested HIV-positive (UNAIDS, 2004a).

Chile and Santiago

The Chilean HIV/AIDS epidemic is similar to that in its neighboring countries: the epidemic is rural and urban, predominantly present among the poor and homo/bisexual men, and increasingly includes women and heterosexuals (CONASIDA, 2001). The first AIDS case was diagnosed in Chile in 1984 (see Table 2), followed by 4,646 AIDS cases and 5,228 HIV-positive cases officially reported between 1984 and December 2001 (CONASIDA, 2001). Rajevic (2000) estimated that there were approximately 20,000 Chileans living with HIV or AIDS, many of whom did not know their HIV status. Also UNAIDS (2004a) estimated that 25,000 adults were living with HIV or AIDS, of whom 8,000 were women. The Chilean Ministry of Health estimated that almost 24,000 Chileans were living with HIV or AIDS by December 31, 2001. Since the first case was reported, 89% of those infected by HIV have been men and 11% women. However, an increase in cases among women is occurring, such that the incidence rate for

Table 2.   Timeline of Sentinel Events in the Chilean HIV/AIDS Epidemic.

Year	Event
1984	First AIDS case diagnosed in Chile
1987	First NGO related to HIV/AIDS prevention founded in Chile
1988	Annual HIV/AIDS incidence rate: 3.8 per 100,000
1990	National Office of AIDS (CONASIDA) founded within Ministry of Health
1997	National coordinator of all NGOs of people living with HIV/AIDS founded
1998	Annual HIV/AIDS incidence rate: 4.6 per 100,000
2002	Chilean AIDS Law passed

women has increased to 14.3% and to 8.9% for men. This change might be related to data collection of HIV seroprevalence among antenatal clinic attendees that began in Santiago and the Southern areas in 1992. The rate among pregnant women has remained below 0.1%.

Between 1984 and 2001, 3,230 HIV/AIDS related deaths were reported. Up to December 2001, the AIDS cumulative incidence was 34.3 per 100,000, with an increasing trend, and a reported annual incidence in 1999 of 4.6 per 100,000 (last reported annual incidence by the Ministry of Health). In 2000, AIDS was the fourth leading cause of death for men between 20 and 44 in the capital, with a national incidence rate of 10 per 100,000 and 14.9 per 100,000 in the Metropolitan region of Santiago. Cumulative AIDS rates are higher in Metropolitan regions, such as Santiago, Valparaíso and Arica (CONASIDA, 2001), indicating that urban areas are more affected. The Metropolitan region of Santiago has the largest number of AIDS cases with an incidence rate of 58 per 100,000. Overall, the appearance of HIV/AIDS in Chile has resulted in loss of human life, HIV financial costs, solitude and fear, due partly to disinformation and a lack of health care responses (Rajevic, 2000; Carmona & Del Valle, 2000).

Sexual transmission accounts for 93.5% of AIDS cases, blood for 5%, and mother to child transmission for 1.5%. There is a known relationship between HIV and other sexually transmitted infections. The annual rate of sexually transmitted infections was 67 per 100,000 in the year 2001 and individuals diagnosed with sexually transmitted infections had prevalence rates of HIV that ranged from 1.3% to 3.5% between 1992 and 1999 (MINSAL, 2001).

In 2002, the first Chilean disease-related law (Law No. 19.779) was passed (see Table 2). It is known as the AIDS Law and it mandates that the government offer adequate HIV/AIDS care to all Chilean citizens and engage in HIV/AIDS prevention. Because the majority of health care providers are employees of the FONASA, this law affects their practice. Despite the existence of the AIDS Law and the presence of an AIDS office (CONASIDA) in the Ministry of Health since 1990, the governmental response and its assurances to address HIV/AIDS appear to be inadequate as reflected in the available epidemic data. UNAIDS (2004a) believes that the national Chilean response has been hampered by insufficient financial resources for the Chilean health system, as well as the cultural element of having a conservative society that impedes HIV prevention efforts. Although CONASIDA was created 6 years after the first diagnosed AIDS case in Chile, there have been limitations placed on its work by society and the government because of the cultural values of Chileans.

CHILEAN PUBLIC HEALTH CARE SYSTEM THROUGH FONASA

Chilean history includes a recent change from socialized medicine to a privatized system. The change has resulted in a modernization of health care, but most noticeably in the care provided by private insurers. Most Chileans work in low-wage sectors and are subscribed to FONASA, which limits their health care options to State-sponsored and subsidized health insurance and health care providers. In other words, FONASA functions as a State-sponsored health network and insurance that includes primary care clinics and their corresponding public hospitals. FONASA is characterized by long waits, limited availability of specialists, and scarce resources for providing treatment (Leon, 2002; Pedersen, 1999; Wallace, 2001). HIV/AIDS services are delivered primarily through FONASA (Bernal, Lukacs, Malebran & Bonacic, 1989).

In 1997, Chile spent an estimated US$3.6 million on health care expenditures, of which US$2.02 million was spent on FONASA for operational expenses of the national health clinics and hospitals. This corresponds to 5.02% of the Chilean national gross product (PAHO, 2001). Although the national health clinics and hospitals both receive national funds, their lines of authority are different. Clinics report to the municipalities, in other words the local governmental bodies, whereas hospitals report to the national Ministry of Health. Nonetheless, clinics and their corresponding hospitals function as an integrated health network. In the national health system, Chileans are assigned to a clinic in their geographical community and, when needed, they are referred to the corresponding hospital for acute care services.

FONASA is a network of 196 general hospitals, 20 high-intensity hospitals, 526 primary care clinics, 1,840 rural health posts and medical stations, and 73 establishments of other kinds, all offering services over a range of intensity and complexity. Chile has approximately 30,000 hospital beds, which is one bed per 5,000 persons or one per 3,000 FONASA members. There is one clinic for approximately 28,500 people, or one per 17,100 FONASA members. In terms of professional human resources, in 1998 Chile had 18 physicians per 10,000 population, but only 8,000 of the country's 18,000 nurses worked in the national health care sector (PAHO, 2001).

The Chilean health system is similar in several ways to other publicly funded and administered national medical systems of its neighboring countries. For example, Argentina, Perú, and Bolivia, all have systems that attempt to be decentralized to the prevention levels; nonetheless the prevention health systems depend on the policies imparted by the National Ministry of Health. Also, the four countries share the characteristic of both having predominantly a public/national system with a much smaller private sector, as in the United Kingdom. This is changing in Chile with a growing private sector, except for people living with HIV or AIDS. When Chileans are diagnosed as living with HIV or AIDS they register in the national health care system, since the private insurances do not cover any HIV/AIDS-related expenses.

In terms of the health sector expenditure and financing for Argentina, in 1997, 55% of health expenditure was public and 60% of it was financed through the social security system and 40% directly from tax revenues. In 1999, the total of health expenditure was estimated at US$23,900 million, which corresponds to per capita expenditure of about US$750. For Perú, in 1998, the country spent 4.3% of its GDP on health. The main sources of financing were household spending, employer contributions, and the national budget. Finally, Bolivia has a national health expenditure amounted to US$422 million in 1998, representing, 5% of the GDP and was equivalent to US$ 46 per capita per annum. Public health expenditures accounted for 65% of the national spending on health (42% to social security; 23% to the public sector) (PAHO, 2002).

CHILEAN CULTURE AND HEALTH CARE PROVISION

The roles of men and women in society are influenced or determined by expectations about their gender. Attributes assigned to each gender are the result of the interaction of innate and learned factors; many of which are exclusively the result of social learning that begins in childhood. In Latino cultures, gender roles are depicted by the concept of *machismo*, which is the idea that men are superior to women in biological, sexual, intellectual, and emotional aspects (Gissi, 1978). In addition, gender roles are depicted in the concepts of *machismo* and *marianismo* in Latino culture. *Marianismo* is the feminine equivalent of machismo (Pinel, 1994). Social expectations are that men should be active and dominant in sexual relations. For instance, if men are unfaithful, their sexual activity confirms their masculinity and sexual role. Consequently, the men who have extramarital relations are not violating social rules as long as they fulfill their roles as protectors and providers for the family. Their sexual relationships outside of marriage are viewed as expressions of virility. In contrast, women are expected to take a passive and subordinate role. If women are unfaithful, their behavior results in strong and negative reactions from the partners and society because they are not assuming the passive female role in sexual matters (Guimaraes, 1994; Prado, 1994; Strait, 1999). The social mores for women does not allow sex just for pleasure or desire or openly showing interest in men (Klein-Alonso, 1996). In addition, in Latin cultures, women and men do not talk openly about sex. The prevalent idea is that one has sex but does not speak about it. Therefore, couples discuss protection in the context of reproduction, and the responsibility is given to the woman (Klein-Alonso, 1996). Men have casual sexual relations with different partners and without protection; hence, the unfaithfulness of the partner puts women at risk to acquire HIV (Navarro, 2000). Homosexuality is also not openly discussed, leading some Latino men to hide their sexual preferences (Diaz, 1998). As noted by Rajevic (2000), Chile is a homophobic country in which homosexuality is not accepted. These cultural values become relevant in understanding the HIV/AIDS epidemic and possible responses to it.

Activism and Change

As people organize around a perceived social problem, groups of individuals generate a social movement around the problematic situation to fight it and to generate social change, usually seeking egalitarian conditions to confront the problematic situation through activism. Social movement was defined by Goodwin and Jasper (2003) as "a collective, organized, sustained, and non-institutional challenge to authorities, power holders, or cultural beliefs, and practices". Social movements in general have relied on groups of ordinary people who construct a social protest and take action concerning that protest in different forms to change some aspect of their society. Understanding social movements helps one to understand human diversity and build upon the understanding of social change, which generally emerge out of civil society (Goodwin & Jasper, 2003).

In the case of HIV/AIDS social movement organizations, their leaders have had experience with other movements (Stockdill, 2003). Thus, the leaders have had good political experience combined with adverse social contexts. The previous involvement has contributed to success in their involvement in the specific movement for change in the era of HIV/AIDS. The overall goal for HIV/AIDS social movement is rooted in activism seeking to convince people in power and in the general society that HIV/AIDS must be prevented and treated. On the other hand, because mostly gay men are the ones who have been affected by HIV/AIDS, additional goals are to recognize the rights of gay men and the value of keeping the human beings alive (Diaz, 1998). In summary, the HIV/AIDS social movement has its roots in multiple forms of inequalities that resulted in a movement of individuals with a need for survival. The HIV/AIDS social movement in Latin America has taken the form of non-governmental organizations (NGOs), where individuals gather together, become organized, and call for social change.

Activism in Chile

One aspect of the Chilean society response towards the appearance of HIV/AIDS was the formation of NGOs. NGOs emerge as the result of community organizing, which in turn results in social movements (Cantu, 2000; Omoto, Odom, & Crain, 1999). NGOs founded in Chile sought to meet the needs created by HIV/AIDS through establishing group connections (Eckstein, 2001). Only after several NGOs were founded in Chile, starting in 1984, did the Ministry of Health create the national office of AIDS, CONASIDA. NGOs continued their efforts during the 1980s. By building coalitions and networks, and establishing the national coordinator of all NGOs of people living with HIV/ADS, they reached the goal of having a law approved by the Chilean congress. The AIDS Law makes the Chilean government responsible for primary, secondary, and tertiary prevention of HIV/AIDS because it is in the health, cultural, and social national interest to not discriminate and to give egalitarian rights to HIV-infected people ("AIDS Law # 19,779," 2001).

Homosexual men have a history of mobilizing to address their community's HIV/AIDS-related needs in Chile, as well as in the United States and Europe. The mobilization comes in the form of claiming access to health services for themselves and others, demanding prevention campaigns, and fighting discrimination. Various authors (Diaz, Ayala, Bein, Henne, & Marin, 2001; Ouellette, Bassel, Maslanka, & Wong, 1995; Ramírez-Valles, 2002; Ramírez-Valles & Brown, 2003; Stockdill, 2003; Wallerstain, 1992; Wilson, 2000) suggest that regardless of sexual orientation, mobilization, as an expression of community organizing fosters the development of a sense of community and social support system, increases feelings of pride and self-esteem, and diminishes psychosocial distress. Such characteristics are both the impetus for and the results of social movements.

In Chile, most social movement strategies related to HIV/AIDS are a reflection of an ongoing struggle by organized groups, usually homosexual men, fighting stigmatization and social death. To clarify, the stigmatization of people with HIV/AIDS occurs from a confluence of certain characteristics within Chilean society that promote the stereotyping and isolating of groups of people associated with the disease. Literally, people are fighting for their survival as they seek to maintain employment, acquire needed medical treatment, and protect family members against discrimination because of the stigma attached to HIV/AIDS. Mainly homosexual men have joined together in an effort to fulfill unsatisfied needs related to HIV/AIDS. These efforts have resulted in a new law, obligating the government to provide universal HIV/AIDS prevention and treatment for people with HIV/AIDS, and for all Chileans who need prevention messages.

METHODS

The two qualitative studies used in this study were conducted between September 2002 and September 2003 by the two authors from Santiago. Both studies shared the epistemological dimension of examining different aspects of the HIV/AIDS epidemic in Chile. The research foci were comprehension and discovery, such that the studies have an ontological perspective of identifying elements and interpreting aspects of reality (Savage & Black, 1995). The qualitative approach was selected for both studies for several reasons consistent with the literature on qualitative methods (Brofman & Gleizaer, 1994; Patton, 2001; Stake, 2000). Both studies sought to have a holistic view of the phenomena, to investigate interpersonal and organizational relationships within a cultural or systems context, and to incorporate consideration of the context in interpretations of the data. Also, both studies sought to have access to immediate reactions of participants, to be closer to participants in terms of creating familiarity and a better sense of confidence, and to be responsive to ethical concerns arising during the study. In addition, qualitative methods are appropriate to be able to effectively describe and understand the uniqueness of individuals' experiences. Individual experiences were the foci of both studies. Individual experiences and views are known to be better captured with a qualitative methodology. Overall, the qualitative approach used in the studies was consistent with the epistemological and ontological perspectives of the researchers.

Study A was a case study, with the case defined as the HIV/AIDS social movement phenomenon in Chile. The study purpose was to identify factors and forces that led the phenomenon of HIV/AIDS social movement in Chile, through understanding of individual perspectives on: the social construction of HIV/AIDS as a problem in Chile, the societal responses toward HIV/AIDS, individual motivations for getting involved in the HIV/AIDS social movement, and outcomes of participation. Thus, Study A was primarily concerned with the HIV/AIDS activists and their relationship to the Chilean health system.

Study B used ethnography to understand the experiences of low-income Chilean women regarding HIV/AIDS. The study sought to understand how Chilean women relate HIV/AIDS to cultural factors, such as *machismo*, *marianismo*, domestic violence, and substance abuse, and whether Chilean women perceive themselves to be at risk for contracting HIV/AIDS. Thus, Study B was primarily concerned with the experiences of a disadvantaged, vulnerable population with the HIV/AIDS care and prevention provided by FONASA.

Data from Studies A and B were used as one data set for two reasons. First, both Studies A and B were based on the same teleological and epistemological perspectives, that of understanding the health system environment created by HIV/AIDS as experienced by users of FONASA. Both groups of interviewees provided detailed information about the Chilean context of HIV/AIDS and their lived experiences. The stories from Studies A and B provide insights into the functioning of FONASA, the factors influencing the organization, and the strategies being used to create health systems change from outside of FONASA. The second reason for combining the data is that the stories are told through different prisms; the activists who are NGO members (Study A) speak as advocates for changing FONASA, whereas the women (Study B) describe FONASA as users of that health care system. Study A is the only research conducted in Chile from the

perspective of activists involved in the first organized response toward HIV/
AIDS. Data from Study A is contextualized by the data from the women in
Study B. In other words, incorporating data from Study B complements the
picture from Study A by providing the perspective of women, one of the
most vulnerable groups in Chile and the heaviest users of the national health
clinics.

Samples

Study A participants were members from two HIV/AIDS-related NGOs in
Chile. These two organizations were selected because of their uniqueness
and well-known organizational trajectory in Chile. A total of 30 NGO
members from the two NGOs were interviewed about their perception of
HIV/AIDS in Chile, the NGO formation and maintenance, as well as, their
motivations and outcomes of participation. The interviewees considered
themselves members of the NGO regardless of whether they were employees
or volunteers.

One of the NGOs was founded in 1997 as a result of a community-based
initiative, and now serves as the national coordinator of all organizations of
people living with HIV/AIDS (see Table 2). The mission is "to build an
answer for the challenges of the epidemic among the people living with HIV
and the society, guiding their actions towards improvement of the quality of
life, through the defense of their civil rights, access to treatment, health
promotion, prevention, and organize and give strength to the net of groups
of people living with HIV/AIDS [translated]." The mission statement of the
other NGO that began in 1987 (see Table 2), 3 years after the first HIV/
AIDS case in Chile, describes itself as "a community, which from an evolutionary perspective centered on human rights, seeks to reduce the impact
of the HIV/AIDS epidemic in the homosexual population [translated]." As
seen from these mission statements, members take an activist stance in relation to the governmental response to HIV/AIDS. Each NGO provides
services aligned with those mission statements. One NGO offers services
related to holistic care, prevention, civilian rights, organizational development, and gender. The other NGO has a community initiative to respond to
the spread of HIV/AIDS among homosexual and bisexual men and is a
service-oriented NGO with a special commitment to the homosexual population. It offers health services, such as promotion of positive life, sexual
orientation, hotline and testing, and education, such as psychosocial workshops, information tables, and community prevention education in places

for public sex. It also provides health services for homosexual individuals. An informant stated: "Since all our environment in Chile is heterosexual, it is good to have an organization that provides good HIV/AIDS care for homosexuals, I'd rather have my peers come here than to any other service." Thus, the members/interviewees have experiences with exposure to being a health care provider.

These two NGOs were founded as a direct outgrowth of the founders' struggles with issues faced by persons living with HIV and AIDS, as well as their family or friends. The interviewees reported fighting for the human rights of people living with HIV/AIDS and of gay people. As any other legal organization in Chile, the organizations are legally enrolled as having a personal jurisdiction: community-based organization and corporation. Both organizations focus their mission on the fight for equality, non-stigmatization, and provision of HIV/AIDS-related care.

In Study A, participants from both NGOs had similar characteristics. Of the 30 interviewees (see Table 3), 24 were men and 21 of them considered them homosexual. Sixteen of the interviewees are employed by the NGO and the others considered their participation to be as a member of the organization.

In Study B, 20 women from one neighborhood in Santiago were selected for participation. The women were between 18 and 49 (see Table 3), and were sexually active with a male partner within the last 3 months although their HIV status was unknown at the time of the interview. They lived in the La Pintana neighborhood of Santiago, a low-income area, and received care at the Health Center of La Pintana, a FONASA clinic. Although most women had not completed primary school, the women were articulate and reflective in telling their stories about their experiences with HIV/AIDS. Seventy-four percent (74%) of the women were currently living with a spouse or partner when the data were collected, for an average of 3.1 years (SD, 1.8). They had 2.2 children on average, with a range from 0 to 6 children. In terms of employment, 56% of were housewives, 26% were unemployed. Of those employed, half were employed as a housekeeper.

Data Collection

Study A included observation, in-depth interviews, and reports reviews about the two NGOs. In-depth interviews were conducted during 2003, in Spanish by the investigator in a place that was comfortable for the participants, and using an interview guide. The investigator spent 3 months

Table 3.   Demographics of Participants in Study A and in Study B.

Sources of Recruitment	Two NGOs Related to HIV/ AIDS in Santiago (Study A, $n = 30$)	Women Attending a National Health Clinic in La Pintana (Study B, $n = 20$)
Demographic characteristics		
Gender	Female 6 (20%)	Female (20) 100%
	Male 24 (80%)	Male 0%
Average age	35	31
Mean income	US$ 615	US$ 54
Education		
Some primary school	0 (50%)	0 (0%)
Some HIV school	1 (35%)	1 (3%)
Completed HIV school	29 (15%)	29 (97%)
Having a stable relationship	17 (57%)	15 (74%)
Catholics	11 (37%)	13 (66%)

visiting the organizations almost every day for field observations. Archives of reports and previous publications were also reviewed in both organizations. Study B included in-depth interviews with 20 women conducted in Spanish by the investigator during 2002. Open-ended questions were asked about their HIV/AIDS knowledge, their experiences of *machismo*, domestic violence, and substance abuse. Probes and follow-up questions were used during the interview to increase the richness and depth of the responses and for clarification. Institutional Review Boards from the University of Illinois at Chicago and from the Pontificia Universidad Católica de Chile approved the procedures used in both studies.

Data Analysis

In both studies interview data were audiotape-recorded and transcribed verbatim in Spanish, and imported into Nudist (N5) software to facilitate data analysis and to assist in data storage, coding, and retrieval. Data were gathered in the form of text. Content analysis was used to recognize, group, and categorize patterns (Patton, 1990). To find meaningful analytical units, and given the emic nature of the data, a combination of concept- and data-based coding methods was used (Gough & Scott, 2000). Data from both studies were first fully analyzed with regard to answering the original studies' research questions. The conceptual frameworks of both studies were used to develop conceptual definitions based on the available literature. The primary data analysis steps were to (1) develop a coding system, (2) code the interview transcripts, and (3) verify the coding system (Weston, Gandell, Beauchamp, McAlpine, & Wiseman, 2001). Following the content analysis process of recognizing, coding, and categorizing patterns from text data (Patton, 1990), the researchers established a set of concepts that were coded. Once all data had been analyzed, three different bilingual individuals reviewed at least 25% of the interviewee transcripts from each study. Each person submitted a report that included the codes found in each interview according to original definitions, as well as additional concepts found. After these reports were combined, differences were discussed until the coders arrived at a consensus. A final codebook was developed based on theoretical explanations and data-driven definitions.

Several findings from both studies appeared related to health services delivery and administration, such as gaps in HIV/AIDS information from providers and unethical behaviors of providers. In other words, participants in both studies volunteered narratives about FONASA providers. Therefore, the data were reanalyzed to answer the question: "What do the experiences of activists and women reveal about FONASA and its response to the HIV/AIDS epidemic?"

To develop the coding system for the secondary analysis of the qualitative data, an iterative process of content analysis and theory building, consistent with the grounded theory approach (Glaser, 1969; Strauss & Corbin, 1990; Charmaz, 2000) was used. An iterative process of model development began by modeling the domains from the stories. The model was then critically compared to the data and modified to more accurately reflect the processes reflected in the stories. The current model was shared with some study participants who agreed that it reflects their experiences. Throughout the coding process, care was taken to identify and include any stories that were unique or dissimilar. However, there was remarkable consistency across the interview data, due in part to the sample selection criteria. The unit of analysis was the sentence within the transcript. This codable unit was chosen since it can have meaning on its own. Furthermore, sentences make it easier to identify categories sufficiently precise to allow different coders to reach the same results using the same data (Silverman, 2001). After an initial set of new codes were defined with a small subset of interviews from both studies, the authors reviewed, identified, and defined the concepts across all interviews. As each interview was reanalyzed, the emerging concepts and theory were modified to accommodate the data. With over half of the interviews re-analyzed, each additional interview served as confirmatory of the data-derived model.

STORIES OF THE REALITIES

The qualitative data from the two primary studies, when interpreted in terms of the health care system, revealed three domains pertaining to problems experienced: personal injustice, practitioner incompetence, and health system inadequacies. A fourth domain, advocacy and activism, describes a response to those problems in terms of strategies to create system change. Stories from each domain are informative about the breadth and depth of issues that currently exist in the national health system. The stories and corresponding domains are summarized in Table 4.

Stories about Personal Injustice with the Health System

The idea that HIV/AIDS started with and is transmitted primarily among homosexual men is dominant in Santiago. Participants used different popular, and sometimes derogatory, terms to refer to homosexual men that are equivalent in English to faggot, queer, and sissy. As in many cultures, being homosexual is associated with discrimination, as one NGO member explained: "I saw young boys throwing stones at a couple of homosexual men. I asked them why are you doing that, they are not bothering you? They answered, 'Because they are queer'". Having HIV/AIDS is also associated with pervasive discrimination. Two women from Study B explained:

> My brother suffers from discrimination, because when people find out that he has HIV, nobody wants to talk to him. Also he was rejected from a place where he was looking for job.
>   When my friend found out that he had AIDS, he only shared it with me, since he was afraid to be rejected or discriminated by his family or friends, because having AIDS is considered worse than having a plague.

Discrimination does not stop at the door of the clinic or the hospital, but directly affects the provision of care. Interviewees describe FONASA as stigmatizing and discriminatory, with uninformed and ignorant health care professionals. As a participant from Study A relayed:

> I saw that man in the hospital, he was very skinny and he impressed me...I asked the nurse does he has cancer? And she said no he has AIDS, because he is a queer and queers are dirty, for that reason he got AIDS.

Other examples of discrimination were found in a book published by one of the activist organizations, "Situations of discrimination that affect people living with HIV/AIDS in Chile" (Vidal et al., 2002). The authors wrote a

Table 4.   List of Domains with Sample Quotes.

Domains	Sample Quote
Personal Injustice Discrimination	"My brother suffers from discrimination, because when people find out that he has HIV, nobody wants to talk to him. Also he was rejected from a place where he was looking for job."
Practitioner Incompetence and Attitudes	"I was able to save money to go to an endocrinologist, of course an endocrinologist [ironic laugh]. And, he said I did not have any problem...'You are not gay because you have pubic hair'."
System Inadequacies	
Inadequate funding	"The health care system does not consider giving money for working on gay-related issues and HIV/AIDS."
Inadequate confidentiality and ethics	"People sign without knowing what they are signing, the doctor says [sign this paper], just for getting the person in, but not to comply with the fundamental principle of an inform consent."
Inadequate provider training	"...The academia and universities have resisted. The best we have gotten in that sector is to have elective courses, but the physicians do not have HIV courses, nor clinical or sensitizing training, that is even less."
Advocacy and Activism	
Information dissemination	"Increasing their sense of belonging, increase self-esteem, increase knowledge and awareness ..."
Legal actions	"Suing the Chilean government for negligence and no commitment to the AIDS law."
Speak out against injustice	"We decided that being treated inhumanly was not acceptable and we chained ourselves in front of congress."
Exert status influence	"I belong to a very influential family, with excellent economic status. Sometimes it has been hard to deal with that, people at the beginning did not felt represented, but now we all understand that that has helped in getting the contacts we need."
Vision driven actions	"The medical model treats the individual as an object, like an item, like an experiment. And we are separated from that medical model. Since the beginning."

section specifically about discrimination in the health system with specific examples of discrimination in the delivery of care, such as segregation and negligence of hospitalized clients, discrimination by specialists in emergency rooms, and in the management of dead bodies. A separate section describes the lack of medical ethics. A very clear example for provider discrimination is the repeated story of dentists not willing to have HIV-positive clients, or having a policy of treating them only at the end of the day.

Stories about Practitioner Incompetence and Attitudes

When attending a clinic, almost none of the participants in either study received any information about HIV or AIDS during a routine health care visit. Interviewees suggested that their search for information is more often directed toward media channels, such as newspaper or TV programs. One participant from Study B explained: "I learned about this disease from the TV, but sometimes the information is contradictory, so I felt confused." In other words, the information obtained from these sources is not accurate or precise. As a result, the women from Study B, especially, had misconceptions about HIV/AIDS. A member from Study A recalled how practitioners also are confused and not well informed in terms of HIV/AIDS and homosexuality. He recalled:

> I was able to save money to go to an endocrinologist, of course an endocrinologist [ironic laugh]. And, he said I did not have any problem…'You are not gay because you have pubic hair'.

Interviewees stated that health care providers appear not to have enough educational preparation nor do they have a positive attitude about working with people living with HIV/AIDS or who have a homosexual orientation. This may explain why participants did not consider health care providers their allies in improving health or gaining a better understanding of their health. Only two participants indicated receiving information from health care providers. One interviewee from Study A relayed that it was because the provider knew he was gay, so "because I was gay it was important for me to know." One NGO member relayed a story of a woman living with HIV/AIDS who went to a public health clinic using her FONASA insurance; "nobody asked that woman anything besides telling her that she could not have a baby, and was asked to sign the consent to be sterilized."

Many participants of both studies were not treated with respect, and referred to the situation that most clients "fear physicians because they can say OK, if you do not follow what I say or if you don't wait for me when I am even 2 hours late, find another place." In other cases one interviewee from Study A noted that patients "who understand their rights and ask for them to be respected, are considered conflictive patients, therefore not desirable to take care of." As mentioned by one of the participants:

> ...Doctors establish relationships only around a scientific ground. They believe theirs is a scientific role, so they point out what needs to be done in that interaction, and they do not suggest any other thing outside what is scientific...they are very pragmatic and very closed minded to the role they believe they have. For example, they are not available to attend a manifestation [rally] with us to fight for the rights of their patients. Also they are going to attend with a great deal of difficulty to a meeting with social components, they are going to have their own circles of conversation, and they are not going to allow the entrance of someone who does not belong to the scientific body: the semi-Olympus. Really, they have done something, but they have circumscribed them to a determined space, in a context very protective of their own role and interests.

Stories about System Inadequacies

Although neither study sought to describe the inadequacies of the Chilean national health system, many of the participants' stories reveal key problems: lack of funding, lack of confidentiality, and inadequate training of providers on HIV/AIDS medical management and prevention.

Inadequate Funding

Participants from both studies noticed a lack of funding for HIV/AIDS health care. They said that the health care system does not "consider giving money for working on gay-related issues and HIV/AIDS." As such, prevention programs or treatment of people living with HIV are scarce, and in general, services are rarely provided or are of low quality. As a participant from Study B recalled: "I tried to call many times the CONASIDA phone hot line, but it was not working or it was busy."

The low funding affects availability of services, and also affects personnel morale. Interviewees from both studies made the direct connection between FONASA funding and staff morale. Two members of the NGOs from Study A recalled:

> Especially people who work in the primary health care settings do not work with HIV motivations and there is a little budget.

Primary health care receives scarce resources through the Ministry of Health; therefore, people who work at it are typically not very motivated due to their low salaries, and usually are the ones with less formal education, keeping the traditional Chilean values in their work and not looking for or willing to work for a change.

Inadequate Confidentiality and Problematic Ethics

Lack of confidentiality was another health system problem described by the participants. They associated the lack of maintaining confidentiality with the spread of HIV/AIDS because they believed that individuals are afraid of getting tested and having their results known in their community. Lack of confidentiality was also related to the lack of accurate information about the disease. One participant from Study A explained:

> ...the problem in the health clinics is that they violate confidentiality, you can always see that, thousands of people from the same neighborhoods that are friends and are afraid of leaks of information...lots of times confidentiality is violated.

Also in relation to ethical issues, one woman with HIV/AIDS talked about how health care providers do not follow international ethics codes for research:

> Research studies in this country in regards with antiretroviral therapy are not yet managed by ethics codes that concur with international standards. People sign without knowing what they are signing, the doctor says [sign this paper], just for getting the person in, but not to comply with the fundamental principle of an informed consent. That has to do with the person extensively understanding in which context he is getting to and what are the pros and cons, its risks...that doesn't exist.

An informed interviewee from one of the HIV/AIDS-related NGOs was particularly articulate and assessed the situation of Chile in the following way:

> It is an anti-value, when you look at professional associations and the analysis they make or their way of actions, really it is a medical association that safeguards the fact of controlling the medical ethics. They want the values attached to medical exercise in their hands, the service provided by medicine is more for them than for their clients, even though they talk eloquently about the incorporation of international values for medical practice, but the ones that have to do with the others, meaning who they take care of are not integrated. And they still keep talking about ethics, I mean they talk about medical ethics in the service of their patients...spectacular contradiction, by knowing just a little of medical ethics they should know how it is for the service of the users or clients.

These ideas are also supported by Vidal et al. (2002), who described transgression of medical ethics in terms of lack of confidentiality and lack of pre- and post-HIV testing and counseling.

Inadequate provider Training

Lack of training and continuing education of health providers seem to be sources of providers' negative attitudes and lack of knowledge regarding HIV and AIDS. Health professionals were not perceived by participants from either study as playing a role in HIV/AIDS education and prevention. This circumstance emphasizes the need to evaluate health professionals' curricula, and to incorporate or modify HIV/AIDS content. One participant was explicit regarding health care practitioners:

> I think that discrimination is a consequence of people's ignorance about AIDS, because they do not know about this disease.

Arguably, the narratives are images of FONASA clients having negative experiences with physicians. Regardless of the professional or technical title, there seems to be a gap in the health providers' education about HIV/AIDS. One interviewee with a health care background suggested:

> ...The academia and universities have resisted. The best we have gotten in that sector is to have elective courses, but the physicians do not have HIV courses, nor clinical or sensitizing training, that is even less. The social workers are as well. Thinking about a broader health care team: physicians don't know, nurses, social workers don't know, psychologists don't know, they are not prepared...and in the University of Chile where I studied, there is nothing.

Stories about Advocacy and Activism

The findings from both studies suggest that HIV/AIDS is a stigmatizing disease, largely as a result of traditional and religious values within the Chilean culture. Although some improvements have occurred in terms of the response towards the epidemic since its appearance, homosexual men and other people affected by HIV have felt motivated to fight the government as many needs have not been addressed by FONASA. Members of both NGOs have changed the environment of FONASA by providing health care, information, and support services. It is through the NGOs that the influence of activists is organized into coherent and consistent actions aimed at changing FONASA. The efforts of the activists have taken four forms: changing the information available about HIV/AIDS, speaking out about and against the injustices inherent in FONASA, taking legal actions to protect individual patients and to hold FONASA providers accountable, and by exerting personal influence based on their HIV status in Santiago society.

Information Dissemination

Interviewees believe that through participation in NGOs individuals acquire life improvement, guidance, information, and empowerment: "People understand their disease", "We guide them to ask for adequate care", "When it got to the point of getting tested and it was positive, here I was taught the way of going up, not succumbing myself, I am still alive," and as the philosophy of "We do not give the fish, instead to teach our members how to fish" are the triggers for changing the current national health care system.

The activities of the NGOs help empower their clients by "increasing their sense of belonging, increase self-esteem, increase knowledge and awareness, and have a better sense of accepting the personal characteristics." As one participant observed, these indirect interactions with hospitals, as well as direct interactions with attending physicians and other providers at the hospitals contribute to a change: "providers of people who become involved in our organization realize that their so quality patients start understanding their rights, start asking more, and they challenged their bad manners and care."

Legal Actions

One organization even had the experience "of suing the Chilean government for negligence and no commitment to the law," referring to the AIDS Law. This was the first law to make the government responsible for massive public service campaigns, and to give people with HIV/AIDS access to respect, confidentiality, and free drug treatment if they were enrolled in FONASA ("AIDS Law # 19,779," 2001). The AIDS Law was partly the result of NGOs' efforts to increase awareness about the disease and demanding that the government assume an active role in primary, secondary, and tertiary HIV/AIDS prevention in Chile.

Speaking out against Injustices

Within both NGOs from Study A, members themselves, as well as their family, friends, or the people they advocate for, experienced injustices within the health care system. Their reactions at initial stages of the epidemic are described as "silent and passive." Although having an initial voiceless response to injustice, the story has changed. Interviewees describe their actions as confrontational and "noisy". For example, an interviewee from Study A recollects:

> We decided that being treated inhumanly was not acceptable and we chained ourselves in front of Congress. The reaction from carabineros (policemen) was nasty and it was hard to be there, but everybody in the country saw us and that necessarily affects society and forced Congressmen and the Ministry of Health to speak and respond to us.

Exerting Status Influence

At least two members in each organization from Study A had an influential sociopolitical positions based on their socioeconomic status, educational background, or international experience. Those personal characteristics gave credibility to the organizations that enabled the individuals and NGOs to be more influential, such that they were able to get the Chilean AIDS Law passed. In situations where individuals from the NGOs did not have status power, they contacted a powerful health care provider who could help safeguard that the NGO, provide updated HIV/AIDS information, and informally suggest what the government was doing in terms of HIV/AIDS care. In these ways, the activists were able to leverage their personal status and the status of supporters of their vision. Some NGO members stated: "Well, I do not represent the typical member of a community based organization; I belong to a very influential family, with excellent economic status. Sometimes it has been hard to deal with that, people at the beginning did not felt represented, but now we all understand that that has helped in getting the contacts we need."

Vision-Driven Actions

Chileans with HIV/AIDS have been dissatisfied with their access to health care for effectively preventing or treating HIV/AIDS. As a result, they initiated and established a social movement in the form of NGOs within Chile.

This social movement is resulting in a growing demand by the HIV/AIDS activists for quality and ethical health care. As a participant from one of the organizations stated: "The medical model treats the individual as an object, like an item, like an experiment. And we are separated from that medical model. Since the beginning." Participants identified a gap between the medical community and the affected individuals, as one woman explained, in which "the relationships cannot be built horizontally; instead they are vertical, like in the case of physicians." Both activist NGOs have missions that pursue the empowerment of Chileans beyond HIV and AIDS, which is reflected in their history and missions. To be an activist requires, to some extent, a vision of a desirable future. The HIV/AIDS activists' actions are based on their vision for a better health system.

FROM STORIES TO MODEL: CONSTRUCTED ENVIRONMENTAL DYNAMISM

The descriptions of issues related to the provision of HIV/AIDS services can be interpreted through the lens of challenges facing health care administrators in FONASA. This perspective led to development of a theoretical description of the forces at work in the organizational environment of FONASA, particularly the key forces generated by the activists and targeted toward specific actors within the FONASA system. The theoretical model provides a heuristic for developing administrative strategies to improve HIV/AIDS care, and health care, in general, in Chile.

Targets and Strategies to Construct Environmental Dynamism

The stories from Santiago revealed that experiences of personal injustice and incompetent and unethical health care by the HIV/AIDS activists led them to take a set of actions directed toward specific stakeholders. In this way, the activists have been able to construct (create) a heightened level of dynamism within the environment of FONASA. Five sets of stakeholders related to FONASA are targeted by the activists, with the expectation that those stakeholders will respond to the changed environment. The activists are affecting these five stakeholders, although each set of stakeholders is acted upon through different strategies.

One set of stakeholders is current and future HIV/AIDS clients, as well as their families and the public at large. These are the constituents of the national and local health care providers. The activists' efforts are particularly directed toward changing the current attitudes of clients living with HIV/AIDS from one of acceptance of their powerlessness, discrimination, and disrespect to one of acceptance of their value and right to health care. Activists achieve this change by altering the informational landscape and speaking out against the injustice. As a Chilean activist suggests, "... our philosophy: We do not give the fish; instead, we teach members how to fish." This process occurs because activists help "people understand their disease" and "guide them to ask for adequate care." Patients "who understand their rights and ask for them to be respected are considered conflictive patients", an indication that the activists are indirectly influencing providers and the environment. Overall, "individuals living with HIV/AIDS feel the right to ask for what they need, they realize that they deserve a better care." Thus, the activists both taught patients about their rights and created an informational jolt to which the health care providers and FONASA must respond.

A second group affected by activists is individual health care practitioners, predominantly physicians. Activists seek to change individual practitioner behaviors from providing low-quality and marginally competent HIV/AIDS care to providing higher quality medical care and HIV/AIDS prevention. They also seek to increase practitioner accountability for quality care and provision of ethical care. Activists realize that the existing organizational environment does not foster accountability, nor is the level of ethical behavior consistent with international standards or the AIDS Law. Activists are making public information about HIV/AIDS, the inadequacies of the system in which the practitioners work, and the lack of ethical behaviors by individual practitioners. This contributes to creating an informational jolt to affect practitioner behavior. The other strategy used by activists is to speak out against injustice, including the injustice of the system in which practitioners work, and the lack of financial rewards for working in the national system. In other words, activists include as an agenda item the motivations of the practitioners as influenced by the institution. A participant stated, "People who work in primary health care settings do not work with high motivation and there is a small budget." That idea needs to be changed and is on the agenda of Chilean activists. One interviewee summarized it by saying, "we do not care if it is through legal actions or what, but physicians need to change their attitude and feel motivated to help their patients."

One route to achieve practitioner behavioral changes is through improved and updated training regarding HIV/AIDS. Therefore, the third group targeted, albeit indirectly, are the educators of health professionals. One consequence of the inadequate education is that health care providers do not have an active role in providing HIV/AIDS care at community clinics, according to the women in Study B who are users of FONASA (Cianelli, 2002). Activists are aware of the need to make changes in the basic education that practitioner receive and thus include professional education as an agenda item in their speaking out. In addition, the informational jolt created around the HIV/AIDS epidemic and health care influences the educators. As described earlier by a participant who is in academe, education for health professionals about HIV/AIDS is lacking.

The fourth set of stakeholders affected by activists is the national hospitals and the municipal clinics. Activists seek to change hospitals' noncompliance with the HIV/AIDS Law, and to increase the level of competent and compassionate hospital care for people living with HIV/AIDS. Activists use two strategies with the hospitals and clinics: speaking out against injustice and exerting influence through the status connections of the privileged activists. HIV/AIDS-related activists in Chile "have established relationships with stakeholders at municipalities and we just speak up when injustice occurs, and they hear us, we can make a lot of noise. Besides, we have good contacts." They also take legal action when necessary to assure access to health care. Lack of confidentiality and providers' unethical behaviors HIV historically exposed clients to hazardous conditions. Before the AIDS Law, confidentiality and ethical behavior of providers were not legally sanctioned under legal code. The existence of the AIDS Law makes providers and hospitals legally liable for patient experiences such as "having their HIV status known by their neighbors and all the people at the hospital." While not a frequently used strategy, activists do take legal actions with hospitals, clinics and the Ministry of Health, which further creates dynamism in the environment of the hospitals, clinics, and national health system.

The last set of stakeholders is the Ministry of Health. The Ministry of Health is responsible for legal oversight and fiscal accountability of the hospitals, and to some degree the local clinics. Activists use two main strategies to influence the Ministry of Health: creating an informational jolt in the environment and exerting their status influence. Use of their status influence is seen in their speaking directly with politicians regarding the inadequate funding for HIV/AIDS primary prevention by the national health system. The informational jolt includes providing users of FONASA with the knowledge and strength to pressure the Ministry of Health and municipalities to actively supervise the HIV/AIDS-related care provided by hospitals and clinics. Testimonies from clients and other Chileans indicate that health care professionals are not promoting individuals' health improvement. After taking their professional oath, health care professionals face no regulation of their professional behavior. This lack of quality control is more apparent in the public arena because of the perception that people "do not have money to pay, [and should] accept what [they] get" and that the national health care system does not "consider giving money for work on gay-related issues and HIV/AIDS."

From Stories to Theoretical Model of Constructed Environmental Dynamism

In general, studies of change processes, including of change processes across organizational, team, and individual levels (Whelan-Berry, Gordon, & Hinings, 2003), minimize or simply assume that organizational processes begin with changes in the organizational environment. Our data suggest that the collective voice of the marginalized who become activists has the potential to reverberate in ways that may force FONASA to change. The role of activists in creating health systems change was in the stories, and, using a grounded theory approach (Glaser & Strauss, 1967), a theoretical model (see Figure 1) emerged of the processes by which the activists are creating a heightened level of dynamism within the Chilean health care sector.

Specifically, the stories point to three elements of a vision for change: high-quality and competent HIV/AIDS care, ethical and equitable HIV/AIDS care, and effective HIV/AIDS prevention programs. The activists not only share this vision, but it is the vision they are seeking to instill in Chilean society and, more immediately, throughout FONASA. The gap between their experiences with FONASA and this vision motivates them to take actions directed toward the five sets of stakeholders previously identified. Activists use four major strategies: creating an informational jolt, speaking out against injustices, taking legal action, and exerting status influence. These strategies have synergistic effects on the five sets of stakeholders who are the targets of their actions. Although each strategy does not equally affect each of the five stakeholders, each strategy does have a primary target. For example, taking legal actions is mostly directed at FONASA and the Ministry of Health. As a synergistic set, the strategies are the means by which activists are constructing dynamism in the environment of FONASA.

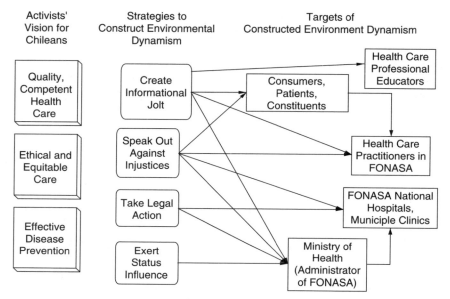

Fig. 1. Model of the Means by which Activists Create Constructed Environmental Dynamism of the Chilean National Health System, FONASA.

Constructed Environmental Dynamism

Activists for HIV/AIDS patients intentionally and explicitly seek to change the organizational environment of health practitioners, the Ministry of Health, and the national hospitals and municipal clinics in Santiago. The processes for change used by the activists involve a set of stakeholders upon whom the activists utilize a set of strategies, thereby creating environmental dynamism. Environmental dynamism within FONASA in Santiago began with the presence of HIV/AIDS, and was enhanced by the acquired voice of HIV/AIDS activists. The stories from Santiago reveal that the organizational environment of FONASA was being constructed. The activists' actions generated constructed environmental dynamism, by which we mean the intentionally created pressures on an organization for change as exerted by key stakeholders of that organization. In this regard dynamism is dissimilar to dynamism as used by Dess and Beard (1984), who stress the uncertainty aspect of dynamism. The concept of constructed environmental dynamism is predicated on the intention and desirability of creating substantive changes to an organization.

To understand constructed environmental dynamism requires that attention is placed on the sources of the forces external to the organization, firm or industry, rather than strictly on the internal modifications and adaptations of an organization. From a force field perspective (Lewin, 1997), the constructed environmental dynamism is one external force being exerted on FONASA. The activists' efforts and resulting increased constructed environmental dynamism must be sufficiently strong to counter the opposing force, namely the inertia for change within Chile and FONASA (Ferrer, 2004). This contrasts with the life cycle theory of organizational change (Van de Ven & Poole, 1995; Dooley & Van de Ven, 1999), which is based on a steady state of equilibrium being the goal and expectation of the organization. Maintaining a steady state, a status quo, is likely the preference of health practitioners and FONASA, precisely those who the activists are intentionally seeking to change. The data suggest that more dynamic processes are at work.

An assumption underlying constructed environmental dynamism is that the portion of the organizational environment in which change is being created is a knowable portion of the organizational environment. This is in contrast to the dominant emphasis in organizational science and business strategy on uncertainty of the organizational environment (Thompson, 1967). In addition, the constructed environmental dynamism that results from activism differs substantively from environmental jolts discussed by Meyer, Brooks, and Goes (1990) or the notion of enacted and perceived environments (Weick, 1979). These organizational theories' frames for understanding environments are predicated on the need to understand organizational responses to the environment, and subsequently, research has focused on organizational responses to environmental changes. For example, Fox-Wolfgramm, Boal, and Hunt (1998) focused on the response of two banks to institutional change, and McKay (2001) identified additional organizational responses to a prevention regulatory change across industries. Such studies typically focus on firm performance, such as profitability, as did Reklitis and Trivellas (2002). But, proprietary performance measures do not have the same relevance to publicly owned and administered organizations, such as FONASA.

Market forces are minimally relevant to a national health system, giving constructed environmental dynamism greater importance. Orsstto and Clegg (1999) acknowledge that national elites play a role in the ability of the state to regulate various industries and in regulatory decisions that can influence the acquisition of capital. Their attention to power, structuration, and political economy is a reminder that in developing nations, organizational change occurs within a dramatically different sociopolitical context from that of highly industrialized, capitalistic Western democracies. The inclusion in the model of exerting status influence as a strategy used by activists is consistent with this awareness.

One other feature of constructed environmental dynamism of the health system in Santiago is that it is predicated on the activists' vision of desirable health systems outcomes. The external imposition of a vision on a public organization contrasts dramatically with the dominant view of organizational strategy development as an internally driven process (Miles & Snow, 1978; Ginter, Swayne, & Duncan, 2002). That the vision for FONASA is held external to the organization raises concerns about how the construction of a dynamic, if not imposing, environment might contribute to resistance to change, resentment, and development of an alternative vision for FONASA.

Notes About the Model

The model was developed specifically around issues faced by a governmental health care system in a developing county. Administrators in these systems would historically have limited experience in strategic planning or thinking. Thus, their skills and experience with broad environmental scanning are also limited. The model provides a rudimentary framework of environmental forces that governmental health system administrators might use to systematically increase their awareness of their organizational environment.

Also, the influential forces in the organizational environment that result from activists' constructed environmental dynamism differ from influential forces, such as market competition, that are studied by scholars of health care systems in highly capitalistic and democratic societies. The changes in the social, ethical, and knowledge landscape of FONASA that activists seek are radical, as might be expected given the historical and cultural context of the Chilean governmental health care system. The extent and degree to which activists actions are radical tend to be much less notable in the health systems of industrialized, democratic Western countries, and thus have received less attention by health services scholars. Nonetheless, the dynamism stemming from activists is critical to health care administrators and scholars in other types of sociopolitical and cultural environments.

Finally, the model stems from the emphasis that activists place on service quality and population health, rather than firm financial performance. These areas of emphasis are consistent with FONASA being under governmental control and with the marginalized status of the persons living with HIV/AIDS in Chile. The concern with service quality is internationally ubiquitous across health care systems. In contrast, the concern with HIV/AIDS prevention has a population health focus, which is aligned with a public health perspective on emergent epidemics. In this regard, the model may have a broader application in terms of addressing public health and global health issues.

Practice Implications for Stakeholders

The activists have a substantive role in shaping the organizational environment of FONASA as both advocates and consumers. Interestingly, Scott, Ruef, Mendel, & Caronna (2000), in their list of six types of social actors involved in the United States health care sector, did not include any mention of advocates or social activists. Huegens, Van Den Bosch, and Van Riel (2002), proposed four types of integration that were based on the theoretical assumption that stakeholder integration is advantageous to organizations. However, given the marginalized status of HIV/AIDS patients and homosexual men who are advocates for HIV/AIDS care, it is unlikely that the Chilean health system will engage in stakeholder integration of this group. By FONASA not engaging in integration of the HIV/AIDS activists, the only course of action for the activists is to become more radical and intensify their use of the four influence strategies. This process creates a reinforcing cycle of activism, non-reaction by FONASA, and greater activism by the activists. As this cycle progresses, the constructed environmental dynamism can be expected to increase.

Aiken, Smith, and Lake (1997) conducted a study of the Chilean response to the AIDS epidemic, focusing on screening and tracking HIV-positive individuals and blood bank procedures. They recommended using the existing health care structure for traditional public health interventions. Their study, however, did not address the subsequent question of how those organizational changes could be implemented, including what system changes need to precede their recommended changes. An approach to organizational change that seems accepted across nationalities and cultures is quality improvement programs (Omaswa, Burnham, Baingana, Mwebesa, & Morrow, 1996), including the use of the Donabedian framework (Camilleri & O'Callaghan,

1998). In addition, Adams, Mosneaga, and Gedik (2003) argue for training hospital managers within a health systems development context.

Although the quality improvement methodologies have appeal in terms of being systems-focused and based on a scientific approach, they do not necessarily take into account cultural influences within or on the structure of health care systems. A word of caution is in order. From a post-colonial perspective (Prasad, 2003), use of quality improvement methodologies could be interpreted as perpetuating the imposition of Western thought and ideology of organizational control (Mir, Mir, & Upandhyaya, 2003). The concept of stakeholder integration also could be viewed as an imposed ideology on post-colonial nations. Many theories and change approaches from the developed world will be applicable internationally; however, organizational scholars ought to be sensitive to the possibility of intellectual hegemony or, more importantly, the perception that they are enabling hegemony. Frameworks for understanding organizational change may need to be adapted to non-Western health systems, and adapted to be more locally and culturally appropriate and acceptable.

An alternative approach to managing stakeholders comes from public health, with its emphasis on involvement of the community. This is distinct from the business model of integrating stakeholders to reduce external costs. By promoting a needs assessment of individuals in the community, roughly equivalent to a market survey, the public health approach actively involves the stakeholders in identifying health needs and in developing programs. The public health approach to developing heath services not only has wide support (NACCHO, 2004), but also can reduce costs by generating support among clients and activists, as well as result in acceptable and effective health services. The process of community engagement results in a collaboration that may benefit FONASA by strengthening its relationship with the activists and the NGOs that are altering its environment. In other words, community involvement provides a means to increase environmental scanning in a manner that is non-threatening.

The culture of Santiago and Chile has been influenced heavily by both the history of authoritarian government and the history of radical intellectualism. Thus, alternatively, the engagement approach (Taylor, Vasquez, & Doorley, 2003) to organizational change may be culturally appropriate. The engagement approach may be useful precisely because it is a key component of an organizational strategy to build relationships with stakeholders in the organization's environment through on-going communication with those stakeholders. This approach is similar to the public health strategies for assessing and developing health care programs. Health administrators have the opportunity to build networks with HIV/AIDS organizations that have expertise and interest in contributing to the improvement of the local public/ national health system. By engaging in dialogue and action with selected advocates and activists, health administrators would have more control over the rate and direction of organizational change that occurs in response to the external environment.

Administrative and Managerial Implications

Focusing on the strategies that result in constructed environmental dynamism, rather than generic characteristics of the environment, has advantages to both health administrators and to activists. For institutions and organizations, knowing that dynamism within the environment can be created suggests a need to scan the environment for manifest evidence of the key strategies used by activists. For activists, being conscious and aware of the processes by which environmental dynamism is constructed enables activists elsewhere to replicate the effective strategies on behalf of other vulnerable and disadvantaged groups.

Personnel development will be critical to FONASA's response to the concerns and vision of the activists. A strictly biomedical approach to health care is not considered an option by the interviewees; they view HIV/AIDS as a complex social problem that affect individuals, families, communities, and society. This will require that health professionals receive training by the hospitals and clinics in Santiago and are provided incentives to incorporate a customer-focus into their practices. This training must be accompanied by changes in the basic content of medical and nursing education. It is clear from the stories that changes in education and workplace training will need to be broad in scope, from ethics to medical aspects of HIV/AIDS, and broad in application, from health administrators to front-line personnel.

A disconnect was expressed by interviewees. Based on their international experience with receiving ethical health care, the expectations of the HIV/ AIDS activists are different from the Chilean national policy reflected in the AIDS Law and the actual practices of health care professionals. The disconnect is validated to some extent by other research, such as that of Frasca (2000) who found a need to make changes in the Chilean health care system that would assure confidentiality. It is a historical and cultural artifact that the provision of the ethical health care does not come easily in Chile, as in many other developing countries. Administrators in FONASA must reconcile system constraints with activists' claims that health care is not ethical by

international conventions, and with the demands for high quality HIV/
AIDS health care services. Attempts to change provider knowledge about
the AIDS Law, about HIV/AIDS, and about bioethics need to be reinforced
and structured into human resource management policies and procedures,
as well as organizational culture.

The interview data point to a need to change national funding streams to
adequately address the needs of persons living with HIV/AIDS and their
care options. It is possible that hospitals, clinics, and the Ministry of Health
will engage in environmental scanning that is sufficiently different. This
could result in each having a different level of awareness of the resources
dilemma. The data do suggest that if hospital and clinic administrators are
aware of external pressures, they lack resources necessary to contemplate,
let alone enact, organizational changes being demanded by the activists. The
activists' awareness of the lack of resources for change and the lack of
incentives for providers to change underscores a dilemma the national
health care organizations face; the dilemma of wanting to change but lacking the means to do so. This type of change in funding allocations is needed
if CONASIDA is to accomplish the goal identified by one participant:
"Seeking efficiency in the use of resources by externalization of services,
alliances with the private sector, and the execution of participative projects
with the national health sector, other sectors of the government, and social
actors trained in the subject". It is unclear whether the vision of the activists
or the forces they are exerting will be sufficient to alter national allocation of
funds.

Future Research

The perceptions of hospital CEOs have been found to be important to a
variety of hospital administration issues. However, studies such as that by
Alexander, Burns, and Morrisey (2001) of hospital CEO perceptions and
competition, have limited applicability to a national, governmental health
system in which there is essentially no competition. Their study does highlight that perceptions and executive attention play a role in the formation of
strategy. What is not known from the data from Study A and Study B is to
what extent administrators in FONASA are aware of the changing
environment created by the HIV/AIDS activists and what would be required to gain their attention.

In their introduction to a special issue emphasizing approaches to organizational change management, Sturdy and Grey (2003) make clear that

the current scholarly emphasis remains on what is change and how to approach it in the context of management. Although some models of change do acknowledge that organizational environmental changes are opportunities (Orlikowski & Hofman, 1997), these models fail to address or typify those environmental changes. Thus, managerial practice remains reactive. There is virtually no attention to change as being intentionally induced from external forces, except in the area of ecology and business. In this area, public relations management seems to be a dominant response to the constructed environmental dynamism of ecology activists. Not evident in our data is the degree to which constructed environmental dynamism leads to organizational change. Longitudinal case studies are needed to understand whether the constructed environmental dynamism being created does, in fact, generate internal organizational changes. In addition, studies that seek to link the external environmental changes to the internal processes of FONASA could yield valuable information about the evolution of national health systems.

One other avenue for future research and theory development is the role of marginalized and socially disregarded, yet active and vocal, stakeholders. The extent to which their actions foster and actually create constructed environmental dynamism that leads to change deserves further attention. Such a line of research would extend and refine the model we have proposed.

CONCLUSION

The activists played a role in shaping the information environment of the Santiago national health system, by increasing health information available and calling attention to the lack of health information coming from the official governmental and professional sources. The information made available by the activists on the unmet health care needs of HIV/AIDS patients, on effective prevention strategies, and on the unethical behavior of providers cannot be ignored by health administrators without experiencing repercussions.

The qualitative data from Santiago embody elements of organizational change and environmental dynamism (Carmona & Valle, 2000) in a way that is novel and potentially informative for creating an international health systems development agenda. The issues identified from the interviewees' experiences hint at the types of organizational and managerial changes and adaptations that are needed to adequately address the HIV/AIDS situation in developing countries. These issues were analyzed from an organizational change perspective, which is congruent with the WHO call for responsiveness by national health systems. In a review of the effectiveness of the AIDS treatment movement, James (1997) found that activists in the United States have been instrumental in sensitizing the medical community to the needs of HIV/AIDS patients, as well as establishing standards for HIV/AIDS care. It seems that the activists in Santiago are striving for similar effects.

Regional administrators and local health care managers in FONASA are faced with a turbulent organizational environment. The specific actions they need to take in order to address and, hopefully, prevent the pending HIV/AIDS epidemic entail deep, fundamental changes that will result in an evolution of FONASA. These changes involve understanding and leveraging opportunities and pressures in new ways that support the provision of equitable, ethical, and accessible health care to groups marginalized in the Chilean society. The events unfolding in Chile can become a model for other developing countries in South America.

REFERENCES

Adams, O., Mosneaga, A., & Gedik, G. (2003). Improving institutional performance by better internal hospital management: A framework for assessing management training needs. *World Hospitals and Health Services: The Official Journal of the International Hospital Federation, 39*(2), 3–10, 41, 43.

AIDS Law # 19,779 (2001). National Congress.

Aiken, L. H., Smith, H. L., & Lake, E. T. (1997). Using existing health care systems to respond to the AIDS epidemic: Research and recommendations for Chile. *International Journal of Health Services, 27*(1), 177–199.

Alexander, J. A., Burns, L. R., & Morrisey, M. A. (2001). CEO perceptions of competition and strategic response in hospital markets. *Medical Care Research and Review, 58*, 162–193.

ARC (1998). *Manual del Instructor sobre el VIH/SIDA [HIV/AIDS Instructors's Manual]*: *American Red Cross*. Unpublished manuscript.

Bernal, J., Lukacs, I., Malebran, A., & Bonacic, H. (1989). Attitudes and knowledge on AIDS in a maternity unit in Santiago de Chile. *Revista Chilean de obstetricia y ginecologia, 54*(3), 151–157.

Brofman, M., & Gleizaer, M. (1994). Participacion comunitaria: Necesidad, excusa o estrategia? O de que hablamos cuando hablamos de participacion comunitaria? *Cadernaos de Saude Publica Rio de Janeiro, 10*(1), 11–122.

Camilleri, D., & O'Callaghan, M. (1998). Comparing public and private hospital care service quality. *International Journal of Health Care Quality Assurance Incorporating Leadership in Health Services, 11*(4–5), 127–133.

Cantu, L. (2000). *Entre hombres/between men: Latino masculinities and homosexualities*. Thousand Oaks, CA: Sage.

Carmona, M., & Valle, C. D. (2000). *SIDA en Chile: La historia desconocida*. Santiago: Andres Bello.

Charmaz, K. (2000). Grounded theory: Objectivist and constructivist methods. In: N. K. Denzin & Y. S. Lincoln (Eds), *Handbook of qualitative research* (2nd ed., pp., 509–535). Thousand Oaks, CA: Sage.

Cianelli, R. (2002). *HIV/AIDS issues among Chilean women: Cultural factors and perception of risk HIV/AIDS acquisition*. Doctoral Dissertation, University of Illinois at Chicago, IL.

CONASIDA (2001). *Boletín epidemiológico semestral (epidemic bulletin) # 14*. Retrieved January 16, 2005, from the World Wide Web: http://www.conasida.cl.

Dayton, J. M., & Merson, M. H. (2000). Global dimensions of the AIDS epidemic: Implications for prevention and care. *Infectious Disease Clinics of North America, 14*, 791–808.

Dess, G. G., & Beard, D. W. (1984). Dimensions of organizational task environments. *Administration Science Quarterly, 29*, 52–73.

Diaz, R. (1998). *Latino gay men and HIV: Culture, sexuality, and risk behavior*. New York: Routledge.

Diaz, R., Ayala, G., Bein, E., Henne, J., & Marin, B. (2001). The impact of homophobia, poverty, and racism on the mental health of gay and bisexual Latino men: Findings from three U.S. cities, *American Journal of Public Health*.

Dooley, K. J., & Van de Ven, A. H. (1999). Explaining complex organizational dynamics. *Organization Science, 10*, 358–373.

Eckstein, S. (2001). Community as a gift-giving: Collectivistic roots of volunteerism. *American Sociological Review, 66*, 829–851.

Ferrer, L. (2004). *NGOs: Communities organizing around HIV/AIDS in Santiago, Chile*. Doctoral Dissertation, University of Illinois at Chicago, IL.

Fox-Wolfgramm, S. J., Boal, K. B., & Hunt, J. G. (1998). Organizational adaptation to institutional change: A comparative study of first-order change in prospector and defender banks. *Administration Science Quarterly, 4*, 87–126.

Frasca, T. (2000). Country watch: Chile. *Sexual Health Exchange, 1*, 9–10.

Frooman, J. (1999). Stakeholders influence strategy. *Academy of Management Review, 24*(2), 191–205.

Ginter, P. M., Swayne, L. E., & Duncan, W. J. (2002). *Strategic management of health care organizations* (4th ed.). Oxford, UK: Blackwell Publishing.

Gissi, J. (1978). El machismo en los dos sexos. In: P. Covarrubias & R. Franco (Eds), *Chile mujer y sociedad* (pp. 550–573). Santiago: Fondo de las Naciones Unidas para la Infancia.

Glaser, B., & Strauss, A. (1967). *The discovery of grounded theory: Strategies for qualitative research*. Chicago: Aldine Publications Co.

Goodwin, J., & Jasper, J. (2003). *The Social movement reader: Cases and concepts*. Oxford, UK: Blackwell Publishing.

Gough, S., & Scott, W. (2000). Exploring the purposes of qualitative data coding in educational enquiry: Insights from recent research. *Educational Studies, 26*(3), 339–354.

Guimaraes, C. (1994). Male bisexuality, gender relations, and AIDS in Brazil. In: P. Wijeyaratne, J. Roberts, J. Kitts & L. Arsenault (Eds), *Gender, health, and sustainable development: A Latin American perspective* (pp. 26–34). Ottawa: International Development Research Center.

Huegens, P., Van Den Bosch, F., & Van Riel, C. (2002). Stakeholders integration: Building mutually enforcing relationships. *Business and Society, 41*, 36–60.

James, J. S. (1997). AIDS treatment activism: Focus on service. *AIDS Treatment News, 21*(267), 4–8.

Klein-Alonso, L. (1996). Women's social representation of sex, sexuality, and IDS in Brasil. In: L. Long & M. Ankrah (Eds), *Women's experiences with HIV/AIDS: An international perspective* (pp. 151–159). New York: Columbia Editor.

Leon, F. (2002). *The case of the Chilean health system, 1983–2000.* PAHO. Retrieved March 11, 2004, from the World Wide Web: http://www.paho.org/English/HDP/HDD/20Fran.pdf.

Levy, J., & Kates, J. (2000). HIV: Challenging the health care delivery system. *American Journal of Public Health, 90*(7), 1033–1036.

Lewin, K. (1997). *Resolving social conflicts. And, field theory in social science.* Washington, DC: American Psychological Association.

McKay, R. B. (2001). Organizational responses to an environmental bill rights. *Organization Studies, 22,* 625–658.

Meyer, A. D., Brooks, G. R., & Goes, J. B. (1990). Environmental jolts and industry revolutions: Organizational responses to discontinuous change. *Strategic Management Journal, 11,* 93–110.

Miles, R., & Snow, C. (1978). *Organizational strategy, structure, and process.* New York: McGraw-Hill.

Ministerio de salud de la nación (2003). Boletín sobre el SIDA en la Argentina. *Programa nacional de lucha contra los retrovirus del humano, SIDA y ETS X* (22). Ministerio Nacional de salud y ambiente de la nación, Argentina.

MINSAL (2001). *Boletín Epidemiológico N°4. Enfermedades de Transmisión Sexual.* Retrieved January 16, 2005, from the World Wide Web: http://www.conasida.cl.

Mir, R. A., Mir, A., & Upandhyaya, P. (2003). Towards a postcolonial reading of organizational control. In: A. Prasad (Ed.), *Postcolonial theory and organizational analysis: A critical engagement.* New York: Palgrave.

NACCHO (National Association of County and City Health Officials) (2004). *Achieving healthier communities through MAPP: A user's handbook.* http://www.naccho.org/project77.cfm (Accessed Equity. 21, 2004).

Navarro, O. (2000). Women and children's at risk of contracting HIV in Costa Rica. In: J. Keenan (Ed.), *Catholic ethicists on HIV/AIDS prevention* (pp. 135–141). New York: Library of Congress Cataloging-in-Publication Data.

Omaswa, F., Burnham, G., Baingana, G., Mwebesa, H., & Morrow, R. (1996). Introducing quality improvement management methods into primary health care services in Uganda. *QA Brief, 5*(1), 12–15.

Omoto, A., Odom, D., & Crain, L. (1999). Helping in hard times: Relationship closeness and the AIDS volunteer experience. In: V. Derlega & A. Barbee (Eds), *HIV and social interaction.* Thousand Oaks, CA: Sage.

Orlikowski, W., & Hofman, J. D. (1997). An improvisational model for change management: The case of groupware technologies. *Sloan Management Review, 38,* 11–21.

Orsstto, R. J., & Clegg, S. R. (1999). The political ecology of organizations: Toward a framework for analyzing business-environment relationships. *Organization & Environment, 12,* 263–279.

Ouellette, S., Bassel, B., Maslanka, H., & Wong, L. (1995). GMHC volunteers and the challenges and hopes for the second decade of AIDS. *AIDS Education and Prevention, 7*(Suppl.), 64–79.

PAHO (2001). *Perfil de Salud de País: Chile*. PAHO. Retrieved March 9, 2004, from the World Wide Web: http://www.paho.org/spanish/sha/prflchi.htm.

PAHO (2002). *Country Health Profiles*. Retrieved December 1, 2004, from the World Wide Web: http://www.paho.org/Project.asp?SEL=HD&LNG=ENG&CD1=&CD=COUNT.

Patton, M. (1990). *Qualitative evaluation and research methods* (2nd ed.). Newbury Park, CA: Sage publications.

Patton, M. (2001). *Qualitative research and methods evaluation* (3rd ed.). London: Sage.

Patz, D., Mazin, R., & Zacarias, F. (1999). *Women and HIV/AIDS: Prevention and care strategies*. Retrieved October 2, 2001, from the World Wide Web: http://www.paho.org/search/DbSReturn.asp.

Pedersen, D. (1999). *The Chilean health care system: From successful socialized medicine to unproven free market reforms*. University of Washington. Retrieved March 10, 2004, from the World Wide Web: http://depts.washington.edu/idpm/pedersen/WritingSample.doc.

Peragallo, N. (1996). Latino women and AIDS risk. *Public Health Nursing, 13*(3), 217–222.

Pinel, A. (1994). Besides carnival and soccer: Reflections about AIDS in Brazil. In: L. Arsenault (Ed.), *Gender, health, and sustainable development: A Latin American perspective* (pp. 61–71). Ottawa: International Development Research Center.

Prado, E. (1994). Love does not protect against AIDS: Reflection about the HIV/AIDS epidemic from a gender perspective. In: L. Arsenault (Ed.), *Gender, health, and sustainable development: A Latin American perspective* (pp. 35–38). Ottawa: International Development Research Center.

Prasad, A. (2003). The gaze of other: Postcolonial theory and organizational analysis. In: A. Prasad (Ed.), *Postcolonial theory and organizational analysis: A critical engagement*. New York: Palgrave.

Rajevic, P. (2000). *El libro abierto del amor y el sexo en Chile (The open book of love and sex in Chile)* (1st ed.). Santiago, Chile: Andros.

Ramírez-Valles, J. (2002). The protective effects of community involvement for HIV risk behavior: A conceptual framework. *Health Education Research, 17*(2), 389–403.

Ramírez-Valles, J., & Brown, A. (2003). Latino's community involvement in HIV/AIDS: Organizational and individual perspectives on volunteering. *AIDS Education and Prevention, 15*(Suppl. A), 90–104.

Reklitis, P., & Trivellas, P. (2002). Performance implications of aligning generic strategies with the business environment. *International Journal of Management and Decision Making, 3*(3/4), 319–336.

Rowley, T. (1997). Moving beyond dyadic ties: A network theory of stakeholders influences. *Academy of Management Review, 22*(4), 887–910.

Savage, G., & Black, J. (1995). Firm-level, entrepreneurship and field research: The studies in their methodological context. *Entrepreneurship Theory and Practice, 19*(3), 25–34.

Scott, W. R., Ruef, M., Mendel, P. J., & Caronna, C. A. (2000). *Institutional change and health care organizations: From professional dominance to managed care*. Chicago: University of Chicago Press.

Silverman, D. (2001). *Interpreting qualitative data* (2nd ed.). Thousand Oaks, CA: Sage.

Stake, R. (2000). Case studies. In: N. Lincoln & L. Denzin (Eds), *Handbook of qualitative research*, (2nd ed.) (pp. 435–454). Thousand Oaks, CA: Sage.

Stockdill, B. (2003). *Activism against AIDS*. London: Lynne Rienner Publishers.

Strait, S. (1999). Drug use among Hispanic youth: Examining common and unique contributing factors. *Hispanic Journal of Behavioral Sciences, 2*(1), 89–103.

Strauss, A., & Corbin, J. (1990). *Basics of qualitative research: Grounded theory procedures and techniques.* Newbury Park, CA: Sage.

Sturdy, A., & Grey, C. (2003). Beneath and beyond organizational change management: Exploring alternatives. *Organization, 10,* 651–662.

Taylor, M., Vasquez, G. M., & Doorley, J. (2003). Merck and AIDS activists: Engagement as a framework for extending issues management. *Public Relations Review, 29*(3), 257–270.

Thompson, J. D. (1967). *Organizations in action: Social science bases of administrative theory.* New York: McGraw-Hill.

UN (2002). *Population/wwp2002.* United Nations. Retrieved June 30, 2003, from the World Wide Web: http://www.un.org/esa/population/publications/wpp2000/annex-tables.pdf.

UNAIDS (2004a). *Report on the global HIV/AIDS epidemic* (00.13E). Geneva, Switzerland: UNAIDS.

UNAIDS (2004b). *Epidemic fact sheets on HIV/AIDS and sexually transmitted infections.* Retrieved October 17, 2004, from the World Wide Web: http://www.who.int/GlobalAtlas/PDFFactory/HIV/EFS_PDFs/EFS2004_AR.pdf.

UNAIDS (2004c). *Epidemic fact sheets on HIV/AIDS and sexually transmitted infections.* Retrieved October 17, 2004, from the World Wide Web: http://HIVinsite.ucsf.edu/pdf/UNAIDS/Bolivia_en.pdf.

UNAIDS (2004d). *Epidemic fact sheets on HIV/AIDS and sexually transmitted infections.* Retrieved October 17, 2004, from the World Wide Web: http://www.who.int/GlobalAtlas/PDFFactory/HIV/EFS_PDFs/EFS2004_PE.pdf.

Van de Ven, A. H., & Poole, M. S. (1995). Explaining development and change in organizations. *Academy of Management Review, 20,* 510–540.

Varas, N., & Toro-Alfonso, J. (2001). Una revision de las politicas en torno al VIH/SIDA en Puerto Rico, Republica Dominicana, Ecuador y Honduras: Tenciones Limitaciones y Logros. *Revista Interamericana de Psicologia, 35*(2), 113–132.

Vidal, F., Zorrilla, S., Donoso, C., Hevia, A., & Pascal, R. (2002). *Situaciones de discriminación que afectan a las personas viviendo con VIH/SIDA en Chile.* Santiago: VIVO POSITIVO.

Wallace, S. P. (2001). Chilean health care as a lesson against the market. Paper presented at the 129th annual meeting of American Public Health Association, Atlanta, GA.

Wallerstain, N. (1992). Powerlessness, empowerment, and health: Implications for health promotion programs. *American Journal of Health Promotion, 5,* 197–205.

Weick, K. (1979). *The social psychology of organizing.* Reading, MA: Addison-Wesley.

Weston, C., Gandell, T., Beauchamp, J., McAlpine, L., Wiseman, C., & Beauchamp, C. (2001). Analyzing interview data: The development and evolution of a coding system. *Qualitative Sociology, 24*(3), 381–400.

Whelan-Berry, K. S., Gordon, J. R., & Hinings, C. R. (2003). Strengthening organizational change processes: Recommendations and implications from a multi-level analysis. *Journal of Applied Behavioral Science, 39,* 186–207.

WHO (2003). *Health systems performance assessment: Debates, methods and empiricism.* World Health Organization. Retrieved January 2004, from the World Wide Web: http://whqlibdoc.who.int/publications/2003/9241562455.pdf.

Wilson, J. (2000). Volunteering. *Annual Review of Sociology, 26,* 215–240.

A COMPARATIVE ANALYSIS OF HOSPITAL MANAGEMENT SYSTEMS IN SOUTH AFRICA

Anne Mills and Jonathan Broomberg

ABSTRACT

This chapter draws on a study conducted in the mid 1990s to compare management differences between three different groups of South African hospitals, in order to understand how these differences might have affected hospital functioning. The groups were public hospitals; contractor hospitals publicly funded but privately managed; and private hospitals owned and run by private companies. Public sector structures made effective management difficult and were highly centralized, with hospital managers enjoying little autonomy. In contrast, contractor and private groups emphasised efficient management and cost containment. These differences appeared to be reflected in cost and quality differences between the groups. The findings suggest that in the context of a country such as South Africa, with a relatively well-developed private sector, there is potential for the government to profit from the management expertise in the private sector by identifying lessons for its own management structures, and by contracting-out service management.

International Health Care Management
Advances in Health Care Management, Volume 5, 73–100
Copyright © 2005 by Elsevier Ltd.
All rights of reproduction in any form reserved
ISSN: 1474-8231/doi:10.1016/S1474-8231(05)05003-2

INTRODUCTION

Management of hospitals has been a key concern in low- and middle-income countries in recent years. It is commonly argued that public hospitals have low levels of efficiency (Preker & Harding, 2003). One policy response has been to seek to increase the autonomy of public hospitals (McPake, 1996), in the belief that greater autonomy will provide the necessary incentives for improved efficiency. Another response has been to suggest that either hospital management services, or the entire provision of hospital services, might be contracted out to the private sector. In the case of hospital autonomy, it is hoped that changing the hospital's incentives and ability to respond to them is sufficient to enable improved performance. In the case of contracting out, it is argued that improved performance is best gained by drawing on the advantages of private ownership, which, it is assumed, provides greater incentives to efficiency than if hospital provision remained within the public sector.

In general terms, frequently discussed approaches to improve the efficiency of publicly-funded hospitals impact on the senior managers of the hospital, and the effect on performance is thus dependent on how those managers translate the incentives inherent in the arrangements to the staff within the hospital. Management systems and structures need to be in place to ensure that the goals of the hospital senior managers can be met through the actions of a large number of staff within the hospital, and such systems and structures need to create the necessary incentives, so that the staff are motivated to help in achieving the hospital goals.

Given this, it is surprising how little attention appears to have been paid to management systems and structures within low- and middle-income country hospitals. In recent years in rich countries, greater attention has been paid to issues of hospital governance and management. For example, questions have been addressed such as whether ownership matters (Duckett, 2001); what should be the appropriate form of governance for health services (Barnett et al., 2001); and whether and how management within hospitals should be decentralized (Aas, 1997). However, the management capacity and funding arrangements of developed country health systems differ greatly from those in less wealthy countries, limiting the extent to which lessons from one can inform the other. In low- and middle-income countries, information is increasing on the relative performance of private versus public facilities in various settings (Bennett et al., 1997), but there has been little detailed exploration of differences in management styles and motivations between publicly and privately owned facilities, and the effect these might have on their functioning. Moreover, it might be expected that contract design will be an important influence on how contracted-out hospitals are managed, but such design features have been barely explored (Mills, 1997). Indeed, Collins & Green (1999) have called for a more open debate around hospital organizational forms.

This chapter compares the differences in management structures, styles and incentives between three different groups of South African hospitals, in order to seek to understand how these differences might be likely to affect hospital functioning. The groups consisted of public hospitals, which were directly managed by provinces; contractor hospitals, of which there were three, providing services similar to those of public hospitals but managed by a private company; and private for-profit hospitals owned and run by private companies. The data were originally collected in 1994/1995 and are now old, but nonetheless they highlight the importance of management structures and processes for hospital functioning. Since the study was done, management reforms have been implemented, especially in the larger public hospitals. However, while some of the detailed management arrangements have changed, the general analysis remains relevant not only to South Africa but also to other countries seeking to address issues of public hospital management.

BACKGROUND AND METHODS

By the standards of the rest of Africa, South Africa has a very well-developed hospital sector. Publicly funded hospitals account for around 81% of total beds, and include both very large tertiary level institutions and smaller provincial and district hospitals. Private hospitals account for the remaining 19% of beds, and are mostly private-for-profit hospitals, which charge fee-for-service and are used primarily by that part of the population (around 20%) with medical scheme or insurance cover. Such hospitals characteristically have a very short length of stay and specialise in acute, especially surgical cases. In addition, at the time of the study, a private commercial company was running three acute district hospitals under contract to local health departments.

The study investigated these three contracted-out acute district hospitals, and for comparison purposes selected three public hospitals each in the same geographical area as a contractor hospital, of similar size and providing similar services. Three private hospitals were also systematically sampled (two run by the same company, and the other by the company with the public sector contracts), again in the same geographical areas though sited in the nearby towns. Table 1 summarises key aspects of the hospitals' workload, showing clearly the more intensive use of facilities in the private hospitals, and the relative similarity in workload between public and contractor hospitals. Private hospitals' workloads consist almost exclusively of those with health insurance, and hence serve the more affluent population groups. As might be expected, surgical cases constituted a much higher, and maternity cases a much lower, proportion of the total admissions than in the other two groups. Although measures of case severity were not available, it is unlikely that case severity was markedly worse at the public and contractor hospitals since these were first-line hospitals, and would refer complex cases elsewhere. However, some element of the difference in length of stay between private hospitals and the other two groups is likely to be accounted for by the greater ability of private hospitals to discharge patients to recover at home. To preserve anonymity, hospitals are referred to in this and subsequent tables and figures by an initial.

One complication in the comparison was that the contractors' role differed between the three contractor hospitals, for historical reasons (Table 2). In one hospital (H), all staff were employed by the contractor, though the hospital was owned by the health department. In the other two, the hospitals had been financed by the contractor, and the contract price included an element of repayment, such that after 20 years the hospitals would pass into government ownership. In one of these (M), medical staff were employed by the government, ostensibly in order to maintain some control over quality of care. In the other (S), only the senior management team was employed by the contractor.

The study sought information on the influence of hospital ownership through a structured interview schedule applied to a total of 41 interviews with senior managers at corporate and hospital levels. At corporate level, the Director-General and one or more Chief Directors were interviewed in

Table 1. Hospital Statistics.

	Contract			Public			Private		
	M	H	S	T	L	B	D	P	N
Beds	178	250	170	322	364	287	138	100	94
Turnover rate	31.7	23.0	32.1	34.1	28.4	43.0	71.1	86.5	99.6
Length of stay (days)	8.2	8.6	9.0	8.3	8.5	5.0	3.7	3.2	3.0
Average bed occupancy rate (%)	71	54	79	78	66	59	71	75	83

Table 2.   Key Features of Contract Design for Contractor Hospitals.

	M	S	H
Contract duration	10 years, renewable for further 10 years	10 years, renewable for further 10 years	5 years; renewed for further 3
Capital resources	Hospital built and equipped by contractor	Hospital built and equipped by contractor	Hospital built and equipped by government
Staff resources	Contractor employed all administrative and nursing staff. Government employed medical staff	Contractor employed only senior management staff. Government employed all other staff	Contractor employed all staff
Reimbursement method	Fixed per diem rate. OPD visit at 1/3 of in-patient day rate	Fixed per diem rate	Fixed per diem rate. OPD visit at 1/3 of in-patient day rate

each of the two relevant Departments of Health, and the Managing Director and several Directors in each of the three head offices of the relevant companies. At hospital level, the actual officials interviewed varied due to the different management structures in place. In the contractor hospitals, the medical superintendent and hospital managers were interviewed; corresponding officials at the public hospitals were the medical superintendent and hospital secretary, while at the private hospitals, they were the hospital managers and assistant managers. These interviews explored the personal motivations and sense of accountability and responsibility of managers, comparing these between the three hospital groups (public, contractor and private) in order to assess their likely implications for hospital performance. Management structures, systems and incentives were also assessed informally in each hospital, through a series of discussions with clinical, nursing, administrative and domestic staff.

On the basis of a review of relevant literature (Boufford, 1991; Enthoven, 1991; Hospital Strategy Project Consortium, 1996; Mills, 1997; OECD, 1992; Walsh, 1995), key factors were identified which were considered likely to affect performance, and used to structure both data collection and analysis:

- The presence or absence of a general management structure at hospital level, and the extent to which the senior management team was able to function as a team.

- The number of layers and grades of staff within the management structures of the hospitals, and hence the extent to which decisions could be taken and implemented quickly.
- The number of the management level(s) above the hospital, and the allocation of responsibilities between hospital and higher management levels, which also affected how quickly decisions could be taken.
- The organisation of the 'head' office (the province or company headquarters) and the extent to which this facilitated support to hospital management.

In addition, specific enquiries were made about three mechanisms, which appeared likely to have an important influence on hospital performance:

- The nature of the hospital management information system (MIS), which determined the information that managers had available to make decisions.
- The methods used by the head office to monitor performance, and the extent to which action was taken on the information received.
- The existence of specific measures to improve staff and managers' efficiency, such as training and performance appraisal, and remuneration levels.

All interviews were recorded manually and subsequently analysed by the same researcher. Additional information was obtained in a series of feedback sessions held with head office and hospital officials from the various government departments and private hospital companies.

Hospital performance was assessed in terms of costs and quality of care. A detailed cost analysis employed a step down cost accounting approach and a combination of data from expenditure reports and primary data collection. Private hospitals did not employ medical staff, or run their own radiology, rehabilitation or laboratory services, so costs were calculated both including and excluding these categories, to ensure comparability across hospital groups. Estimates were adjusted for service mix using an indirect standardisation approach based on the mean service-mix profile of all hospitals; unadjusted figures are provided here, since adjustment made little difference.

Quality of care was assessed by evaluating structural aspects and the quality of nursing care. Structure assessment used a survey instrument incorporating 132 measurement criteria and associated standards, grouped into appropriate categories and functional clusters (Broomberg & Mills, 2004a). The instrument was developed through a process of consultations with an expert group. The nine clusters represent the major functional divisions within a hospital, and most were divided into the standard categories of staff, functions/services, supplies and equipment and buildings. A scoring and weighting system was developed through consultation with the experts, in order to aggregate scores by category and cluster. Individual criteria were scored, and weighted in order to reflect the relative impact of each category in its cluster. Similarly, the weighting of clusters reflected the relative impact of each cluster on overall quality of care. Hospitals were rated by a single researcher, using information from structured interviews with senior managers, a questionnaire distributed to all medical staff, and direct observation.

Evaluation of quality of nursing care used a survey instrument structured along similar lines, developed by two nursing experts (Broomberg & Mills, 2004b). The instrument evaluated various aspects of nursing care against a set of pre-defined criteria and standards, drawing on the methodological literature on explicit process of care assessment (Ashton et al., 1994). It covered both clinical nursing and nursing management, with standards based on a combination of existing public sector standards and, where they did not exist, the opinions of the experts. Several elements of the nursing care cluster were based on a particular model of appropriate nursing care, in which a nurse makes an assessment and diagnosis of each patient on admission, followed by the development and implementation of a nursing care plan, and adjustments to it if the patient's circumstances change. The final instrument consisted of 29 separate criteria grouped into two broad clusters – nursing care and nursing management. Data collection was done by the experts, using direct observation and interviews with nursing service manager and medical superintendents.

The analysis considers first the influence of ownership on the motivations and priorities of senior managers. It then analyses management structures and styles at the hospital level, the corporate level and the interface between these levels. Next it examines the specific mechanisms and systems, including information systems, which the private companies explicitly used to encourage good hospital performance. The performance data are then presented, and conclusions drawn on the extent to which ownership and management arrangements facilitated the efficient provision of hospital services. Policy implications are identified for the public sector.

THE ROLE OF HOSPITAL OWNERSHIP

In the contractor and private groups, corporate-level managers perceived themselves to be clearly accountable to the owners of the company, represented by the Board of Directors, for ensuring adequate returns to shareholders, and secondly to the employees of the company who needed to be kept satisfied and well motivated. In the case of the contractor company, senior managers also perceived some degree of accountability to the government as the purchaser of services, and to the communities served by the hospitals.

There was less consistency between these two hospital groups in views expressed at hospital level. All private hospital managers were well aware of the ownership structure of their company and the need to ensure good returns to shareholders. This imperative translated into specific operational requirements including maximizing revenues through increased throughput and occupancy rates, and minimizing costs wherever possible. These managers were acutely aware of the essential role played by medical staff in determining hospital revenues, and devoted substantial energies to ensure good relationships as well as to attracting new medical staff.[1] It thus seemed clear that the private ownership structure and the need to ensure returns to shareholders were among the primary motivators of management behaviour.

The situation was different in the case of the contractor hospitals. Hospital managers had little information regarding the actual shareholding of the company, and perceived themselves as accountable to their immediate superiors and ultimately to the senior company executives rather than to the shareholders. None of the managers cited the need to increase returns to shareholders as one of their objectives or priorities, focusing instead on the need to control costs, ensure good quality of care and manage and motivate hospital staff.

In the case of the public hospitals, there was some variation among head office officials in their perceptions of their lines of accountability. Some officials perceived themselves to be accountable to higher levels in the public sector bureaucracy and thereafter to the elected political representatives, while others understood themselves to be accountable more directly to the communities which they served. None of the officials regarded themselves as directly accountable to hospital staff. In some cases, specific responsibilities were only vaguely defined in terms of the orderly running of the hospitals, with some mention made of the quality of patient care. Other officials had more detailed notions of their responsibilities, and listed among them the smooth running of the hospitals, ensuring adequate quality of patient care, ensuring that staff were motivated and satisfied, and that budgets were adhered to.

Hospital-level managers in the public hospitals generally had similarly variable and vague notions of their own lines of accountability and responsibilities. In most cases, these managers regarded themselves as accountable directly to the head office, and not to either hospital staff or the community. In relation to their specific responsibilities, most managers cited a similar list to those of the head office officials. The public hospitals were thus almost at the opposite extreme from the private and contractor hospitals in relation to the motivations and perceived responsibilities of senior managers. Public ownership was associated with very diffuse and vague notions of accountability and responsibility.

MANAGEMENT STRUCTURE AND STYLES AT HOSPITAL LEVEL

General Management Structures

Fig. 1 provides a schematic illustration of the management structures at hospital and corporate level in the three hospital groups. An essential difference between the three groups at hospital level concerned the presence or absence of a general management structure, and the corresponding degree of integration (or lack thereof) in the senior management team. In the case of public hospitals, the figure demonstrates what has been termed the 'hierarchical silo' management model (Hospital Strategy Project Consortium, 1996), where there was a complete separation between the management of nursing, administrative and medical services, with no general management structure and very limited integration and coordination between the three functional divisions. While the medical superintendent was nominally regarded as the most senior manager in the hospital, in effect he/she had very limited jurisdiction over the areas of responsibility of the nursing service manager or the hospital secretary.

In contrast, all three private hospitals had a small, integrated general management structure and all reporting to the corporate level occurred via the hospital managers. Hospital medical staff were not the hospital employees, and therefore did not form part of the formal management structure.

Management structures at contractor hospitals lay between these two extremes. They also used a general management structure, with all functions ultimately reporting to the hospital managers. There were, however, two constraints on the degree of integration in the top management team. The first was an arrangement whereby the nursing service manager in the

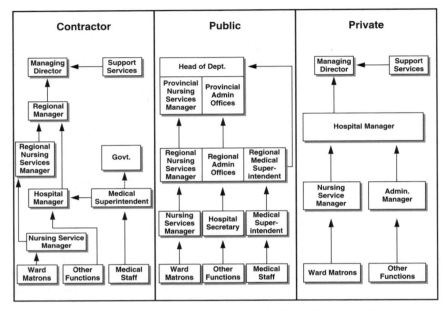

Fig. 1. Management Structures at Hospital and Corporate Level.

hospital reported to the regional nursing service manager as well as to the hospital manager, thus undermining the authority of the hospital manager to some extent. The second constraint was a result of the integration of these hospitals into public sector management arrangements. At hospitals M and S, the medical staff reported to their superiors in the government rather than to the hospital managers, while at hospital S this arrangement affected both medical and nursing staff.

Complexity of Hospital Management Structures

In addition to the presence or absence of a general management structure, hospital-level management structures differed significantly in terms of scale and complexity. Even allowing for hospital size differences, the management cadre at the public hospitals comprised far more categories of staff within each functional area than did both other groups, as well as much greater numbers of staff within each category. Contractor and private hospitals had very few categories of management staff, and relatively few staff per category.[2]

These differences in management structures were reflected in the functioning of the management teams. Public officials at both hospital and corporate levels perceived the management teams at all three public hospitals to function extremely poorly, and to be characterised by minimal coordination between different functions, slow, ineffective decision-making, an inappropriate degree of formality, poor implementation and a pervasive lack of morale and initiative. In this situation, even highly motivated managers faced severe constraints to effective action. For example, two medical superintendents were recognised by their superiors as highly motivated and competent, but unable to achieve their full potential given managerial structures and systems.

In contrast, the management teams at all three private hospitals appeared to function in small, tight-knit teams, which operated on a relatively informal and flexible basis, emphasised a participative approach to management, and were able to take decisions rapidly and to implement quickly and effectively. These teams also seemed to enjoy a high level of motivation and job satisfaction.

The picture at the contractor hospitals was more variable, and was affected by their differing management arrangements. At hospital H, for example, where all staff were employed by the contractor, the management team appeared to function in a similar way to those in the private hospitals. In the case of hospital M the situation was similar, with a motivated and flexible top management team, which emphasised participation and a relatively informal style. Relationships between the government-employed doctors and management team were good. In both these hospitals, however, managers noted that the nursing management teams functioned in a bureaucratic and rigid way. They attributed this mainly to the fact that the senior nurses had been recruited after long careers in the public sector, and had imported public sector nursing management systems into the contractor hospitals. The managers acknowledged that the company had not worked sufficiently hard to overcome the 'public sector' culture among the nursing staff, and that this problem was aggravated by the requirement that these nurses report to the regional nursing service managers as well as to the hospital managers.

The 'dual employment' situation at hospital S created substantial fragmentation, tension and conflict between senior managers. Both the contractor and government officials reported a serious split between the two management teams at the hospital, with the hospital managers (employed by the contractor) functioning in an apparently effective team with the other contractor-employed management staff, but with an entirely separate management structure, under the control of the medical superintendent and nursing service manager, governing the publicly employed nursing and medical staff.

MANAGEMENT STRUCTURE AND FUNCTIONS AT THE CORPORATE LEVEL AND HOSPITAL INTERFACE

In the case of the public sector, Fig. 1 showed a corporate management structure characterised by two management levels, with hospital management reporting to a regional office (which in turn reported to the head office). At both levels, the management structures had large numbers of staff, and were complex and unintegrated, with multiple divisions dealing with different management functions. Several critical functions, such as transport, maintenance and procurement, were located outside of the health department in other government departments.

This bureaucracy created considerable difficulties in communication between the corporate and hospital levels. Hospital managers often had to communicate with multiple officials to resolve even simple issues, and uniformly complained about the often extreme delays by the head office in responding to requests for assistance. Interviews suggested that the complex organisational structure and external location of key functions were key explanatory factors. Other explanations included the lack of skills and capacity among many officials, and the existence of many vacant posts (due to lack of suitable candidates).

These problems were aggravated by the lack of autonomy granted to hospital managers within the public sector regulatory framework, which placed authority for almost all critical management functions in the hands of very senior officials at head office level, severely disempowering hospital-level managers (Hospital Strategy Consortium, 1996). For example, hospital officials had no authority over any key personnel management functions, including establishment levels, hiring and firing of staff, salary and bonus levels and staff discipline; no authority to procure any goods or services on their own except for very low value items; and no power to shift resources across budget lines. They did make submissions regarding the hospital budget, but these were not taken into account and the budget often bore no resemblance to hospital expenditure patterns. Deficits were always funded from elsewhere in the Departmental budget and surpluses could not be used.

This combination of unrealistic budgeting, soft budget constraints and lack of accountability and responsibility meant that hospital-level officials had no effective role in the financial management of their hospitals.

Interviews with hospital managers and head office officials also highlighted a culture which failed to reward initiative, and instead encouraged risk aversion and rule-bound behaviour. This managerial culture and system effectively prevented hospital managers from 'managing' their institutions in any real sense of the word, and instead they functioned as 'administrators' of a set of rules which were not of their making, and which they had no power to influence. Not surprisingly, this system was perceived to lead to severe 'undermanagement' of public hospitals, and to undermine morale.

The corporate structure and functions in both private hospital companies differed substantially from those of the public sector. In both cases, there was a single corporate head office structure, which was lean and simple with relatively few divisions dedicated to specific functions and with an apparently high degree of integration between divisions. Both groups were also characterised by simple, effective lines of communication between the hospital managers and corporate officials. Hospital managers in both companies perceived themselves to be well supported by their head offices, which they consistently described as responding rapidly and effectively to all requests. In both companies, there appeared to have been careful thought as to the most effective division of labour between the corporate and hospital levels, and specifically to where scale economies could be achieved by centralized productivity management functions. Both companies had, for example, developed strong capacity in procurement, industrial relations and personnel management, MIS, and the provision of medico-legal advice.

This effective support system co-existed with a high degree of autonomy for hospital managers. Officials at both private companies believed in granting hospital managers maximum possible autonomy to manage their own institutions, within a context of intensive corporate support and supervision and strong requirements for accountability. In all three private hospitals, managers controlled critical personnel and financial functions, and as a result, were highly focused on issues of personnel productivity and sound financial management. Despite strong centralized procurement capacity, hospital managers could purchase outside if they could do so more cost-effectively.

The contractor company occupied a position somewhere between the two extremes defined by the public and private hospitals, but somewhat closer to the private than to the public end of the spectrum. As Fig. 1 showed, hospital managers reported to regional managers, and via that line, to the corporate head office. The corporate structure, like that of the private hospital groups, was small in scale, simple and integrated in structure and set up to support hospitals in areas where scale economies could be attained. The company had extensive expertise in procurement, industrial relations and personnel management, and clinical/medical support and was perceived by hospital managers to provide effective and rapid assistance. Unlike the private hospitals, however, the contractor hospital managers perceived the corporate level to have limited MIS capacity, and to have systematically under-invested in this area. Two of the managers also noted that the corporate decision-making process could be slow for decisions on capital expenditures.

Autonomy at hospital level was more constrained than was the case in the private hospitals. For personnel management, for example, the corporate level controlled more tightly the size and composition of staff establishments, salary scales and appointments than did the private hospital companies, though the hospital manager's could make recommendations on hiring and firing of staff, and promotions and bonuses. Similarly, hospital managers enjoyed constrained autonomy over financial management, for example having some freedom to manage funds across line items, and being held accountable for ensuring that expenditure and revenues matched budget projections. However, much hospital expenditure occurred at head office level (e.g. staff salaries, procurement of most supplies) and this information did not appear to be adequately or speedily shared with hospital managers.

The general picture in the contractor hospitals was thus of theoretical commitment to substantial autonomy, but in practice a higher degree of centralized control and less autonomy than hospital managers would prefer. The situation did however appear to be a dynamic one, with a general tendency to grant increased autonomy to hospital managers over time. One possible explanation for this pattern, expressed by some head office officials, was that several of the key managers in the corporate team responsible for the contractor hospitals came from public sector management positions and were more comfortable running an operation that resembled, at least to some extent, the public sector environment. This was noted to contrast with the corporate team responsible for the portfolio of private hospitals run by the same company. In this case, the team had been drawn from various private sector positions and tended to grant their hospital managers far greater autonomy.

MECHANISMS AND SYSTEMS FOR ENCOURAGING GOOD HOSPITAL PERFORMANCE

Over and above the impact of these management structures and styles, a number of other mechanisms used within the three hospital groups appeared likely to affect hospital performance. These included the MIS, mechanisms for monitoring hospital performance, and the use of specific incentives for managerial and staff efficiency.

Management Information Systems

The public hospitals used a very limited MIS which was entirely manual, and consisted of paper patient records and collated statistics covering numbers of admissions, patient days, theatre cases and OPD visits. Hospital staff received no training in the use of management information, and the collated statistics were not used in any managerial or clinical decision-making. As a result, data quality was often poor, and patient records frequently lost.

In contrast, all three private hospitals had sophisticated, computerized MIS which collected detailed management and patient demographic and clinical data. Staff received detailed training and hospital managers made extensive use of the management information to guide decisions within the hospital, and to provide regular reports to the head office. The only deficiency was that the clinical information was collected for billing purposes only, and was not used to guide management decisions.

The contractor hospitals appeared more like public than private hospitals in terms of the availability and use of MIS. The corporate head office used an outdated, inefficient MIS, which was not standardized with or linked to the hospital system and which continually needed updating and maintenance. At hospital level, all systems remained manual and collected very limited utilization data, and no relevant clinical or management information. As at the public hospitals, staff were not trained in the use of the MIS nor motivated to ensure good data collection. As a result, the managers were anxious about the quality of the data, and in one case, the managers had instituted a nightly headcount of patients to corroborate MIS information.

Monitoring of Hospital Performance

Monitoring of public hospital performance by regional and head office officials appeared to be unsystematic and irregular despite recognition of the need for systematic monitoring. All hospital officials believed that the reports they submitted were simply filed at head office, and never used for management purposes. Head office officials did appear to monitor budgetary performance although this tended to occur retrospectively and often two or three months in arrears, thus undermining its value.

In all three private hospitals, in contrast, ongoing, highly systematic monitoring was built into the management system. There were live computer links with the head office, allowing daily monitoring of key parameters such as patient utilization and financial performance. Regular patient surveys were conducted and results sent to head office. All exceptions to normal parameters were identified, explanations requested from managers, and where required, interventions or solutions implemented. In addition, the relative performance of all company hospitals was analysed, and this information passed regularly to hospital managers.

The contractor company monitored the performance of its hospitals much more closely and effectively than was the case with the public hospitals, but somewhat less so than for the private hospitals. Detailed monthly management reports were submitted by hospital managers covering patient statistics, staff and other input to output ratios and budgetary performance, although they did not cover quality of care nor information on patient satisfaction. Head office officials clearly used the information submitted, and all variances from expected performance were identified and communicated back to hospital officials for explanation and correction. Similarly, the relative performance of hospitals was analysed and fed back to hospital management staff.

Individual Incentives for Efficiency

Managers and staff at public hospitals appeared to have little incentive to improve efficiency. Training was focused almost exclusively on nurses and controlled by nursing service managers. Some interviewees suggested that training opportunities for nurses might be used as rewards for friends or for loyalty, and not as part of a systematic approach to staff development. Neither managers nor staff had their performance monitored or reviewed systematically, and there were no systems for linking remuneration to performance for any categories of staff. The public service did in theory have a merit-based promotion system, but in practice all promotions were based only on seniority and tenure. Many categories of staff appeared to face specific disincentives to efficient behaviour. In the case of managers, these included the extremely bureaucratic restrictions under which they operated, the lack of any management authority, and their recognition that even extreme 'management failures', such as budget overspends or quality of care problems, were likely to go unmarked and certainly to go unpunished. In the case of other hospital staff, disincentives included the rigid, hierarchical management style within the hospital (particularly for nurses) and the lack of flexibility in the system regarding inter-hospital transfers or other employment conditions.

In terms of remuneration levels and benefit packages, interviews elicited a mixed picture. In the case of nursing staff in particular, take-home pay was widely regarded as too low although non-cash benefits, including housing and education allowances, were considered acceptable. Similar sentiments were expressed by administrative and management staff. Under these conditions, it is not surprising that all interviewees regarded morale amongst hospital staff as extremely low, and recognised the intimate linkage between these problems of morale and poor hospital efficiency.

The private hospital companies and the contractor company placed substantial emphasis on staff training, and included all staff in their training programmes. Managers and officials acknowledged the value of investments in training, and the impact of this investment on the long-term productivity of their staff.

Managerial and staff incentives at the private hospitals differed somewhat between the two companies. In one hospital, a detailed performance evaluation system measured the performance of each staff member, including the hospital managers, against customised performance targets on a two monthly basis. Successful performance against these targets was directly linked to pay increases. Interviewees at the hospital felt this system was effective in influencing staff morale and productivity among all categories of hospital staff. While the systems in use at the other two hospitals appeared less formalised, there was nevertheless a clear linkage in the minds of hospital staff between performance and remuneration, and a strong sense that staff performance was evaluated by management on a regular basis and good performance rewarded. In all three hospitals, nursing and management staff appeared generally satisfied with remuneration and benefit levels, which were perceived to be superior to those in the public hospital system, the benchmark used for comparison, particularly by nurses.

In the contractor hospitals, managers were aware that their performance was monitored and remuneration somehow linked to performance, but they were unclear on the precise linkage between performance and pay. This linkage was much clearer for other hospital staff, who had an annual performance review. Most officials felt this system assisted with morale and improved staff productivity. Nursing staff cash salaries were higher than those in the public sector, but non-cash benefits were regarded as inferior, which was cause for some dissatisfaction in spite of recognition that transfer and promotion policies were much more flexible than in the public sector. On the basis of the interviews, staff morale and motivation at the contractor hospitals appeared to be superior to that observed in the public hospitals but inferior to that seen in the private hospitals. Hospital S was an exception to this pattern, with nursing and other staff employed by the government expressing fairly high degrees of dissatisfaction with their conditions of employment in contrast to the views of the contractor staff, who were generally happy with employment conditions.

PERFORMANCE

Selective performance data only are presented here, for reasons of space. Fig. 2 shows cost per admission adjusted to ensure comparability between hospital groups[3]; detailed cost data are provided in the appendix. The small sample size means that generalizations should be made cautiously, but the differences between hospital groups are suggestive. Individual hospitals ranked almost completely consistently by group, with contractor hospitals the lowest cost, followed by public and then private, though one public hospital was just below the cost of the highest contractor hospital, and one private hospital was below two of the three public hospitals. Adjusted costs were around 95% of total costs, except for the highest and lowest public hospitals, where they were around 90%. Adjustment therefore made public hospitals appear less costly relative to the other groups. Cost per inpatient day showed a similar pattern between the groups. It should be emphasized that incentives for cost containment differed between the groups: public hospitals received a global budget; contractor hospitals were funded per day; and private hospitals received a fixed payment per day for hotel costs, and reimbursement with a percentage mark-up for drugs and medical supplies. In addition, they were dependent on attracting external physicians to admit patients to the hospitals, so needed excellent medical facilities (hence the high theatre and capital costs).

Data on the composition of costs (see the appendix) supported the argument that contractor hospitals were in general able to manage resources better than public hospitals. In particular this was achieved through more effective allocation and management of staff resources, and specifically by

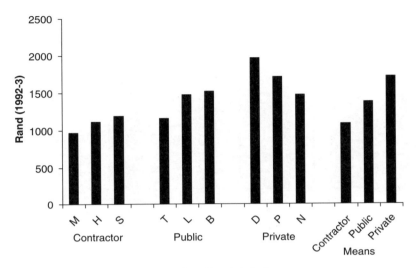

Fig. 2. Cost Per Admission.

obtaining higher levels of productivity from smaller numbers of more highly skilled and better paid nurses than was the case in the public hospitals. The data on administration costs show that the external administration costs of contractor hospitals were less than half of those of the public hospitals, but internal administration costs were much higher (with the exception of one public hospital that showed a different pattern). Total administration costs of the private group were higher than those of contractors, but not consistently higher than the public group.

The lower contractor costs were not in general obtained at the expense of quality of care in terms of structure and process indicators. Fig. 3 and Table 3 show mean scores for structural quality and for nursing quality, respectively (individual hospital data are not shown since these were largely consistent with the means; they are available in Broomberg & Mills, 2004a, b). Public hospitals were in general better equipped and staffed, but had worse standards of maintenance and cleanliness than contractor hospitals. Nursing quality was systematically better in the contractor hospitals. As would be expected, given their costs and clientele, private hospitals scored highest except, interestingly, for staff where public hospitals scored highest.

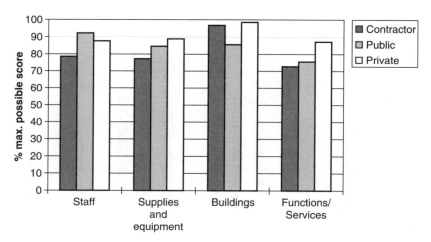

Fig. 3. Mean Structural Quality Scores.

Table 3. Nursing Quality (% of Maximum Possible Score).

	Contractor	Public	Private
Nursing care: all wards			
Nursing assessment/diagnosis	53	26	84
Nursing care planning/monitoring/control	48	37	76
Equipment	40	25	90
Diet	72	50	100
Total	50	33	82
Nursing management	48	51	83
Overall Total	50	39	83

DISCUSSION

Methodological caveats must precede any discussion of the implications of these findings. The public hospital group represented a tiny sample of all public hospitals, and performance data showed great variability between the public hospitals (though management structures and regulations would be common across all public hospitals). The contractor group represented the only three hospitals of this type within South Africa, and were run by only one company. Public hospitals were purposively selected to be as comparable as possible to contractor hospitals with respect to possible confounding factors, such as patterns of service delivery, scale, or location. There was indeed relative similarity between the contractor and public hospitals in regard to patterns of service delivery and scale, although some specific differences in these dimensions were apparent in that the public hospitals were larger than the contractor hospitals, and in some cases, provided specialized services not available in the contractor hospitals. These differences were, however, adjusted for in several of the analyses, and these factors are thus unlikely to be important confounders in the comparison of the contractor and public hospitals. This is less likely to be the case for the private hospitals, which had markedly different patterns of service delivery and utilization to the other two groups. The three private hospitals represented a hospital sector serving a very different population group, and with different sources of income from either public or contractor hospitals. Data on outcomes of care were largely unavailable and so conclusive comparisons of relative efficiency cannot be made. Thus while the performance data are suggestive, the real value of this study lies in the qualitative differences rather than in strict quantitative comparisons.

Despite these methodological concerns, there did seem to be some clear differences in performance between public, contractor and private hospital groups, which appeared to be associated with hospital ownership and management structures, styles and incentives. Management approaches in the public sector head offices and hospitals were not such as to encourage good hospital performance. Public ownership was associated with diffuse and vague notions of accountability, responsibility and objectives. The corporate structure and head office–hospital relationships reflected bureaucratic imperatives rather than those of efficient production of hospital services. Perhaps, most importantly, public sector management structures and systems were characterised by a high degree of centralization, with hospital managers enjoying virtually no autonomy over most key management functions, thus ensuring that even well-motivated and competent hospital managers were unable to compensate for the extremely weak central support provided to them. Despite spending almost as much on management as the private group, management performance was clearly worse.

In contrast, in the contractor company and within the contractor hospitals themselves, there was a pervasive emphasis on efficiency, which can be associated with the impact of the for-profit ownership structure on the perceptions and motivations of corporate officials and hospital managers. Corporate officials perceived themselves as motivated primarily by the need to ensure profitability and delivery of high-quality and cost-effective care. While these motivations were not consistently communicated to the hospital managers, this group nevertheless perceived themselves as directly account-able to their superiors, and responsible for ensuring control of costs and good quality of care. The hospital managers also demonstrated a clear un-derstanding of the key determinants of hospital cost, and of the extent and limits of their capacities to influence such costs.

These clearly articulated motivations of ensuring profitability and hence low costs were reflected in (and in part attributable to) the corporate struc-ture and capabilities of the contractor company, and the interaction between corporate and hospital levels. The corporate structure, for example, was small, functioned well, had good capabilities in critical support functions and particularly emphasised efficient management of staff resources. The high level of corporate support to the hospitals was accompanied by close scrutiny of hospital performance. Despite this strong central role, hospital managerial were given fairly substantial autonomy over several key areas of managerial decision-making, although within fairly tight constraints. This better management performance was achieved at a cost per inpatient day for administration that was almost half of that of the public hospitals.

The study also identified some instances, however, where the emphasis on cost containment in contractor hospitals appeared to have been taken too far, with detrimental effects. This was seen, for example, in the poor man-agement information infrastructure available at both corporate and hospital levels, suggesting that contract specification needed to pay greater attention to information system requirements.

Further issues on contract design arose from the differences between the contracts in staff employment conditions and their implications for the management of the hospitals. The management task in hospital S, where only the senior management staff were employed by the contractor, was made very difficult by the division in staff loyalties. This experience suggests that contracting out the senior management function, while retaining other staff in public employment, may not be desirable.

Given that the same company ran both the contractor hospitals and one of the private for-profit hospitals, and yet there were distinct differences between them in management structures and styles, an obvious question is why these differences existed. One possibility is that the contract business was not perceived to be sufficiently secure to warrant investment in expen-sive support systems such as MIS, and that in any case in the long term all contractor hospitals would come under government ownership, thus further reducing incentives to invest in information systems. Another possibility is that the business, despite relatively generous contract terms (Broomberg et al., 1997), was not sufficiently profitable to warrant extending the standard private hospital management systems to these contractor hospitals. A third possibility is that the provision of hospital services to the general public was seen to be a distinctly different business from that of providing private hospital services, and hence managers were recruited from the public sector who brought with them a 'public' style of management.

While the private hospital management structures and styles reflected what was possible with better trained and qualified managers, higher pay and greater administrative expenditure, they also provided some lessons. These hospitals were not always more expensive per patient treated than public hospitals because they were able to obtain very high levels of staff productivity. Moreover, they had extremely effective systems of cost control where the payment system encouraged them to minimize costs (e.g. because hotel costs were reimbursed at a fixed per day fee). Conversely, they were very effective at generating revenue where such cost controls were not imposed (e.g. drugs were reimbursed at cost price plus a fixed percentage mark-up, explaining the very high per patient drug costs). However, given the small numbers of hospitals involved in this study, conclusions must be tentative on the extent to which their experience can be drawn on to inform public hospital management reform.

POLICY IMPLICATIONS

Drawing on this study and on other investigations of the public hospital system in South Africa (Hospital Strategy Project Consortium, 1996), this section suggests some approaches to improving the management of publicly funded hospital services.

The findings from this study support the arguments made by public sector managers, since the early 1990s, for radical reform of public hospital management in South Africa. The management structures and systems applied in the private sector encourage reflection on what mechanisms might be considered to improve the performance of public hospitals. One such mechanism is the decentralization of substantial management authority to the hospital level, including most of the key management functions such as financial and personnel management and procurement. This has been a common reform prescription elsewhere (Preker & Harding, 2003). In the South African setting, it would help address the numerous problems attributable to over centralized authority in the public hospital system.

However, it would require significant legislative reform, as well as substantial investment in developing adequate managerial capacity (Hospital Strategy Project Consortium, 1996).

Some other mechanisms, including changes to the structure and functioning of management teams at both the hospital and head office level, could be more rapidly applied. The contractor and private hospital company structures suggest that management teams at both levels in the public system might be smaller and simpler and could function in an integrated manner with a single locus of executive authority. In addition, there is a need to redefine the role of the head office team. Rather than being engaged in day to day management of hospitals, a more appropriate role, and one more consonant with modern management approaches, would be to provide support and leadership, on a defined set of issues, to hospital level management. These changes would require careful selection of appropriate officials to lead and operate within these management teams, substantial improvements in the skills of officials at all levels, and the development of adequate information systems.

In addition, the study suggests that greater attention might be paid to the incentives facing hospital and head office managers. As with traditional public sector bureaucracies in many countries, the public service arrangements studied discouraged risk-taking and encouraged rule-bound, inefficient behavior. In this setting, the introduction of performance-based contracts for senior management may have a role to play in linking reimbursement and performance. The development of systematic performance review mechanisms, such as those in the private hospital companies and to a lesser extent the contractor company, could also help hold hospital managers accountable for good performance while allowing the delegation of sufficient responsibilities to enable effective hospital management.

Together, these suggested reforms to management structures and systems would help address the inefficiency of the management of the public hospital system of South Africa. If more radical reform is considered desirable, such as a much greater degree of decentralized or hospital autonomy, or the creation of UK-style independent hospital trusts, these initial reforms would be essential in providing the basis for more complex reforms to be feasible and effective.

Since this study was done, a number of changes have been introduced in public hospital management though there is still perceived to be scope for further improvements. There is a greater decentralization of management responsibilities, even at district hospital level. There have been efforts to break down the 'hierarchical silo' structure, and many hospitals now have chief executives, often not medically qualified, with a small component of performance-related pay. A large investment in management training has been made across the public sector. However, some important functions, particularly maintenance, still remain outside direct hospital control.

Apart from the issue of improving public hospital management, this study also sheds light on the potential value of contractual arrangements. The evidence from the contractor hospitals suggests that in the context of a country such as South Africa, with a relatively well-developed private sector, there may be potential for the government to profit from the management expertise in the private sector to deliver services on its behalf. However, the study suggests that careful thought needs to be given to the design of contracts, and in particular to the range of responsibilities given to the contractor and to performance monitoring. Analysis of other aspects of the contractual arrangements emphasises also the importance of ensuring that the government has sufficient capacity to monitor the performance and prevent opportunistic behaviour by contractors (Broomberg et al., 1997).

The literature on hospital reform in developing countries has to date given greater attention to issues of decentralization and hospital autonomy than to those of internal management structures (Preker and Harding, 2003). This study suggests there would be value in building up a literature on the internal organisation of hospital management functions in resource-poor settings, so that contractors have available to them better evidence on which to consider improvements in hospital management.

From a more global perspective, this study adds to the evidence on the role of ownership in influencing performance, and on the potential value of contractual relationships. In the developed world context, the evidence that the private sector can manage hospitals better than the public sector is mixed: there does not appear to be a clear efficiency difference between for profit and other forms of hospital ownership (Duckett, 2001). Indeed Ducket has suggested that ownership is probably a 'policy distraction'. In the developing world, however, the market is highly segmented, with different types of hospital serving very different population groups, and being paid and managed in very different ways. It might be expected, therefore, that performance differences would be much greater. Given the very small samples of hospitals in this study, the findings are more indicative and suggestive than conclusive. However, the study does provide some evidence that confirms suspicions of the inefficiencies of traditional public bureaucracies, and suggests that expertise may reside in the private sector that could be drawn on to benefit public hospital users, whether through learning from their management methods, or contracting their management skills.

However, the performance of private and contractor hospitals reflects the context they work within, and especially the financial incentives. A capable private hospital company, contracted to provide hospital care to the state, needs to be balanced by a purchaser with sufficient capacity and expertise to manage and monitor the contractual relationship. In this case the public purchaser did not benefit as much as it might have done from the contractual arrangements because it neither drove a hard enough bargain, nor monitored the contract adequately. In contract with lesser capacity than South Africa, contracting with commercial companies is likely to carry greater risks. In other settings, this has led to identification of non-government organisations (NGOs) as suitable service providers, given the likely greater identity of values and motivations between NGOs and governments.

NOTES

1. Medical staff were not employees in private hospitals, but were key in ensuring a flow of patients to the hospital
2. Hospital S was an exception to this observation, since its nursing management structures were those of the public sector
3. in other words to remove costs which did not fall on the private hospitals' budgets, such as radiology

ACKNOWLEDGEMENTS

The research reported here was funded by the UK Department for International Development (DfID) through a grant to the Health Economics and Financing Programme, Health Policy Unit, London School of Hygiene and Tropical Medicine. However, the DfID can accept no responsibility for any information provided or views expressed. The authors acknowledge the generous co-operation of Lifecare Group Holdings, and the management and nursing staff at all nine of the study hospitals.

REFERENCES

Aas, I. H. M. (1997). Organisational change: Decentralization in hospitals. *International Journal of Health Planning and Management*, *12*, 103–114.

Ashton, C. M., Kuykendall, D. H., Johnson, M. L., Chuan, C. W., Wray, N. P., Carr, M. J., Slater, C. H., Wu, L., & Bush, G. R. W. (1994). A method of developing and weighting explicit process of care criteria for quality assessment. *Medical Care, 32*(8), 755–770.

Barnett, P., Perkins, R., & Powell, M. (2001). On a hiding to nothing? Assessing the corporate governance of hospitals and health services in New Zealand 1993–1998. *International Journal of Health Planning and Management, 16*, 139–154.

Bennett, S., McPake, B., & Mills, A. (Eds) (1997). *Private health providers in developing countries: Serving the public interest?* London: Zed Press.

Boufford, J. I. (1991). Managing the unmanageable: Public hospital systems. *International Journal of Health Planning and Management, 6*, 143–154.

Broomberg, J., & Mills, A. (2004a). *Quality of care in contracted-out and directly provided public hospital services in South Africa: Evaluation of structural aspects.* London: Health Economics and Financing Programme, London School of Hygiene and Tropical Medicine http://www.lshtm.ac.uk/publications/downloads/working-paper/02_04.pdf.

Broomberg, J., & Mills, A. (2004b). *Evaluating the quality of nursing care in the context of a comparison of contracted-out South African hospitals.* London: Health Economics and Financing Programme, London School of Hygiene and Tropical Medicine http://www.lshtm.ac.uk/publications/downloads/working-paper/03_04.pdf.

Broomberg, J., Masobe, P., & Mills, A. (1997). To purchase or to provide? The relative efficiency of contracting out versus the direct public provision of hospital services in South Africa. In: S. Bennett, B. McPake & A. Mills (Eds), *Private health providers in developing countries: Serving the public interest?* (pp. 214–236). London: Zed Press.

Collins, C., & Green, A. (1999). Public sector hospitals and organisational change: An agenda for policy action. *International Journal of Health Planning and Management, 14*, 107–128.

Duckett, S. (2001). Does it matter who owns health facilities? *Journal of Health Services Research and Policy, 6*(1), 59–62.

Enthoven, A. C. (1991). Internal market reform of the British NHS. *Health Affairs, 10*(3), 60–70.

Hospital Strategy Project Consortium. (1996). *Towards equity and efficiency in South Africa's public hospital system.* Shortened Final Report of the Hospital Strategy Project. Johannesburg: Hospital Strategy Project Consortium.

McPake, B. (1996). Public autonomy hospitals in sub-Saharan African. *Health Policy, 35*, 155–177.

Mills, A. (1997). Improving the efficiency of public sector health services in developing contract: Bureaucratic versus market approaches. In: C. Colclough (Ed.), *Marketizing education and health in developing contract: Miracle or mirage?* (pp. 245–274). Oxford: Clarendon Press.

OECD. (1992). *The reform of health care. A comparative analysis of seven OECD contract.* Health Policy Series No. 2. Paris: OECD.

Preker, A., & Harding, A. (Eds) (2003). *Innovations in health service delivery. The corporatisation of public hospitals.* Washington DC: The World Bank.

Walsh, K. (1995). *Public services and market mechanisms: Competition, contracting and the new public management.* London: Macmillan Press.

APPENDIX

Detailed Cost Data (Rand, 1992/1993, per admission)

	Contractor			Public			Private			Mean		
	M	H	S	T	L	B	D	P	N	Contractor	Public	Private
External administration	58.14	37.41	67.95	108.65	158.95	78.30	62.38	59.65	57.24	54.50	115.30	59.76
Internal administration	22.71	20.64	17.46	2.99	4.59	32.65	104.64	65.09	57.54	20.27	13.41	75.75
Admin. Total	80.85	58.05	85.41	111.64	163.54	110.95	167.02	124.74	114.78	74.77	128.71	135.51
Transport	20.91	28.55	82.44	54.95	58.91	19.50	37.26	2.08	6.39	43.97	44.45	15.24
Laundry	56.74	44.46	67.95	44.74	44.88	96.25	11.77	13.09	14.19	56.39	61.96	13.01
Catering	98.56	75.34	116.64	91.88	147.31	136.30	60.35	82.53	84.72	96.85	125.16	75.87
Housekeeping/maintenance	45.35	85.66	116.46	94.37	193.38	178.10	89.54	104.13	83.64	82.49	155.28	92.44
Domestic services total	221.56	234.01	383.49	285.94	444.47	430.15	198.91	201.82	188.94	279.69	386.85	196.56
Pharmacy	66.01	88.75	50.49	62.58	74.21	57.45	215.45	620.64	449.01	68.42	64.75	428.37
Radiology	5.25	26.14	23.76	9.13	8.25	5.25	0.00	0.00	0.00	18.38	7.54	0.00
Rehabilitation services	4.51	1.89	15.39	14.53	15.56	25.75	0.00	0.00	0.00	7.26	18.61	0.00
Laboratory	22.63	16.68	9.09	18.09	90.02	18.65	0.00	0.00	0.00	16.14	42.25	0.00
Operating theatres	175.89	144.39	187.29	188.83	223.89	193.95	649.68	304.42	294.66	169.19	202.22	416.25
Clinical support services total	274.29	277.87	286.02	293.16	411.91	301.05	865.13	925.06	743.67	279.39	335.37	844.62
Adjusted total[a]	241.90	233.15	237.78	251.41	298.10	251.40	865.13	925.06	743.64	237.61	266.97	844.61
Nursing Staff	358.09	494.93	435.60	445.63	512.55	648.75	624.34	388.90	360.39	429.54	535.64	457.87
Medical Staff	13.61	16.08	12.60	69.06	45.39	21.95	0.00	0.00	0.00	14.10	45.47	0.00
Staff total	371.71	511.01	448.20	514.68	557.94	670.70	624.34	388.90	360.39	443.64	581.11	457.87
Adjusted total[a]	358.09	494.93	435.60	445.63	512.55	648.75	624.34	392.42	363.60	429.54	535.64	460.12
Capital costs	66.67	96.06	53.28	63.25	61.80	79.10	117.48	73.47	64.35	72.00	68.05	85.10
Total costs per admission	1015.08	1177.00	1256.40	1268.66	1639.65	1591.95	1972.88	1713.98	1472.13	1149.49	1500.09	1719.66
Adjusted costs per admission	969.08	1116.19	1195.56	1157.85	1480.45	1520.35	1972.88	1717.50	1475.31	1093.61	1386.22	1721.90
Adjusted as % of total	95%	95%	95%	91%	90%	96%	100%	100%	100%	95%	92%	100%
Adjusted costs per IP day[a]	118.18	129.79	132.84	139.50	174.17	304.07	533.21	536.72	491.77	126.94	205.91	520.57

[a] Adjusted so costs are comparable across all three groups.

AMERICAN HOSPITAL FIRMS AND THE BURGEONING CHINESE PRIVATE HEALTH MARKET

Blair D. Gifford and David Wood

ABSTRACT

Globalization of health care services is becoming an alternative or com-plementary strategy for some U.S. health care organizations due to in-creased competition, a stagnant health care market, and nationally imposed cost constraints in the U.S. Additionally, entrepreneurial U.S. firms may see globalization as an opportunity to promote their services in new countries with increasing demand for advanced technological services. If an ambitious American health care firm decides to globalize its product or service lines, what might be some of the primary strategies it would use to enter an international market? To investigate this question, this chapter considers the strategies of two American firms that have entered the Beijing and Shanghai markets since 2000. We conducted numerous tel-ephone conversations and interviews with executives of these firms in an attempt to understand their market entry and early development strat-egies. These firms' market entry strategies range from "greenfield" op-erations, where the hospital does little to change its corporate and managerial style from what it uses domestically, to a "glocalization" strategy, where the firm is quite sensitive to fitting into the Chinese culture and being accepted by the Chinese government. The strategic challenges

International Health Care Management
Advances in Health Care Management, Volume 5, 101–115
ISSN: 1474-8231/doi:10.1016/S1474-8231(05)05004-4

for international hospital organization developments in China are many, but the potential rewards from becoming among the leading firms in a large nation with an expanding economy are tremendous. What we learn from the experiences of enterprising American hospital firms in Chinese may well portend the future for international developments by many other American-based health organizations.

INTRODUCTION

This chapter is about the differing market entry strategies into the Chinese hospital market by two American-based hospital development companies. Both of these companies have executives with similar, extensive backgrounds in the U.S. private hospital industry, and both have international joint venture organizations with Chinese firms that are based in Hong Kong. Both companies are aiming at large, but different, urban areas – Beijing and Shanghai – for market entry, and both have plans to expand to other major urban areas within months. And, both firms expect that their western standard quality care management and customer service will give them a distinct competitive advantage in the market places they enter.

The similarities between these firms are striking. However, their market entry and marketing strategies differ widely. The first firm is building an "international hospital" that caters to expatriates from other nations and upper class Chinese. Its hospital model, which is based on the top international hospital in Asia, Bumrungrad Hospital in Bangkok, Thailand (Balfour, Kripalani, Capell, & Cohn, 2004), could be located almost anywhere in Asia. Even though the hospital will have Western and Eastern (i.e., Traditional Chinese Medicine) medicine wings, there is little effort being made to localize the culture and management of this facility. The intention is to become an international destination hospital in Beijing for all nationalities. The second firm is taking a "glocalization" approach to market entry. Glocalization, which means thinking globally but acting locally, implies an optimal mix of parental control and local initiative and product development. In effect, a glocalization strategy means that local managers will have some freedom to develop their own implementation plans for products, marketing and production that are consistent with local political, economic, legal and cultural demands (Phatak, 1992). The second firm will be opening private units within existing Chinese public hospitals. Marketing of their services will be aimed at the emerging Chinese middle class, while also providing the subtleties of care expected by expatriates and upper class Chinese. Their goal is not to be the top international hospital in Chinese, but to become a brand name for international quality of care standards throughout China in coming years.

BACKGROUND

The Growth of International Health Services

The health care sector is among the most rapidly growing business sectors in the world economy. The size of the sector is estimated at about US \$3 trillion (Health and the International Economy, 2002) in the Organization for Economic Co-operation and Development countries alone and is expected to rise to US \$4 trillion by 2005 (Zarilli & Kinnon, 1998, p. 55). Health and related services have become increasingly tradable due to a variety of economic, social, technological, and global institutional factors, although the sector is also subject to a wide range of tariff and non-tariff protections for health-related commodities and inputs across developing countries. In recent years, there has been significant growth in trade and investment opportunities both within the health services sector and in related services, such as health insurance, across developed and developing countries.

The General Agreement on Trade in Services Treaty (GATS) characterizes services as being traded via four modes of supply: (1) consumption abroad, (2) commercial presence, (3) movement of persons, and (4) cross-border supply. Of these, commercial presence will be the primary subject of this chapter. However, one should note that the other modes of supply do have growing health industry applications. For example, consumption abroad – or the movement of patients to receive treatment in foreign markets – is growing quickly, especially among neighboring countries and within regional trading blocks (Chandra, 2002; Freeman & Frank, 1995). The movement of health personnel, including doctors, nurses, paramedics, technicians, consultants, and health management personnel, has been discouraged by host countries, but is a growing phenomenon as health workers continue to seek better wages and working conditions (Zarilli & Kinnon, 1998). Finally, the cross-border supply of health services reflects the growth in telemedicine and cross-border delivery of medical samples and diagnosis. For example, Mathur (2001) discusses the potential of information technology for revolutionizing health care design and delivery by influencing wide-ranging aspects of health care, from the development of new medicines based on biotechnology to distance supervision of patients and the transfer of medical information to the health care insurance companies and health care administration.

The emergence of international health service delivery is being driven by a number of developments. First, the cross-border training and movement of health professionals has made high-quality health care available in most nations of the world. Second, advanced quality of telecommunications has allowed physicians to consult on procedures that are happening in real time thousands of miles away. Third, the increasing availability of high-speed transportation has made it such that a 24 hour or less air flight will get you half the way around the world. Fourth, the concept of overseas hospitals should be attractive to governments, employers, insurance companies and HMOs in the U.S. and other western nations who carry the primary burden of rising costs of medical care.

An emerging commercial presence in the health sector has grown in importance because of the increasingly liberal attitude of countries toward foreign direct investment and toward collaboration with foreign companies in the form of joint ventures, alliances, and management tie-ups. Developing countries, in particular, are becoming increasingly aware that they must learn to capitalize on their advantage of low-cost skilled human resources in the global market. This advantage is particularly important in the labor-intensive field of medical care. Those countries that have a ready supply of well-trained health workers, language and cultural proficiency, good government, and a need for foreign investment in their health care system (there are many such countries) are taking a proactive posture in persuading foreign governments and corporations to shift their medical care services to their shores. One high-quality, medium-size foreign hospital could bring an investment of tens of millions of dollars per year (Jain, 2003).

The Chinese Hospital System

The Chinese government is looking for joint venture clinics and hospitals with foreign firms to help with the long-term development and advancement of China's health care system (Wood, 2004). Exclusively foreign-invested medical institutions are still denied access to the Chinese market. Joint ventures can set their own prices for medical services, are exempt from business tax for the first 3 years operation, and their self-made drugs are exempted from value-added tax for the same period. Since all hospitals participating in the medical insurance system must be state-owned, private clinics including joint ventures may receive only self-funded patients.

The demand for international caliber health care in Chinese has been best reflected in the growth of international standard clinics and outpatient facilities operated by foreign-invested enterprises. Since the first Sino-foreign hospital was founded in 1989, almost 200 joint venture or cooperative venture hospitals or clinics of various types have been established in China. However, 50% of these clinics and hospitals have investment of less than US $2 million, and only about 10% have funding of more than $10 million. Most are clinics without in-patient beds, and less than 20% of the hospitals have more than 200 beds (Wood, 2004). They are currently regulated as for-profit health care service providers.

Although China's health system is classified by most as having developing world conditions, it is quickly evolving. China's hospital system provides care to 1.3 billion citizens under a system of national health insurance that is funded primarily by the government, but with some contributions from its citizens through a self-pay mechanism for those individuals not covered by the national insurance plans. Currently, there are three national health insurance plans in China, but they only cover relatively few (approximately 15% of the populations citizens).

Healthcare expenditures are especially low in the rural areas of China, with per capita health care expenditure per year of US $45. In comparison, per capita health care expenditure per year is US $2,908 in Japan (highest amount in Asia), and US $4,737 in the U.S. (Final Update, 2003). Life expectancy differences are as follows: China is 62.8 years, Japan is 73.5 years (highest in Asia), and the U.S. is 77 years (By The Numbers, 2002).

Seventy percent, or 900 million, of China's 1.3 billion people live in rural areas. This 70% only uses about 20% of China's health care resources (Chen, 2003). The urban population of Chinese, in comparison, has broad access to health care, both in the quantity of hospitals and clinics available and the quality of health services that are offered. Recent studies have suggested that there are more than 23 million 'affluent' households in China, where affluence is defined as sufficient income to allow discretionary spending power. In 2000, 8.4% of urban households were projected to meet this criterion (Executive Summary, 1999). Significantly, affluent households spend four times as much on health care as non-affluent households (Executive Summary, 2001).

The actual number of hospitals in China and their distribution is difficult to assess with precision. The definition of a hospital is not clearly delineated in government documents, and often sub-acute and extended care facilities, nursing homes, etc., are included as "hospitals." Of some reliability is the number of large-bed facilities which may with some confidence be considered acute care facilities. The official count of hospitals in China, as of 2002, is 17,148. A major role for hospitals in China is provision of primary care. Of the 17,148 official hospitals, only 8,849 are classified as acute care facilities. According to the Ministry of Health (2003), the breakdown of acute care facilities by bed size is as follows: hospitals over 500 beds, 977; hospitals between 250 and 500 beds, 5,198; and hospitals less than 250 beds, 2,674.

The physical plants of Chinese hospitals vary in their quality and appearance, with large urban hospitals built in the last 25 years appearing, in many respects, to be equivalent to those found in Western countries. However, even in these facilities, the level of maintenance is strikingly poor, with inadequate hygiene, dirty floors and walls, torn and shabby furniture, and inadequate toilets and restrooms. Equipment is often the latest generation, international brands, but it is often poorly maintained and calibrated. Typically, the large urban centers have very few upper-tier hospitals with reasonable standards. The other urban hospitals and most of the rural hospitals are wholly inadequate by international standards. Further, Chinese hospitals have rudimentary management systems. Most managers are nonprofessional and physician managers with little, if any, business training and experience. Typically, organizations do not have organization charts, and joint management/medical staff committees and board governance is nonexistent. Many hospitals do not have a chief financial officer and do not utilize cost-center budgeting, have no reimbursement or accounts receivable functions, and have minimal IT support of financial functions (Wood, 2004).

In May 2000, the Ministry of Health announced that China would establish new health care service management policies in an effort to make high-quality medical care available to all Chinese. Competition between hospitals is being introduced to improve the distribution, efficiency, and quality of services. Patients now have to pay a user fee to attend a hospital, and they can choose which hospital to attend. The Ministry of Health also announced that medical service organizations would be divided into for-profit and not-for-profit units and that patients would be able choose their hospitals on their own. Not-for-profit providers still predominate in China. They receive preferential tax policies and must adhere to government guidelines on prices. Alternatively, for-profit hospitals (about 11% of all hospitals in 2004) are allowed to set their own prices and they pay taxes.

RESEARCH AND METHODS

In return for providing strategic and proprietary information on their activities for use in this chapter, the lead author promised the organizations that their identities would remain confidential. Firms that are in the market entry stage are generally very private about their strategies and do not want their intentions publicized. The summary information provided herein comes from a series of interviews, telephone conversations and document exchanges between the lead author and each of these case study organizations over the last 3 years.

The second author of this chapter, due to his former position as CEO of Beijing United Hospital and current position as president and senior partner of China Care Group (Beijing) and due to the proprietary nature of the information provided by the case organizations, was not involved in information exchange with either of the case study hospitals and has never talked to representatives from either organization. The second author's primary role in this chapter has been to critique the plans of the two case organizations. His comments regarding both firms' market entry strategies are interspersed throughout the following text.

The lead author communicated, at the beginning of his association with both organizations, that he would eventually write a summary piece of this nature and that he would construct his own analysis and critique of each organization's strategies. A draft of this chapter was delivered to both organizations for comments, corrections, and changes prior to publication. Note that the lead author has felt no pressure from either organization to alter or not report the information that was divulged in the interviews and the documents provided by the organizations. Conversations with 'Chinese International Partnership Hospital' (CIPH, an alias name for this chapter) started in September 2002 and have been as recent as July 2005. Conversations with 'International Hospital in China' (IHC, an alias name for this chapter) were initiated in February 2003 and have been as recent as october 2004.

CASE STUDIES

Chinese International Partnership Hospital

CIPH was initiated as a U.S. corporation in 2002 and is the principal firm in CIPH International (alias), a joint venture organization based in Hong

Kong. Like all other international hospitals in China, CIPH focuses on providing high-quality and state-of-the-art medical services and technologies. However, CIPH differentiates itself from other international hospitals by targeting middle-class Chinese citizens, focusing on being the high-quality provider of just one service – maternity care, and by not starting greenfield hospital operations in China, but opening up its own private "VIP" units within existing hospitals.

CIPH's focus on state-of-the-art service allows it to market services to middle and upper class Chinese and expatriate populations. Clinical quality of care is managed at CIPH through a clinical training contract with a top medical school on the east coast of the U.S. According to the CEO of CIPH, the University entered into an exclusive contract (7 initial years, plus 5 years renewable), non-compete contract in China with CIPH. However, the authors believe that this University has arrangements with other Western health facilities in China. It is not clear how CIPH's contract with the University might differ from other contractual relations by the University in China.

CIPH also focuses on having an immediate cash flow without having high capital risk and risk of liability. This strategy entails starting with small, profitable projects and then developing market share. For example, CIPH opens small units (11–13 beds) within Chinese women's and children's hospitals. After contracting a partnership, CIPH opens its own floor within the hospital, housing private rooms and VIP services, and then expanding its units to other floors of the hospital as demand increases. This development strategy has less risk of failure and capital loss, while providing a quality brand for the partnering Chinese hospital. As a result, consumers are less likely to see CIPH as a profiteering international hospital, and more likely to see it as a Chinese hospital with high-quality Western services. This culturally sensitive approach to international hospital development is supported by Chinese government officials.

CIPH's focus is on maternity care, although it expects to move into other services in coming years. CIPH estimates that there are about 600,000 babies born annually to middle-class Chinese, and that this number will increase to about 1,200,000 babies in 3–5 years as the Chinese middle class grows. CIPH's goal is to capture 1–2% of births to middle class Chinese in the next couple of years, and 5% of these births in 5 years. According to the CEO of CIPH, there are three primary reasons why they chose to focus on high-quality obstetrical care as a strategy. These reasons include:

1. Chinese women have a tradition of being their families' gatekeepers to health care services. CIPH will offer other hospital-based services in

coming years, and it expects women who have given birth in one of its obstetrical units to come back to use other services at CIPH.

2. There is vast opportunity for Western-based obstetrical services in China. Due to the one-child family policy in China , the Chinese are willing to expend considerable costs to assure the best standards of care for birthing. Also, obstetrical care services in China are about "20 years behind Western standards." Obstetric units in Chinese hospitals generally hold 4–8 patients, with a shared bathroom or a bathroom down the hall. The hallway is dark, and families wait outside in small waiting areas; it often takes hours for families to hear about the childbirth outcome.

3. Compared to other service lines, Chinese obstetrical physicians and mid-wives are quite well trained. Introductory training of Chinese health professionals for CIPH can be done in 1 or 2 months at the U.S. medical university with which CIPH has contracted. In comparison, cardiology or oncology training of Chinese physicians would be substantially longer and more complex.

CIPH's focus on the middle-class Chinese market is supported in the pricing structure of its maternity services. Currently, CIPH charges from US $2,500 to $3,500 per delivery. These prices are about one-half to one-third the costs of childbirth at other international hospitals. For example, Beijing United (a 50-bed maternity hospital in Beijing) caters to the expatriate market and charges US $8,000 for a natural childbirth and up to US $12,000 for a complicated childbirth.

As of mid-2004, CIPH had a small maternity unit (13 beds) operating in a leading Shanghai hospital, was about to open another unit in a Guangzhou hospital, and had plans to open three smaller units within existing hospitals in three large Chinese cities in the next 6 months. There are other high-quality international hospital obstetrical units in Beijing and Shanghai, but not in any of the cities where CIPH will soon be starting operations. Note that the Shanghai-based obstetrical unit, which opened in October 2002, generates high revenue per month and will soon expand capacity to handle increasing demand for service. The expansion of the unit was delayed for months due to the SARS crisis in spring 2003, but construction will soon begin on an additional 30 beds.

According to the CEO, CIPH will continue to differentiate itself from competitors in the long term by: (a) providing well-known brand name recognition in urban China, (b) partnering with well-established Chinese hospital partners, and (c) further developing Western-based management systems, including advanced information technology for medical records and clinical care protocols.

International Hospitals in China

Established in 2001, IHC is a Hong Kong Corporation with offices in the U.S. and Beijing. IHC is owned by IHC Intl, which manages five international clinics: two in New York and one each in Chicago, Atlanta, and San Diego. These clinics integrate Eastern and Western medicines. IHC's corporate vision is to develop the first health care network capable of delivering "U.S. standard" medical care in leading economic and trade centers throughout China. This capability includes providing leading technology solutions and global resources to health care professionals.

IHC has aggressive growth plans for building full-service hospitals and referring clinics in Bejing first, and other major Chinese metropolitan areas in coming years. IHC's facilities will provide primary, secondary, and tertiary care services through partnerships with Chinese joint venture hospitals and clinics. IHC will own controlling interests in each joint venture hospital and supporting clinic. Each hospital will operate 250 beds and have Eastern and Western primary-care clinical services. Secondary services will be provided through a variety of sources – from sophisticated preventative and diagnostic services to surgical and interventional procedures.

IHC will develop Centers of Excellence (COE) in each IHC hospital by meeting the standards of the top U.S. teaching hospitals. For example, one IHC hospital will be a cardiovascular COE, another an orthopedic COE, and so on. Additionally, U.S. health care partners will provide remote consultations, provide on-site rotational services, teach Continuing Medical Education (CME) course for Chinese physicians, and provide training opportunities for Chinese physicians in the U.S. IHC has partnership arrangements with nationally renowned teaching hospitals in the U.S. to administer CME courses.

IHC will "target cash-paying customers such as expatriates, tourists, and high-income patients." Based on market studies, IHC believes there are about 4.92 million Chinese citizens in its target markets. Note that 4.92 million is much larger than other marketing surveys have indicated for high-end health service market users. Target customers will pay U.S. market rates on an upfront fee-for-service basis. Qualified customers (such as multi-national corporations) will pay an annual network access fee to use an IHC facility. According to IHC, "ninety-five percent of payments will occur in advance of the treatment, thus there will be very little need for a billing and collection operation, and virtually no bad debt." However, there is no precedent for such a high volume of out-of-pocket pay in China. Other Western hospital firms rely on insurers' payments to cover the costs of care for expatriates and tourists.

The management team of IHC is well rounded and has excellent experience in hospital industry. The executive team includes managers who have been serving the health care industry for over 30 years in the U.S. and for over 15 years in Asia. Their combination of hospital operational expertise and health care technology expertise are "unsurpassed by any competitor," as stated in their business plan, and should be seen by future investors as a competitive advantage of IHC. In particular, the management team of IHC has expertise in hospital construction, health system development, customization of health information technologies and international business. Although the leaders of the management team are new to the development of hospitals in international markets, and, in particular, the Chinese private health market, their perseverance, financial wherewithal and other resources may be enough to bring them success in China.

Other key competitive advantages of IHC include:

1. *Patient-focused health care solutions.* Hospitals will be designed to focus on patient's physical and mental health to limit administrative duties for health professionals so that they can concentrate on patient care.
2. *Combination of Eastern and Western medicine.* IHC believes that traditional Chinese medicine (TCM) and Western medicine complement each other, thereby empowering patients to control, alleviate, and prevent many chronic conditions.
3. *U.S. hospital partnerships.* IHC has the means to access the most recent clinical information and cutting-edge procedures, treatments, and technology. IHC has established relationships with over 200 of the major teaching hospitals and academic medical centers in the U.S.
4. *U.S. and International Healthcare Standards.* According to IHC, all of "their hospitals will be designed and operated according to U.S. codes and standards." However, the authors note that there is no way to operate on U.S. codes and standards in China. China does not have the infrastructure to allow implementation of U.S. codes and standards and will not have the necessary infrastructure for years to come. Also, the idea of having similar strategies running for multiple organizations on centralized administration will be a new concept within the Chinese health system, and management of such will take a large investment.

5. *Technology solutions.* IHC has tremendous experience in Health Information Systems including partnerships with PeopleSoft, Lawson, SAP, HBOC, Oracle and over 60 health care organizations. IHC is confident that its "electronic solutions, developed in conjunction with leading U.S. technology partners, will have tremendous resale value throughout Chinese." However, the authors note that the transfer of Western-based health IT solutions is very difficult in China. All Western IT systems have to be rewritten in pinyin or Chinese characters, and the financial systems have to be adapted to the Chinese accounting system to meet the claims of IHC's management. Further, the IHC's financial systems will have to be approved by the Chinese government before they would have any resale value.

6. *Supply chain solutions.* IHC has significant experience in creating new directions for health care supply chain models and logistical transportation practices. IHC's fully integrated supply chain solutions – developed in collaboration with materials managers, nurses, physicians, vendors, and technology partners – address the complexities inherent in the procurement process, reduce costs, and increase organizational efficiency.

CONCLUDING REMARKS

Summary

Most nations in the world have a private segment in their national health systems, and most of these private segments are increasing in size as international trade policies open up markets and consumers begin to demand health care in accordance with international standards. It can be argued that U.S. hospital firms have a distinct advantage over hospital firms from other nations in these emerging private markets. U.S. hospital firms have tremendous managerial experience in competitive markets, and they understand the necessity for providing the highest quality and technological care to gain hospital market share. Furthermore, the hospital industry in the U.S. has pockets of opportunity, but on the whole it is a mature industry with heightened competition for small profit margins. Heightened profits in foreign hospital markets have become alluring enough in recent years to attract some American-based firms to put forward the tremendous investment of time, energy, and capital to move into overseas market developments.

As shown by the two enterprising firms discussed in this chapter, there is no one model for entering an overseas hospital market, or at least, not the Chinese hospital market. Although the case study firms are quite similar in managerial experience, competencies, and structure (in terms of partnership development), their market entry strategies are divergent. IHC is attempting to build an international hospital system in the Beijing area. Its system is designed to serve expatriates and the wealthiest Chinese as is symbolized by its choice of location for the first hospital: next to the 2008 Beijing Olympics village. This hospital is being built in Beijing because the demand for Western-based private hospital services may be the greatest in Beijing of all Chinese markets. In contrast, CIPH is building private units within existing public hospitals in China. CIPH's strategy is to develop market penetration and name brand recognition by middle- and upper-class Chinese. It will do this by focusing on Western-based maternity care services, a service line which is of critical interest in China due to the one child policy. CIPH is not building an "international" hospital like IHC; it is bringing Western techniques and standards into China's existing hospital system.

The efforts of these firms over the next few years will be watched and scrutinized by many. Because their marketing strategies are so different and the markets in China are so large, it is possible that both firms will not compete head-to-head and will thrive. Yet, it is also possible that one of these strategies will win out over the other. As the Chinese economy quickly expands and Chinese citizens, in turn, begin to appreciate and seek health care services that meet international standards, there is tremendous profit potential for the winners of the race into the burgeoning private health markets in China.

Toward a Theory of International Health Strategic Management

The rapid development of international health service trade calls for the development of an international health strategic management perspective. Such a perspective will provide a cognitive and conceptual framework to managers who are considering international health developments. This exercise, however, will require more than a simple consideration of which theories are most applicable in foreign health service markets. For example, U.S. health care service organizations, in particular, will encounter some barriers that organizations in other industries may not encounter as international strategies are implemented. In most other countries, health care is believed to be a fundamental need and right, and governments ensure equal access to health services for all people. This social welfare state orientation leads government to play a strong role in the delivery of health care services. Foreign governments don't just oversee but are involved in the management of different delivery and reimbursement mechanisms. Also, foreign governments can be directly involved in financing health care and setting overall fee schedules for physicians and annual budgets for hospitals. Developing strong governmental relations, as well as understanding reimbursement policies, are crucial for the successful implementation and management of organizational strategies.

Other hurdles which will temper the development of international health strategy theories include:

1. *Regulation* — For example, in the U.S., citizens are generally precluded from obtaining health care anywhere they want without paying a substantial amount above their monthly insurance premium.
2. *Licensure* — Licensed health practitioners in one nation may not have legal permission to offer care in another. Even if they do, the liability risks might make providing such care economically risky, creating a substantial disincentive to practice medicine across national lines.
3. *Information* — There are no international standards in health care nomenclature, making it difficult to share data.
4. *Culture* — In many cultures, a patient's immediate family members will not just accompany the patient to a hospital, but will stay with him or her, handling such chores as cooking, bathing and laundry. One can imagine that this cultural convention suggests a much different approach to hospital design as well as communication channels between health professionals and patients.

REFERENCES

Balfour, F., Kripalani, M., Capell, K., & Cohn, L. (2004). Sand, sun and surgery: Asian hospitals are luring more patients from around the world. *Business Week*, (February 16): 48–49.

By the Numbers. (2002). *Modern healthcare*. December 23rd.

Chandra, R. (2002). *Globalization of services: India's opportunities and constraints*. New Delhi: Oxford University Press.

Chen, N. (2003). *Reform of health insurance system in Chinese.* Healthcare Insurance Conference, Bangkok, Thailand.

Executive Summary. (1999). *Current and expected expenditure patterns of Chinese households.* December 12th.

Executive Summary. (2001). *Projected growth of affluent hospitals.* Asian Demographics Ltd.

Final Update. (2003). *Chinese Briefing.* May 21.

Freeman, A. G. -D., & Frank, J. (Eds) (1995). *Health systems in an era of globalization: Challenges and opportunities for North America.* Washington, DC, Mexico City: Institute of Medicine and National Academy of Medicine.

Health and the International Economy. (2002). The Report of Working Group 4 of the Commission on Macroeconomics and Health. World Health Organization.

Jain, S. C. (2003). Globalization of medical services: Antidote for rising costs. *Healthcare Papers, 4*(2), 39–45.

Mathur, A. (2001). *The role of information technology in designs of healthcare trade.* Background paper prepared for Working Group 4 of The Commission on Macroeconomics and Health. Geneva: World Health Organization.

Ministry of Health, People's Republic of Chinese. (2003). www.moh.gov.cn

Phatak, A. V. (1992). *International dimensions of management.* Belmont, CA: Wadsworth Publishing Co.

Wood, D. (2004). *Hospital Development in the People's Republic of Chinese.* Working Paper, The Chinese Care Group Consultants, Beijing, Chinese. See www.Chinacaregroup.com

Zarilli, S., & Kinnon, C. (Eds) (1998). *International trade in health services: A development perspective.* Geneva: UNCTAD/WHO.

INTEGRATED HEALTH CARE DELIVERY BASED ON TRANSACTION COST ECONOMICS: EXPERIENCES FROM CALIFORNIA AND CROSS-NATIONAL IMPLICATIONS

Katharina Janus and Volker Amelung

ABSTRACT

Integrated health care delivery (IHCD), as a major issue of managed care, was considered the panacea to rising health care costs. In theory it would simultaneously provide high-quality and continuous care. However, owing to the backlash of managed care at the turn of the century many health care providers today refrain from using further integrative activities. Based on transaction cost economics, this chapter investigates why IHCD is deemed appropriate in certain circumstances and why it failed in the past. It explores the new understanding of IHCD, which focuses on actual integration through virtual integration instead of aggregation of health care entities. Current success factors of virtually integrated hybrid structures, which have been evaluated in a long-term case study conducted in the San Francisco Bay Area from July 2001 to September 2002, will

International Health Care Management
Advances in Health Care Management, Volume 5, 117–156
ISSN: 1474-8231/doi:10.1016/S1474-8231(05)05005-6

elucidate the further development of IHCD and the implications for other
industrialized countries, such as Germany.

Health care delivery in all major industrialized countries is faced with the
rising cost of health care. Increasingly, sophisticated health care consumers
demand high-quality and flexible health care (Draper, Hurley, Lesser, &
Strunk, 2002). Moreover, the needs of an aging population and advanced
medical technology further drive up these costs (Thorpe, Florence, & Joski,
2004). Consequently, these countries are struggling with escalating costs
threatening their citizens' access to the highest quality of health care.

Health care expenditures in the U.S. amounting to 14.6% of Gross Domestic Product (GDP) in 2002 (Organization for Economic Cooperation
and Development (OECD), 2004) make the U.S. health care system the
most expensive in the world, implying that it is not recommended in general
to be taken as a reference model for health reform in other industrialized
countries. Nevertheless, the U.S. health care market provides innovative
approaches to integrated care delivery, which emerged as a result of the
coordination of health care provision and financing through mainly *private*
organizations. Most of these organizations have similar goals: higher quality, lower costs, greater competitive advantage, and increased market share.
Despite sharing the same objectives, these experiments offer a wide range of
market circumstances, approaches, and opportunities to learn (Coddington,
Moore, & Fischer, 1996). In particular the *San Francisco Bay Area*, being
the second largest metropolitan area in the largest managed care market of
the United States, offers examples of almost every different kind of organizational approach to integrated health care delivery (IHCD).

Therefore, a long-term research project (Janus, 2003) has been conducted in
the San Francisco Bay Area. Twenty organizations have been evaluated regarding issues such as incentive and control mechanisms, dispute settlement capabilities, adaptation and flexibility, communication and information technology
(IT), confidence and culture within the respective organizations, and the general
management of the organizations. The research encompassed general questions
regarding the specifics of each organizations and their historical development in
order to account for changes in organizational structures and their effects.

Structured interviews were conducted face-to-face with 80 health care professionals. The number of interviewees per organization was based on the
degree of integration, ranging from 1–6. This proceeding was chosen because
a higher degree of integration implies the necessity to consider the perspectives of different parts of the system. The majority of interviews were done in
(sometimes) several sessions in the period of time from July 2001 to

September 2002. Table 1 provides an overview of the surveyed organizations, their main business activity, their geographic orientation, their customers/members, and the number of their affiliated physicians and hospitals.

The study focused on the dynamic organizational developments in IHCD in the Bay Area, which have been primarily driven by managed care in the mid-1990s and its backlash at the turn of the century. Although the enrollment in health maintenance organizations (HMOs) as the indicator for managed care penetration (amounting to 48.6% in 2002 (Aventis Pharmaceuticals, 2003, p. 18)) remains the highest in California in comparison to all other States, the rush toward consolidation slowed down. Today it is regarded as an "over-expansion pitfall" because a number of integrative efforts failed. Most organizations are currently focusing on their core competencies and core markets.

Organizations in the Bay Area are largely refraining from further integrative activities after their experience in managed care, which encompasses the application of management concepts, the (at least) partial integration of health care provision and financing and the selective contracting of payers with preferred providers (Amelung & Schumacher, 2004), since it has not achieved the desired objectives to provide high-quality and cost-efficient health care. Thus, the question is raised whether IHCD can be considered as an "outdated" model and, if not, *how* IHCD *can* be implemented in other industrialized countries such as Germany to overcome the shortcomings that occurred in the Bay Area health care market. It remains to be evaluated which issues of the U.S. case study can and should be transferred abroad, and how they could be applied to the German health care system.

Based on the reasoning of transaction cost economics, the following section will shed light on the issues why IHCD failed to provide health care efficiently in the San Francisco Bay Area but why it is still deemed appropriate. The "new" understanding of IHCD, focusing on virtual integration, provides a possible solution to this contradiction. The success factors for integrated care delivery in today's health care market will be presented in more detail. Taking these experiences into account implications for Germany will be discussed.

INTEGRATED HEALTH CARE DELIVERY

Reasons for Providing Health Care in Integrated Delivery Systems (IDSs)

Transaction cost economics as an economic theory sets the basis for integrating care delivery in hierarchical organizations instead of providing care through non-integrated market organizations.

Table 1. Basic Facts about Interviewed Organizations.

Organization	Main Business	Geographic Orientation	Customers/Members	No. of Physicians/Hospitals (if applicable)
Acordia	Insurance broker	National	450 companies employing more than 500,000 employees	—
Aetna	Insurance/Health plan	National	13.9 million medical, 11.9 million dental, 11.7 million group insurance customers	Networks with 539,000 health care service providers
Alta Bates Medical Group	IPA	Regional to local	90,000 lives	600 physicians (400 speciality and 200 primary care physicians)
Brown & Toland	IPA	Regional to local	237,000 lives	1600–1700 physicians
Blue Shield of California	Insurance/Health plan	State-wide	2.8 million members	—
Children's First Healthcare Network	PHO	Local	30,000 Medical members	170 PCPs, 250 specialists, 1 hospital, and research center
San Francisco Mental Health Plan	Health plan	Local	106,818 Medical beneficiaries, 5,200 healthy family members, 3,500 healthy workers, over 100,000 indigent, and uninsured residents	Affiliated with the General Hospital and outpatient providers
California Pacific Medical Center	Academic medical center	Regional	—	—
Catholic Healthcare West	Hospital system	West Coast	—	37 hospitals, 9,144 staffed bed
Daughters of Charity Health System	Hospital system	State-wide	—	7 hospitals, (northern and southern California)

Health Net of California	Insurance/Health plan	State-wide	2.5 million members	Networks with more than 49,000 physicians and hospitals
Hill Physicians Medical Group	IPA	Regional	300,000 lives	2,200 physicians
John Muir Mt. Diablo Health System	Health network	Local	80,000 lives	268 physicians, 2 hospitals
Kaiser Permanente	Integrated delivery system	National	8.1 million members	11,345 physicians, 29 hospitals
Palo Alto Medical Foundation	Health network (medical foundation)	Local	500,000 lives	About 500 physicians organized in 3 medical groups, contracts with 4 hospitals
Permanente Medical Group(s)	Medical group	Local	8.1 million lives	11,345 physicians (all groups)
San Francisco Magnetic Resonance Center	Magnetic resonance center	Local	—	—
Stanford Hospital & Clinics	Academic medical center	Local, national, and international	—	980 fulltime faculty physicians, 100 IPA physicians (Standford Clinics)
Sutter Health	Health network	Regional	—	26 hospitals, 5,000 physicians
University of California San Francisco Medical Center	Academic medical center	Local, national, and international	—	—

IPA: Independent Practice Organization; PHO: Physician-Hospital Organization.

Williamson begins his explanations regarding the transaction costs theory by noting that "…the transaction is the ultimate unit of microeconomic analysis" (Williamson, 1975, XI) whereas the transaction itself is considered not to be the exchange of goods and services, but the transfer of property rights across a technologically separable interface. One stage of activity terminates and another begins (Scholz, 1997; Williamson, 1985, 1986).Transaction costs include all sacrifices and disadvantages of the exchange partners associated with the realization of the transfer of these property rights (Stiles, Mick, & Wise, 2001). Their magnitude, then, affects the ways in which economic activity is organized and carried out. Included within the general category of transaction costs are *ex ante* costs, such as search and information costs, bargaining and decision costs, and *ex post* costs, such as executing, policing, and enforcement costs (Dietrich, 1993; Dugger, 1993; Furubotn & Richter, 1997; Picot, Dietl, & Franck, 1997; Williamson, 1986) as shown in Fig. 1.

Owing to the fact that transaction costs are rarely measured directly, a comparative approach is taken by transaction cost economics, which "…entails an examination of the comparative costs of planning, adapting, and monitoring task completion under alternative governance structures" (Williamson, 1996, p. 58) (such as markets or hierarchies).

The *discriminating alignment hypothesis* then holds that transactions, which differ in their attributes, are aligned with governance structures, which differ in their costs and competencies, in a discriminating – mainly transaction cost economizing way (Williamson, 1990, 1996). Williamson thus suggests to select a governance structure, which entails the lowest transaction costs after having assessed the *specificity* (see Appendix A for a detailed discussion of asset specificity with respect to health care transactions), the *frequency*, and the *uncertainty* of the transactions while taking

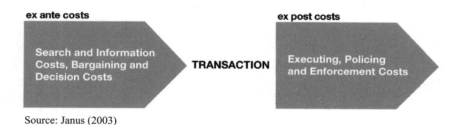

Source: Janus (2003)

Fig. 1. Transaction Costs.

into account the *behavioral* (bounded rationality and opportunism) and the *environmental assumptions.*

Increased specificity entails different forms of organization (Picot, Reichwald, & Wigand, 2001). As the costs of organizing transactions in the market rise due to higher monitoring and control activities, the tendency to organize transactions through hierarchies gains prominence (Williamson, 1996).

As a consequence, the organization of health care transactions in integrated delivery systems (IDSs) (hierarchies) is favored due to, in general, high asset specificity, uncertainty, and indeterminable frequency, taking environmental and behavioral conditions into account.

The Meaning of Integrated Health Care Delivery and its Purpose

Integrated health care delivery purports that health care transactions are organized in modes of governance that are close to hierarchies (contractual relationships) or actually are hierarchies (ownership) if full integration has occurred. The organizational mode of hierarchy states that transactions are placed under unified ownership (buyer and supplier are in the same enterprise) and [are] subject to administrative controls (an authority relation, to include fiat) (Williamson, 1996, p. 378).

Such partnerships can entail both horizontal integration (consolidation within each sector, e.g., hospitals) and vertical integration (featuring relationships across sectors). Horizontal integration is referred to as a combination of several similar organizations, such as independent hospitals, in one system (The Institute for the Future, 2000, p. 57). Nevertheless, the horizontal merging activity of hospitals did not ensure a continuous patient flow. It is illegal for hospitals and other non-physician entities to employ physicians in California (Robinson, 1999). As a consequence, they have to work continuously on the relationship with physicians or physician groups in order to limit transaction costs. Horizontal integration created *hospital systems* out of sole-standing *hospitals.* Hospitals' efforts to reduce transaction costs between themselves and their physicians have led to a closer integration of physician and hospital services, which implies a shift from *hospital system* to *health system* (Buckley, McKenna, & Merlino, 1999). This is referred to as vertical integration.

The process of vertical integration is considered to be a strategy of incorporating products or services that are related to the firm's existing activities and that have usually been developed and offered by others to the marketplace (Berkowitz, 1996, p. 397). The result of a vertical integration process is the formation of an IDS, sometimes also referred to as an organized delivery system (ODS). It is defined as a network of organizations (e.g., ambulatory care clinics, physician groups, diagnostic centers, hospital, nursing homes, and home health care agencies) usually under common ownership, which provides, or arranges to provide, a coordinated continuum of services to a defined population and is willing to be held clinically and fiscally responsible for the health status of that population. These systems often own or are closely aligned with an insurance product. As the definition suggests, ODSs are primarily pursuing a vertical integration strategy (often in a defined geographic region), and, therefore, are frequently referred to as vertically integrated (regional) systems. While ODSs utilize horizontal integration strategies as well, vertical integration strategies are emphasized to differentiate them from multi-hospital systems or other chains providing services at a single stage of the delivery process (Devers, Shortell, Anderson, Mitchell, & Erickson, 1996, p. 122). Fig. 2 provides an overview of an integrated delivery approach to ensure seamless care provision.

With respect to transaction costs, vertical integration seems to be advantageous as it reduces uncertainty, cuts back opportunism, makes information more easily and readily available (Riordan, 1990), and thereby diminishes the need for "excessive" coordination. Therefore, one important reason for the formation (evolution) of hierarchies is that information is not a free good. It needs to be produced (discovered, invented, searched, or found out by bargaining) and, under certain conditions, can be exchanged.

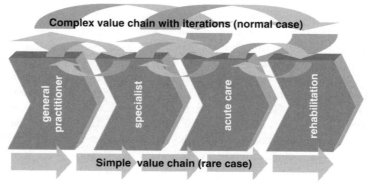

Fig. 2.   Vertical Integration and Seamless Care Delivery.

Inter alia, it needs to be made credible or trustworthy. In fact, the way information is produced, transferred, and made credible are characteristic features of hierarchical organizations (Hart, 1995; Furubotn & Richter, 1997). Ideally, when individual organizations are merged, a central mission is created that permeates the entire organization (Bea, 1996). As a consequence, information, negotiation, contracting, control, and adaptation costs are lower, and vertically integrated systems can be considered as more efficient forms of organization with respect to the provision of health care transactions.

Failure of Integrated Health Care Delivery Systems

It can be derived from the preceding that the advantages of internalization reside in the fact that a hierarchy's *ex post* access to the relevant data is superior, it attenuates the incentives to exploit uncertainty opportunistically, and the control machinery that the firm is able to activate is more selective (Williamson, 1986). This is due to the fact that the external labor market has been replaced by an internal labor market, which can be seen as a response to opportunism. In the internal labor market the wage rate attaches to the job, not the worker. This reduces individual bargaining and thus opportunism (Pitelis, 1991). However, any attempt to change institutional arrangements while at the same time holding incentives constant is likely to fail (Furubotn & Richter, 1997). Similar to market failure, hierarchy failure can be attributed to contract failure, namely the failure of employment contracts.

Efforts to "hold incentives constant," thereby to effect incentive neutrality in hierarchies, thus turn out to be delusional. Internalizing the incremented transaction leads to incentive disabilities, and as a consequence transaction costs – or "added bureaucratic costs" – arise (Williamson, 1985, 1996).

The distorted incentives prevalent in hierarchies allow for opportunism in the form of using the resources of the organization to pursue subgoals (Williamson, 1975, 1985). If pecuniary incentives in firms are weaker than those in markets, then political games and preferences have greater sway (Williamson, 1985). Ford, Wells, and Bailey (2004) analyzed sustainable network advantages in a game theoretic approach, and came to the conclusion that mutual cooperation was not automatic and that member organizations might pursue strategies that are individually rational but collectively suboptimal. Thus, a key problem for organizational economics is to determine how to motivate individuals so that they will, in fact, work toward collective interests and make the firm successful (Furubotn & Richter, 1997).

The reasoning concerning distorted incentives and their implications casts doubt on the advantages of IHCD. It seems as if opportunism and bounded rationality also cause relational contracts like the employment contract to fail. In addition, although uncertainty disappeared in the environment, it reappears in the organization, which is unable to deal with it (Bauer and Cohen, 1983). This is of particular concern the larger the organization gets. Knight brought the maxim of "diminishing returns to management or entrepreneurship" into discussion (Knight, 1965). If uncertainty reappears and increases within a hierarchy, problems of organization become increasingly more complex and bounds on cognitive competence are reached (Williamson, 1985). This causes limited spans of control because transmitting information across hierarchical levels involves losses of information and added costs, which are cumulative and arguably exponential in form. As firm size increases and successive levels of organization are added, the effects of control loss eventually exceed the gains. This "excessive laddering" implies that information passes through too many people and too many levels, which smothers effective leadership (Jaques, 1990; Wigand, Picot, & Reichwald, 1997).

As a result, incentive distortion becomes even worse and transactional diseconomies are incurred along with the size of a hierarchy (Williamson, 1975). Thus, as transaction costs associated with administrative coordination appear to be severe as well, recourse to a less integrated mode of organization seems to be promising (Williamson, 1986).

The "New" Understanding of Integrated Health Care Delivery

As a consequence of the rather likely failure of hierarchies, it remains questionable whether hierarchical organization of health care delivery is preferable. Virtual integration, which is referred to as a combination of various care-delivery services provided by separate organizations that offer services under contract to each other and are organized seamlessly (The Institute for the Future, 2000, p. 57), is the result of the emergence of IT and the trend toward maintaining loose, but coordinated, relationships.

Virtually integrated health systems can be considered as *hybrid* forms of organization. The term *hybrid* describes an umbrella term encompassing the multifaceted spectrum of modes of governance located in between market and hierarchy featuring characteristics of both to a certain extent. Hybrids consist of (more or less) autonomous units that have joined together to achieve a common purpose (Alexander, Lee, & Bazzoli, 2003). They can be defined as long-term contractual relations that preserve autonomy, but provide added transaction-specific safeguards, compared with the market (Williamson, 1996). Table 2 provides an overview of the advantages and disadvantages of hybrids.

Hybrids range from loose cooperations and close-to-market organizations to centralized networking organizations that are close to hierarchies. With respect to IHCD, the focus is clearly on hybrids of a higher degree of integration. While IHCD with respect to ownership models may have topped out after managed care did not achieve the desired objectives, IHCD based on contractual relations has gained prominence and seems to be a promising future strategy as it allows for actual integration more easily.

Virtual Integration Instead of Vertical Integration to Achieve Actual Integration

California's experience of the past 15 years suggests that coordination of health care does not necessarily require unified ownership (Robinson and Casalino, 1996). An integrated system can also achieve its objectives by building networks and developing contractual relationships (Shortell, Gillies, & Anderson, 1994). After having experienced failure with IDSs in the 1990s, most systems today are moving toward mixtures or hybrid forms that entail both ownership and contractual relationships while focusing on their core competencies. The combination of a marketplace in rapid

Table 2. Hybrid Organization – Advantages and Disadvantages.

Advantages	Disadvantages
• Adaptive flexibility • Reduces current and future uncertainty • Contributes to the formation of rational expectations • Creates signaling opportunities • Allows for decentralized coordination • Combines autonomy and control	• Reconciliation of ideas and interests of different parties • Risk of free riding and increased resource consumption • Negative externalities • Abuse of acquired information by opportunistic network participants

Legal Independence of the Participating Organizations

transition and a blossoming variety of organizational forms has led to a debate on both the merits of attaining various levels of integration and on the ability to attain them through contractual or networking relationships as opposed to ownership and employment relationships (Zelman, 1996).

The premise of *virtual integration* is that many of the same benefits can be achieved by linking organizations in networks connected by contracts and information systems instead of merging multiple organizations into a single entity (Kongstvedt, Plocher, & Stanford, 2001; The Institute for the Future, 1999). Virtually integrated organizations comply with the demand for seamless care delivery but retain their own identities (Zelman, 1996). Furthermore, Reve (1990) argues that economies of integration can often be more efficiently obtained through vertical corporate agreements than through vertical integration by ownership. Vertical control (administrative- or incentive-based) is decisive rather than ownership. Full vertical integration ties up capital resources, increases complexity, and creates management problems as the organization gets involved in successive stages of distribution where it has little experience.

As a consequence, actual integration is essential to a successful management of hybrid forms of integration. So far, consolidation in health care systems has come more easily than actual integration (Zelman, 1996). However, there is reason to believe that hybrid forms of organization represent a mechanism to achieve integration without the necessity of ownership of all components. These "integrative" organizations will likely prove especially important in the context of a constantly changing environment and will allow the participants to work cooperatively with one another, yet hold onto a significant measure of autonomy to a certain degree (Friedman and Goes, 2001).

The ability of ODSs to achieve actual integration in order to economize on transaction costs and add value may thus depend more on certain competencies and capabilities than on ownership models. The three capabilities *functional*, *physician*, and *clinical* integration have to be attained. Beginning with functional integration, the tightening of an organization will be enhanced by an increased integration and participation of physicians within the network in order to achieve sophisticated clinical integration (Shortell, Gillies, Anderson, Erickson, & Mitchell, 2000). Physician integration is reflected in the extent to which physicians are economically linked to a system, use its facilities and services, and actively participate in its planning, management, and governance (Scott, Ruef, Mendel, & Caronna, 2000). If actual integration in terms of functional, physician, and clinical integration can be achieved, hybrid modes of organization enjoy the advantages of hierarchies without incurring hierarchical dysfunctionalities.

INTEGRATED HEALTH CARE DELIVERY IN THE BAY AREA AND IMPLICATIONS FOR GERMANY

The case study conducted in the Bay Area (Janus, 2003) evaluated how organizations should be organized in more detail based on experiences from the past. The answers of the interviewees have been aggregated and success factors for actually IDSs will be derived. However, Appendix B provides an example of a question and the interviewees' responses in order to provide an insight into the proceeding of aggregation when evaluating the success factors. In addition, recommendations regarding a future proceeding will be evaluated and conclusions for IHCD in Germany will be considered in more detail in order to shed light on cross-national implications.

Current "Success Factors" in the Bay Area Health Care Market

As mentioned, the Bay Area health care market offers examples for all different kinds of organizations, ranging from less integrated to completely IDSs. Fig. 3 provides an overview of the interviewed organizations and their degree of integration. While highly integrated organizations focus on the primary care physician (PCP) as the gatekeeper and case manager for the patient, lower integrated systems are rather specialty dominated.

Kaiser Permanente provides an example for a fully integrated and "hierarchical" delivery system. The application of managed care in its original form (integrated financing and delivery of health care) can only be pursued successfully in IDS because otherwise the economics are different. The reason is that care management with respect to both quality and affordability can be pursued most efficiently and effectively if patients stay for a longer period of time with their providers and their health plan. The average member stays for 12 years with Kaiser Permanente while the average member stays with other HMOs only for 30 months. As a consequence, quality care that also includes preventive care and care management "pays off" and quality and affordability go hand-in-hand. The flip-side of hierarchy in the form of added bureaucratic costs resulting in hierarchy failure is not prevalent in the system currently (but was 5 years ago) due to tight management, enabling the organization to take advantage of a hierarchy without facing the disadvantages. The system is thus able to react quickly to any kind of health care news and market changes as it has organized its care management thoroughly and based on sophisticated data management. The

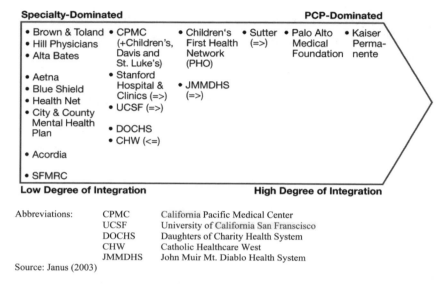

Specialty-Dominated   **PCP-Dominated**

• Brown & Toland	• CPMC	• Children's	• Sutter	• Palo Alto	• Kaiser
• Hill Physicians	(+Children's,	First Health	(=>)	Medical	Perma-
• Alta Bates	Davis and	Network		Foundation	nente
	St. Luke's)	(PHO)			
• Aetna	• Stanford				
• Blue Shield	Hospital &	• JMMDHS			
• Health Net	Clinics (=>)	(=>)			
• City & County	• UCSF (=>)				
Mental Health					
Plan	• DOCHS				
	• CHW (<=)				
• Acordia					
• SFMRC					

Low Degree of Integration   **High Degree of Integration**

Abbreviations:	CPMC	California Pacific Medical Center
	UCSF	University of California San Franscisco
	DOCHS	Daughters of Charity Health System
	CHW	Catholic Healthcare West
	JMMDHS	John Muir Mt. Diablo Health System

Source: Janus (2003)

Fig. 3. The Bay Area Health Care Market and Its Major Players.

standardization achieved in the field of care management at Kaiser Permanente facilitates health care provision and thereby economizes on transaction costs.

However, since by and large managed care has failed to achieve its objectives most of the surveyed organizations today follow a hybrid mode of organization that complies with the assumption that hybrid forms of organization provide incentive and control mechanisms of both markets and hierarchies as well as adaptive capabilities in both autonomous and cooperative respects (which makes sense due to the unique and highly complex character of health care transactions). The general objective in today's health care market is to establish a decentralized networking structure, focusing on core competencies and core markets. This trend has also been analyzed by Dubbs, Bazzoli, Shortell, and Kralovec (2004). An analysis of organizational configurations conducted in 1994 and 1998 shows a shift from centralized to decentralized coordination in order to allow for greater independence and autonomy for organizations to respond quickly to local market changes. For example, Kaiser Permanente withdrew from a market where the delivery system was not working well with the health plan. A hybrid like Sutter Health does not plan to expand out of Northern California. Within its market, the system is thus able to respond flexibly and quickly without adding bureaucratic costs. A hybrid mode of organization like Sutter Health allows its affiliates to share interests but preserve a certain degree of autonomy. The last issue is in particular important with respect to physicians who always fear a loss of control. Several success factors for hybrids are illustrated in Fig. 4 and will be explained in more detail in the following sections.

The Dynamic Tension of Centralized and Decentralized Coordination

The majority of organizations indicated that they preferred decentralized coordination over focal coordination; however, most of them used both ways to coordinate activities. Additionally, those organizations that mentioned that they were either more centralized or more decentralized usually added that they planned to move closer to the other form of coordination to finally use both mechanisms according to the saying "Think globally, act locally." Moreover, several informants of organizations (e.g., California Pacific Medical Center (CPMC) and Hill Physicians) pointed out that they used more centralized coordination due to turnaround activities, but moved or planned to move toward a decentralized structure as this was considered important in a growth face.

At Sutter Health, the system sets objectives and the overall strategic direction centrally (shape what the market is), but leaves room for flexibility and local execution to allow for market orientation. Only some functions

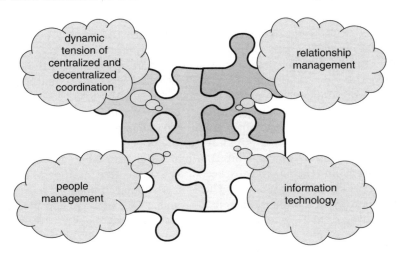

Fig. 4. Success Factors of Integrated Delivery Systems.

have been centralized. Therefore, the organization is very market-driven from an affiliate standpoint and gives the affiliates leeway to act and react independently. Sutter Health aims at being an operating and a holding company at the same time. For example, the whole IT initiative is driven regionally, but implemented locally. This business strategy created a situation of dynamic tension between ~80% decentralized coordination and 20% centralized management. The tension is managed by internal councils that act as mediators within the organization. Moreover, there are meetings several times a year and a 3-day symposium is held every year to educate the CEOs of the affiliates about everything and to foster interaction. A two-way evaluation of the relationships rounds off this proceeding: Report cards are used in both directions, the affiliate rates the system and the system rates the affiliate, for example, with respect to leadership, expertise, and responsiveness. Each board has obligations, but the system has obligations as well. The tension of centralized and decentralized coordination drives the whole system. It is a "tight–loose–tight" approach, which means that the top (the system) defines the goals (tight) and passes them down to boards or affiliates (loose) that execute and implement them locally. The system then controls the results (tight).

The examples have shown that the dynamic tension of centralized and decentralized coordination drives a hybrid and underlines a coopetition (featuring cooperation and competition simultaneously) approach based on confidence and power respectively. Decentralized coordination tends to rely on confidence as a mechanism while centralized management employs power to accomplish objectives. Although hybrids usually employ both modes of coordination in order to be able to adapt autonomously and cooperatively, coordination by power is in general more prevalent on the administrative side of an organization while the clinical side could only be managed by confidence as power is a non-starter with respect to physicians. Owing to the inherent characteristics of a hybrid (more ties among participants than in the market, but less authority than within hierarchies), it is then able to create and maintain a status of coopetition that stabilizes itself. Transparency of actions and informational exchange while still remaining independent and being able to keep confidential information allows for efficient health care transactions. This is in particular important with respect to the coordination of physician relationships, as they always fear the loss of control when entering a larger system. In addition, health care is local (Dubbs et al., 2004) and community-based with respect to decision-making, which has enticed health systems to focus on core competencies and core markets, following the adage "same store growth." Nevertheless, with respect to certain issues, for example, IT which is considered a "change agent" for hybrids, cooperations should be centralized and systemwide to allow for standardization.

Relationship Management
Relationship building and maintaining is critical to economize on transaction costs within a hybrid mode of organization as it cuts back opportunism, avoids or ends prolonged disputes, and smoothes health care transactions in general. Relationship management refers to internal and external relationships respectively and is usually supported by certain divisions (e.g., Sutter Connect at Sutter Health) or parts of an organization that facilitate the relationships with other parts of the system, such as physicians, or with "external players," such as pharmaceutical companies, disease management companies, or independent institutions, for example, The Leapfrog Group. Brown & Toland (B&T) has created a physician relations department in addition to the customer services department. While the former is proactive and deals with bigger issues, the latter is occupied with daily issues of patients and physicians and is more reactive. This proceeding has smoothed out the transactions with physicians and customers considerably.

Some of the surveyed health care organizations pursue relationship building with other market players in order to enhance the relationship with patients. They have begun to see disease management as a cooperative service for patients, which is provided by a health system in cooperation with health plans and disease management companies. The objective is to set up critical pathways and guidelines to enhance effectiveness by following a comprehensive approach to health care provision.

In this context, *bilateral dependency* has an impact on the durability of the cooperative arrangement. It arises due to the medium to highly specific character of health care transactions and can be seen as an incentive substitute because it enhances cooperation among entities of a system. This is due to the fact that it cuts back opportunism and fosters stable and reciprocal relationships.

In general, bilateral dependency increases with the degree of integration of a health system. This explains why informants at Kaiser Permanente pointed out that bilateral dependency was total and, thus, provided an effective mechanism for cooperation. Less-integrated systems stated that bilateral dependency always depended on the amount of business a certain entity did with a system and how strong its financial position was. If it is likely that the parties will meet again and the future has a sufficiently large shadow, tighter relationships based on trust are supported. At Sutter

Health, each service area has one main hospital and the others act as feeders that send patients into these hospitals. The main hospitals would be unable to exist without the feeder hospitals and vice versa because certain services are only provided at the main hospitals in every service area with the intention to build centers of excellence and avoid duplication of high-cost services as high volumes have to be achieved in these fields of medical care.

With respect to less-integrated systems, such as Catholic Healthcare West (CHW) or Daughters of Charity Health System (DOCHS), hospitals are dependent on each other for financial resources. They usually do not refer business to each other (except for certain services at the DOCHS) because of different cultures and a less tight organization. Entities of looser integrated systems therefore see themselves not as bilaterally dependent entities, but as partners that "coordinate" business and have no intense cooperation.

Bilateral dependency is closely related and positively correlated to *informal organization*. Although everything that has to be formally organized is formally organized since managed care, informal organization, which is rather prevalent on the clinical than on the administrative site, is extremely important. It enhances spontaneous action, creativity, and individuality. Moreover, it is critical for the sharing of information and for the creation of an information-driven organization. Even formal committees are basically more informal and thereby enhance trust and relationship building and, thus, cut back opportunism. Finally, informal organization is in particular essential in hospitals and in dealing with physicians who prefer autonomy and less "formal" control.

The consequence of successful relationship building is the creation of a *reputation*, which in turn enhances further relationship building. Three modes of reputation are crucial:

- with respect to health plans a reputation as a *tough negotiator* is important,
- with respect to patients and employers a *quality* reputation is indispensable, and
- with respect to physicians a *value* reputation is crucial.

These three modes of reputation impact future relationship building to a large degree and reduce uncertainty with respect to health care transactions.

People Management
Besides relationship building, hybrids put an emphasis on the role of talented people (human capital) who are able to manage and strengthen these relationships. People management is in particular important as hybrids

employ a complex mix of social and monetary mechanisms to allow for autonomous and cooperative coordination respectively. Although the majority of the surveyed organizations still rely on monetary incentives, for example, the development of performance-based reimbursement methodologies, the focus is increasingly shifting toward social mechanisms, emphasizing corporate *culture, communication,* and *trust.* In particular, hybrid organizations rely on these immaterial incentives as the glue of collective action, rather than on ownership or consolidated balance sheets (Alexander et al., 2003). These immaterial incentives have been neglected for a long time; however, they increasingly gain in importance as studies question the effectiveness of monetary incentives (Baker, Jensen, & Murphy, 1988; Robinson, 2001; Mays, Claxton, & White, 2004; Frey and Osterloh, 2000). A structural and cultural fit among the partners makes social mechanisms work and facilitates the alignment of physician and hospital incentives, which contributes to an efficient coordination of health care transactions.

In general, hybrid forms of organization face more difficulties in establishing a common *culture* within their organizations than a completely IDS. In addition, hybrids usually attain a common culture in administration, while it is more difficult to achieve a common culture among (loosely) affiliated physicians, in particular if there is a clash of entirely different cultures. Nevertheless, some key issues enable a hybrid to set up a cohesive corporate culture. Similar to the management of hybrid forms of organization, they rely on a mix of cooperative and competitive culture. At Sutter Health, this has resulted in an umbrella culture (system culture), which overlaps each individual culture (autonomous culture of the affiliate). This umbrella culture is evolving at an increasing pace and fosters the understanding as a system, in particular as it is supported by IT and human resources (HR). This implies that culture has to be designed as a systemwide initiative and its power should never be underestimated because "culture eats strategy for lunch every day" as an informant at Kaiser Permanente mentioned. Culture has a tremendous impact on whether an organization succeeds or fails to organize health care transactions efficiently. A strong culture will promote a system perspective and provide a platform for cooperation among the participants as it serves as an "immaterial" incentive system.

Creating a corporate culture is only possible if a certain degree of *trust/confidence* has been achieved among the partners. Conversely, culture supports an atmosphere of trust if successfully implemented. Confidence reduces opportunistic behavior and, thus, cuts back transaction costs. It therefore serves as a major mechanism for coordination and also enhances a proactive approach to information exchange. It can thus be considered the "underlying glue" for hybrids and increases the "systemness" and the seamless interoperability within the organization together with IT, which can be seen as the technical counterpart to trust.

An atmosphere of trust is based on meaningful *communication* within the organization. The organization has to have "glass ceilings and glass floors" as an informant at CPMC mentioned. The top management has to listen to the people and explain strategies to "open the door." One has to "sell services each and every time again" to make people feel that they are part of the game. Then, resistance is getting less, in particular if people see the benefits of the changes and if they take a long-term instead of a short-term perspective. If the people of the organization communicate among each other and share the vision, the health system becomes "tighter" and actual integration is achieved.

Information Technology

IT is the "glue" that holds a hybrid together and it is simultaneously the prerequisite and the consequence of the development of a health system as it fosters actual integration. Hybrid organizations rely more heavily on IT than fully IDSs due to their looser structure. In order to maintain a stable cooperation within a hybrid, a sophisticated technological infrastructure is indispensable, which, in turn, has a significant impact on the transactional atmosphere. This is a result of the overwhelming necessity to transfer and exchange information, which is very diverse in content, format, and size. There is a plethora of information available in all organizations, but there is still the need for more efficient and effective communication as it is important that the right information is exchanged and that it is understood. Although it can be considered more difficult for a hybrid organization than for an IDS to successfully carry out IT strategies, it sets the basis for change with respect to a hybrid, and networks are continuously changing as new affiliates join the system. At Sutter Health, the IT department acts as a change agent for the whole company. The dynamic tension allows affiliates to be pushed into the same direction with respect to IT systems. While IT at Sutter Health gets more and more centralized, an emphasis is put on achieving joint agreements on standards and on sustaining the individual flexibility of affiliates. This is accomplished by treating every affiliate as a "customer," which drives efficiency and prevents the emergence of bureaucratic structures.

Contrary to current literature (Picot et al., 2001), the majority of hybrid organizations reported that the development of new technologies enhanced integration and allowed for a tighter integration over a large area due to improved communication. Although there is currently no hybrid in the Bay

Area health care market that can be considered to be perfectly "wired," new technologies so far have helped organizations to achieve coherence within the system and to tighten the organization. It becomes clear that if new technologies have an impact on the creation of a trend toward integration or market organizations, they will rather facilitate the emergence of more *integrated* systems. However, it has been stated that the majority of organizations have moved away from integration and focus on core competencies and markets since the failure of managed care to meet its objectives. This raises the question how the current development of tighter networking boosted by IT corresponds to the idea of "less-integrated" hybrids, focusing on core competencies. The following outlook provides a possible solution to this issue.

Future Issues in Integrated Health Care Delivery

First, it has to be contemplated that the "over-expansion pitfall" of managed care in the mid-1990s, which resulted in the organization of health care transactions mainly in highly integrated hybrids or IDSs, for the most part did not involve *actual integration*. There was very often no sound strategy and health care organizations rushed into mergers and acquisitions without thinking through the consequences. As a result, they are more careful now before embarking on a new "adventure."

Second, health systems focus on core competencies *and* simultaneously the majority of them moves toward a higher degree of actual integration supported by increasingly sophisticated infrastructure. This does not necessarily involve vertical integration, but rather enhanced cooperation, be it in the form of contractual arrangements or ownership (depending on the respective transaction).

Achieving actual integration is crucial to the efficient and effective provision of health care due to three reasons: *the relationship to physicians*, *a continuum of health care provision*, and *the nature of health care transactions*. Kaiser Permanente provides an example for efficient and effective care delivery in a continuum. Managing costs as well as managing the quality of care is most easily possible within a completely IDS as incentives can be aligned compatibly among the parts of the system. Separate contracting involves different economics and also "frictional losses" in the form of additional transaction costs. However, if a completely IDS entails added bureaucratic costs, which involve hierarchy failure as described, these advantages may be more than offset and a hybrid form of organization provides more flexibility and the benefits of actual integration. Furthermore, the nature of health care transactions demands for care coordination because they are of an interdependent and reciprocal character, which involves multiple interactions of health care market players in order to achieve a healthy state of well-being. In addition, health care transactions are in general of medium to high asset specificity, which calls for the organization within a more highly integrated form of organization. Finally, relationships to physicians are crucial for a health system as they "feed" the hospital with patients and have the primary contact to the patient, which influences the degree to which patients trust the whole organization. Clinical and functional integration is insufficient; only if physician–system integration is achieved, the health system achieves actual integration. This does not necessarily involve complete vertical integration, but at least results in hybrid forms of organization that are closer to hierarchical organization than to market organization in order to allow for care provision in a continuum. As discussed, *actual integration* can sometimes be achieved more easily through *virtual integration* than through vertical integration. More flexibility and less bureaucratic distortions are the benefits.

Except for very few systems, which currently refrain from "integration," the majority of hybrids state that they are "integrating, and not integrated." They pursue the tightening of the network very carefully; however, they aim at extending it to include other organizations according to a more comprehensive view of health care provision. For example, hybrids that were further integrated in the mid-1990s and withdrew themselves from including the risk-taking health plan function in their system have learned that they have to build the delivery system first before taking risk and integrating further, otherwise no actual integration could be achieved. CHW is even disintegrating and does not plan to further integrate other entities. Patrick E. Fry, the chief operating officer (COO) of Sutter Health, mentioned that the system was not yet "integrated" enough to support a health plan. This means that the relationship among different physician groups was not close enough yet. As a response, the system advances physician alliances by fostering the sharing of best practices and standards among different groups. For example, comprehensive and systemwide case and disease management supports actual integration and, thus, economizes on transaction costs.

Implications for the German Health Care Market

The Bay Area health care market has been taken as an example of examination because it offers a wide range of private organizations providing and financing health care. An overview of the current system is provided in the following in order to highlight the issues the German health care system is faced with. Taking experiences made in the Bay Area into account, implications for the German health care market will be derived.

Basic Ideas of the German Health Care System
The rise of Germany's modern health care system dates back to 1883 when the parliament made nationwide health insurance compulsory (Oberender and Fleischmann, 2002; Amelung, Glied, & Topan, 2003). Germany is recognized as the first country to have introduced a national social security system. In the following decades the principle of statutory social insurance, called the *Bismarck system*, was also applied to alleviate the risks of work-related accidents and invalidity (1884), old age and disability (1889), unemployment (1927), and the need for long-term nursing care (1994). The prominence and structural continuity of social insurance is one of the key features of the historical development of Germany's health care system to the present day (European Observatory on Health Care Systems, 2000).

Statutory health insurance (SHI) was created to provide coverage of expenditures in case of illness, encompassing direct costs related to illness as well as indirect costs caused by a loss of productivity. It has been set up based on the idea of solidarity which implies that the contributions (equally shared by the employer and the employee) are not actuarially based, but always represent a certain percentage of gross income, depending on the respective sickness fund the person is a member of (Oberender and Fleischmann, 2002). In addition, non-earning spouses and children are covered as well without any surcharges. Currently, 88% of the population are members of the SHI, 2% are covered by free governmental health care (soldiers, police officers, etc.), and 9% of the population have opted out of the SHI and joined a private (and actuarially based) health insurance (European Observatory on Health Care Systems, 2000). This is mainly due to the fact that sickness fund membership is optional for employees whose income exceeds EUR 3,487.50 (gross) per month in 2004. They can (but are not obliged to) become a member of a private health insurance.

The basic principle behind "German-style" cost containment was an income-orientated expenditure policy to guarantee stable contribution rates. This was (and still is) an important objective in a time of economic restructuring and growing international competition, since the contributions are jointly paid by employers and employees. Therefore, increases in contribution rates were (and still are) perceived to be a question of weakening the international competitiveness of Germany (Amelung et al., 2003). Fig. 5 provides an overview of the structure of the German health care system.

Reforms and Recent Developments in the German Health Care Market
The drive for cost containment (and quality-enhancement), which intensified after reunification, was realized through a long series of legislation. While the Health Care Reform Act (Gesundheitsreformgesetz) of 1989 primarily focused on cost containment, the Health Care Structure Act (Gesundheitsstrukturgesetz) of 1993 and the following 1st and 2nd Statutory Health Insurance Restructuring Acts (Neuordnungsgesetze) shifted the emphasis to quality-orientated issues and increasingly focused on IHCD and care coordination. In particular, the 1st and 2nd Statutory Health Insurance Restructuring Acts dealt with rather market-orientated reform tools and new ways of organizing health care transactions instead of focusing on costs. Thus, selective contracting between sickness funds and providers of care became a feasible option, and horizontal integration of physicians was enhanced by the introduction of §63 and §73a Code of Social Law (Sozialgesetzbuch (SGB)) V.

The Reform Act of Statutory Health Insurance 2000 (Gesundheitsreform 2000) introduced §§140 a–h SGB V, which extended the former merely horizontal forms of cooperation to include vertical cooperation in order to achieve "integrated health care delivery." Since then, physician networks are allowed to collaborate with hospitals and other health care providers, which are licensed by the SHI system. In addition, such measures as the introduction of PCP gatekeeper system and the possibility to take over the budget responsibility for an IDS became feasible. The objective was to overcome the strict separation between the ambulatory and inpatient care sectors and provide health care in a continuum in order to enhance quality of care while simultaneously containing costs.

Although the above-mentioned legislation provided the framework for new forms of cooperation, no actual integration of health care delivery happened. The most prominent form of new health care delivery was the formation of between 300 and 400 physician networks, of which some achieved considerable improvements with respect to an efficient and effective organization of health care transactions. However, the majority of these networks were only existent for a short period as they employed neither sufficient incentives nor sophisticated management capabilities.

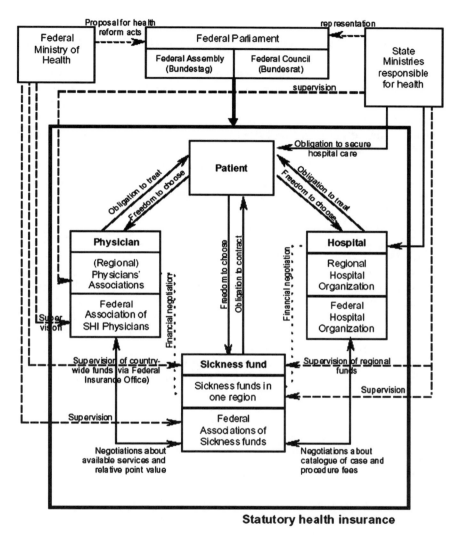

Fig. 5. The Structure of the German Health Care System. *Source*: European Observatory on Health Care Systems (2000).

Managed Care and the Necessity for Privatization
The idea of IHCD in Germany was based to a large degree on managed care. However, while managed care focused on the integration of insurance and provider functions in order to manage costs and simultaneously ensure the quality of care, IHCD in Germany put an emphasis on the cross-sectoral cooperation of providers rather than the integration of financing and risk-sharing. Both elements impact each other as they aim at the same objective: providing high-quality and efficient health care in order to achieve a status of health and well-being.

Nevertheless, while managed care penetrated the Bay Area health care market (and also other markets in the U.S. although to sometimes a lesser degree) and finally underwent the further development to "light" managed care after its backlash, IHCD never really took off in Germany. This raises the question *why* there were no activities in this direction, *whether* any initiatives could be expected in the future and, if yes, *how* they should be approached.

Although §140 SGB V provided for new forms of health care delivery, it cannot be compared with the managed care movement and the rush of private organizations to provide health care in IDSs. Cooperation became possible in Germany, but they were still highly regulated and always involved public bodies. Acting like a private organization while facing public restrictions has impeded "integrated health care delivery" to a large degree. Nonetheless, as the German health care system was approaching a crisis condition with respect to its financing, new legislation was passed to enhance in particular IHCD.

The Health Care Modernization Act
The Health Care Modernization Act *(Gesundheitsmodernisierungsgesetz (GMG))*, which became effective at the beginning of 2004 as a non-partisan legislative approach, was designed to lower labor costs in Germany by reducing the percentage of health insurance contribution that is deducted from gross salaries (Janus, 2004). This implies that private households will take on a larger percentage of health care costs and become more responsible for their health care. The Act explicitly recognizes that health care consumers are entitled to have a say in health care delivery. This empowerment of the consumer was accompanied by incentives for changes on the institutional side. An emphasis is put on integrating the highly fragmented sectors of health care delivery in Germany in order to enhance the – sometimes conflicting – goals efficiency and quality in health care. Therefore, §§140 a–h SGB V have been modified (Orlowski & Wasem, 2003).

According to §140 SGB V, integrated care delivery is a targeted cooperation of organizationally and financially independent providers (hospitals, physicians, medical clinics, etc.) of health care across sectors of care delivery. IHCD aims at ending the era of fragmented care delivery by organizing medical and economic responsibility across sectors and along the value chain.

The conditions for integrated delivery laid down in the legislation encompass the following main issues:

- The core idea is selective contracting between two or more providers of different sectors with one or more sickness funds.
- In comparison to previous legislation the involvement of physicians' associations is not anymore mandatory, but explicitly excluded.
- The sickness funds have to convince their members to participate in such a project. Therefore, they are able to offer the insured bonus programs such as deductions of co-payments.
- Up to 1% (amounting to 680 million Euro per year approximately) of the total budget of the sickness funds for the ambulatory care sector and up to 1% of the invoices billed by hospitals could be withheld for services delivered under contracts of integrated delivery. This is designed only as a start-up financing for the first two years. Starting from 2007 this rule will not apply anymore. Fig. 6 provides an overview of the proceeding.

As a result of less bureaucratic regulations and the planned 3-year start-up financing, the interest into IHCD has grown considerably. Some sickness funds have already agreed upon bonus models for their customers, which reward the participation in IHCD. Intense and comprehensive negotiations across sectors are happening, ranging from population-based approaches to indication-based plans as shown in Fig. 7.

Currently, there exist about 200 contracts in Germany for IHCD approaches; however, the majority of these contracts do not cover all sectors of health care delivery and very often only cover certain specific diseases. Very few systems represent "total budget approaches" by taking over part of the financial risk for providing health services.

Although the Health Care Modernization Act provides opportunities for seamless care delivery in IDSs, there are obstacles that will impede fast structural changes. There is a danger that as there is the financial incentive of the 1% of payments from sickness funds that will be withheld and only paid to integrated care delivery approaches everybody will rush into integration contracts without thinking through the consequences and without carefully designing contracts. These "quick and dirty" contracts will lack

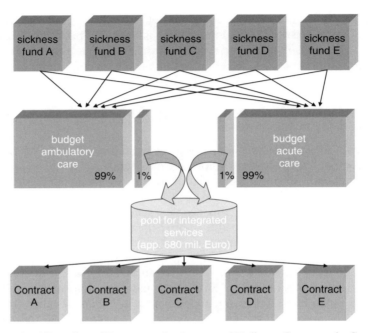

Fig. 6.   The Allocation of Resources for Integrated Delivery Contracts in Germany.

sophistication and will not be conducive to the further development of in-tegrated care delivery. Rather, they will impede the development of care delivery because the partners will be bound to the contract. It is unlikely that they will be exchanged by more sophisticated contracts soon.

Furthermore, it is insufficient to focus on the "1% incentive." The establishment of an IDS requires much more investment (capital *and* hu-man) to sustain as a long-term system. In addition, the "1% incentive" will exist only until 2006. The legitimate question is what happens with IHCD in 2007. On the one hand, this short-term perspective increases uncertainty among stakeholders and, thus, complicates transactions. On the other hand, it also implies that a long-term approach to integrated care delivery has to have a pay-off without considering "the 1%." It rather requires a focus on "the 99%" of the budget and how these can be reorganized and will be re-shifted. If a rearrangement of the 99% does not show any cost savings, the undertaking cannot be considered promising in general.

Moreover, a certain volume is needed with respect to both the size of the sickness fund(s) and the lives for which care is provided. This is of particular

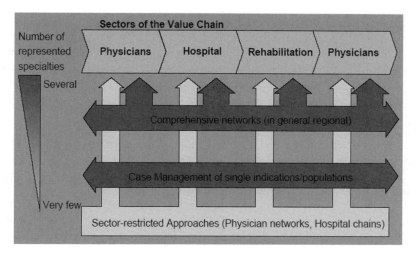

Fig. 7. Possible Approaches to Integrated Health Care Delivery.

importance in order to assess the risk an integrated system is taking over. While medical innovations pose a permanent financial challenge to a system, morbidity risks of the enrolled population can be reduced if the number of lives is increased. This gains in significance if the IDS takes over full budget responsibility.

Furthermore, as providers fear price dumping in competition they focus on costs to influence their risk. However, in order to take a long-term approach to integrated care, quality should be considered as a competitive advantage as it is a much more flexible tool for (re)designing and improving care delivery. In addition, it offers the opportunity to implement techno-cratic decision procedures and thereby develop standards of care. In this case, quality and efficiency complements each other as improved quality or quality indicators very often translate into enhanced efficiency.

The question remains how to redesign care delivery according to the Health Care Modernization Act in order to provide high-quality and ef-ficient care. The new legislation has set the basis for privatization in health care. Based on demographic forecasts and the further development of med-ical technology, researchers expect that more services will be gradually ex-cluded from the SHI coverage.

This suggests a shift toward private provision and financing of health, while some "basic services" will remain to be covered by social health insurance. As the private provision of services increasingly takes hold, the organization of health care transactions in private organizations may gain in importance in Germany and will push the trend toward "integrated health care delivery." The extent to which this development will actually penetrate the market remains to be seen. However, the cost pressure is there and will become more severe due to demographic reasons and advances in medical technology.

Organizing Health Care Delivery in Private Organizations: Applying U.S. Success Factors and Management Concepts
In Germany, the revised §§140 a–h enhanced the movement toward integration of provision and financing of care; however, IHCD is still in its infancy. With respect to organizing health care transactions in private organizations in order to economize on transaction costs while simultaneously providing quality of care and value, the presented success factors of the Bay Area study should be considered because private organizations in Germany are now faced with the same challenges, which organizations in the Bay Area had to cope with in the 1990s. However, German health care organizations have the unique opportunity to avoid making the same mistakes. Therefore, any approach to integration of health care delivery should always focus on achieving *"actual integration,"* instead of pursuing only *aggregation* (Amelung, 1999, p. 66). This is sometimes easier to achieve by organizing health care transactions in a hybrid mode (instead of integrating them into one system) as the hybrid offers more flexibility and adaptation capabilities in both autonomous and cooperative respects. The organization of health care transactions in (actually integrated) hybrid modes of organization can be considered as the further development of managed care. This can only be achieved if the structures comply with the overarching strategy of the organization and if the focus shifts from a piecemeal approach to a global perspective. Although there is the "1%" and short-term incentive for integration, Germany could still make a leap from today's market to this new way of health care delivery, avoiding the rush toward integration for integration's sake and other pitfalls of managed care, which impeded and impede actual integration in the U.S. In order to achieve actual integration in private organizations, the evaluated success factors for hybrids have to be taken into account and assessed according to their applicability to German conditions.

Managing People. In Germany, leadership cultures are highly specialized and are oriented toward a head of a department or other authorities.

Nevertheless, the establishment and the operation of an IDS require all different constituencies of the system to focus on a common goal in the first place. Every participant of the system has his or her position in the value chain of health care delivery and has to give up not only a certain degree of autonomy, but also has to shift the focus from an authority toward a system goal. For this purpose, German health care decision-makers have to heavily invest in HR to enhance communication and cooperation (soft skills). In this respect, physician integration is critical. While hospitals are allowed to employ physicians in Germany and, thus, are not faced with the same restrictions as hospitals in some states of the U.S., there still remains the issue of integrating locally based physicians into a health network or an IDS. Cultural differences have to be reconciled and incentive structures (material and immaterial) have to be set up and aligned with other entities of a health system (Janus and Amelung, 2004a). The abolishment of sectoral budgets, which were a result of a highly fragmented industry, becomes absolutely essential to allow for IHCD in the German health care system. This sets the basis for comprehensive corporate cultures, which in turn support integrative strategies in hybrid forms of organization. The coherence of material and immaterial incentive structures then allows for clinical integration, the last step to achieve actual integration. Finally, a whole new "breed" of health care professionals who drive and manage the process of integration has to be trained and recruited as management departments, such as managed care departments in U.S. organizations, are not yet existent in German health care organizations.

Managing Relationships. The external dealing with partners and affiliates is so far difficult due to the different sectors of the German health care system; however, this will improve as the sectoral structure is continuously abolished. Health care market participants experience a learning process as far as successful business relationships are concerned. In this respect, particular emphasis should be put on employing incentives to entice cooperation (or at least coopetition) rather than competition and resentment. Certain services such as disease management can be outsourced easily or provided in cooperation with other organizations. The exchange of best practices and evidence-based guidelines will be enhanced and the quality of care ameliorates as a consequence of integrated care delivery in actually integrated health systems.

Information Technology. In Germany, hospitals uses different kinds of IT systems, which are not compatible with one another. Therefore, a complete turnaround is needed that requires a high volume of investments on the one hand, and a careful consideration of data privacy requirements and the ownership of personal data on the other. Finally, a certain degree of reliability on legislation and its changes can be considered a prerequisite for the willingness to commit to a large investment to wire health care organizations. Nevertheless, comprehensive IT structures have to be implemented to support virtual integration (Janus and Amelung, 2004b). This will facilitate not only relationship management, but also help to achieve a tension between decentralized and centralized coordination.

Dynamic Tension between Centralized and Decentralized Coordination. So far, local approaches to IHCD with a decentralized coordination based on autonomous physicians prevail in Germany. A lack of centralized coordination and goal-setting causes a large number of approaches to fail. This is also due to insufficient management capabilities, which could enhance the process of centralization that is needed in a turnaround mode as revealed by the Bay Area study. However, the creation of franchised IDSs is beginning to take off based on contracts according to §§140 a–h SGB V. In addition, the tightening of the European Union will further drive the creation of IDSs. Nevertheless, the development of centralized structures has to be monitored as decentralized coordination and local presence is essential to account for community-driven health care and local health care needs in the long term.

Considering the described success factors for organizing health care transactions in actually integrated hybrid modes of organization, the Health Care Modernization Act has set the basis for a more proactive approach to integrated care delivery. It remains to be seen whether German health care market participants will be enticed to pursue long-term structural changes instead of just "hunting for the 1%." This "trouble-shooting" strategy initiated by health care policy makers in Germany is comparable to the rush to integration in California in the mid-1990s and does not enhance long-term health system design. Rather, German health care market participants should consider and assess the evaluated success factors thoroughly when designing their IDSs.

CONCLUSION

Based on the findings in the San Francisco Bay Area health care market, it can be concluded that IHCD should not be considered an outdated model if pursued according to its new understanding, focusing on *actual* integration.

Although organizations in the Bay Area faced difficulties with respect to integrative activities, the basic reason for providing care in integrated systems, *continuous care delivery*, remains to be valid and economizes on transaction costs. However, fully integrated care delivery systems easily incur hierarchical dysfunctionalities and although the nature of health care transactions favors hierarchical organization due to the interdependent and highly complex character of health care transactions, "virtual" integration in the form of a hybrid mode of governance is preferred as it can achieve actual integration more easily and simultaneously provides flexibility. Therefore, it seems to be appropriate that almost all surveyed organizations in the Bay Area health care market today follow a hybrid form of organization, which is closer to a hierarchical than to a market organization. However, the derived success factors such as the tension between centralized and decentralized coordination, relationship and people management, and the sophisticated implementation of IT are decisive to a successful undertaking of IHCD.

Based on these experiences, Germany has been taken as an example to elucidate cross-national implications of the Bay Area study. After a long period of public restrictions the Health Care Modernization Act, which became effective January 1, 2004, sets the basis for a comprehensive approach to IHCD. It also implies that privatization in the health care sector will take off and that if German market participants aim at long-term structural changes they could employ the success factors derived from the Bay Area study. If they took these success factors for organizing health care transactions into account, they could avoid the pitfalls associated with managed care in the U.S. and, thus, they could make a leap to optimizing IHCD in the future, focusing on actual integration in hybrid modes of organization. However, building sophisticated organizational structures in health care requires appropriate management capabilities, which are not yet in place in almost all German health care institutions. They are still administrated rather than properly managed. For this reason, building IDSs will require a significant amount of time and capital resources in the future.

REFERENCES

Alexander, J. A., Lee, S.-Y. D., & Bazzoli, G. J. (2003). Governance forms in health systems and health networks. *Health Care Management Review, 28*(3), 228–242.

Amelung, V. E. (1999). Managed Care: Organisationen im Wandel – Produktdifferenzierung und Mehr-Produkt-Unternehmen [Managed care: Organizations in transition – Product differentiation and differentiated companies]. *ZfB-Ergänzungsheft, 5/99*, 51–79.

Amelung, V. E., Glied, S., & Topan, A. (2003). Health care and the labor market: Learning from the German experience. *Journal of Health Policy, Politics and Law, 28*(4), 693–714.

Amelung, V. E., & Schumacher, H. (2004). *Managed Care – Neue Wege im Gesundheitsmanagement [Managed care – New approaches to health care management]* (3rd ed). Wiesbaden: Gabler.

Aventis Pharmaceuticals (Ed.) (2003). *Managed care digest series 2000 – HMO PPO/Medicare-Medicaid digest.* Aventis Bridgewater, NJ.

Baker, G. P., Jensen, M. C., & Murphy, K. J. (1988). Compensation and incentives: Practice vs. theory. *The Journal of Finance, XLIII*(3), 592–616.

Bauer, M., & Cohen, E. (1983). The invisibility of power in economics: Beyond markets and hierarchies. In: A. Francis, J. Turk & P. Willman (Eds), *Power, efficiency and institutions – A critical appraisal of the 'markets and hierarchies' paradigm* (pp. 81–104). London: Heinemann.

Bea, J. R. (1996). Components of a vertically integrated system. In: P. Boland (Ed.), *The capitation sourcebook* (pp. 18–32). Berkeley, CA: Boland Healthcare.

Berkowitz, E. N. (1996). *Essentials of healthcare marketing.* Gaithersburg, Maryland: Aspen.

Buckley, M. P., McKenna, Q. L., & Merlino, D. J. (1999). Managed care: Past, present, future. In: J. William (Ed.), *Integrated healthcare: Lessons learned* (pp. 179–191).

Coddington, D. C., Moore, K. D., & Fischer, E. A. (1996). *Making integrated health care work.* San Francisco: Jossey-Bass.

Devers, K. J., Shortell, S. M., Anderson, D. A., Mitchell, J. B., & Erickson, K. M. (1996). Implementing organized delivery systems: An integration scorecard. In: M. Brown (Ed.), *Integrated health care delivery – Theory, practice, evaluation, and prognosis* (pp. 121–134). Gaithersburg, Maryland: Aspen.

Dietrich, M. (1993). Transaction costs and revenues. In: C. Pitelis (Ed.), *Transaction costs, markets and hierarchies* (pp. 166–187). Oxford, UK: Blackwell.

Dranove, D. (2000). *The economic evolution of American health care – From Marcus Welby to managed care.* Princeton, New Jersey: Princeton University Press.

Draper, D. A., Hurley, R. E., Lesser, C. S., & Strunk, B. C. (2002). The changing face of managed care. *Health Affairs, January/February*, 11–23.

Dubbs, N. L., Bazzoli, G. J., Shortell, S. M., & Kralovec, P. D. (2004). Reexamining organizational configurations: An update, validation, and expansion of the taxonomy of health networks and systems. *Health Services Research, 39*(1), 207–220.

Dugger, W. M. (1993). Transaction cost economics and the state. In: C. Pitelis (Ed.), *Transaction costs, markets and hierarchies* (pp. 188–216). Oxford: Basil Blackwell.

European Observatory on Health Care Systems (2000). *Health care systems in transition – Germany.*

Ford, E. W., Wells, R., & Bailey, B. (2004). Sustainable network advantages: A game theoretic approach to community-based health care coalitions. *Health Care Management Review, 29*(2), 159–169.

Frey, B. S., & Osterloh, M. (2000). Pay for performance – Immer empfehlenswert? [Pay for performance – Always recommendable?] *Zfo*, 69. Jg., H. 2, 64–69.

Friedman, L., & Goes, J. (2001). Why integrated health networks have failed. *Frontiers of Health Services Management, 17*(Summer), 3–54.

Furubotn, E., & Richter, R. (1997). *Institutions and economic theory – The contribution of new institutional economics.* Ann Arbor, MI: The University of Michigan Press.

Hart, O. (1995). *Firms, contracts, and financial structure.* New York: Oxford University Press.

Janus, K. (2003). *Managing health care in private organizations – Transaction costs, cooperation and modes of organization in the value chain.* Frankfurt: Peter Lang Publishing.

Janus, K. (2004). La legge per la "modernizzazione dell'assistenza sanitaria". Effetti di breve termine e sfide a lungo termine per gli attori del mercato dell'assisstenza sanitaria in Germania [Health Care Modernization Act. Short-term effects and long-term challenges for health care]. In: V. Atella, A. Donia Sofio, F. S. Mennini & F. Spandonaro (Eds), *Rapporto CEIS – Sanità 2004 – Sostenibilità, equità e ricerca dell'efficienza* (pp. 363–387). Rome: Italpromo Esis Publishing.

Janus, K., & Amelung, V. E. (2004a). Integrierte Versorgung im Gesundheitswesen – Anreizorientierte Vergütungssysteme für Ärzte [Integrated health care delivery – Incentive based reimbursment systems for physicians]. *zfo*, 6/2004, 73. Jg., 304–311.

Janus, K., & Amelung, V. E. (2004b). Integrierte Versorgungssysteme in Kalifornien – Erfolgs- und Mißerfolgsfaktoren der ersten 10 Jahre und Impulse für Deutschland [Integrated delivery systems in California – Ten years of experience and implications for Germany]. *Das Gesundheitswesen, 66*, 649–655.

Jaques, E. (1990). In praise of hierarchy. In: J. M. Shafritz & J. S. Ott (Eds), *Classics of organization theory* (pp. 245–263). Orlando, FL: Harcourt Brace College.

Kay, N. M. (1993). Markets, false hierarchies and the role of asset specificity. In: C. Pitelis (Ed.), *Transaction costs, markets and hierarchies* (pp. 242–261). Oxford, UK: Blackwell.

Knight, F. (1965). *Risk, uncertainty and profit.* New York: Houghton Mifflin.

Kongstvedt, P. R., Plocher, D. W., & Stanford, J. C. (2001). Integrated health care delivery systems. In: P. R. Kongstvedt (Ed.), *Essentials of managed health care* (pp. 42–71). Gaithersburg, MD: Aspen.

Mays, G. P., Claxton, G., & White, J. (2004). Managed care rebound? Recent changes in health plans' cost containment strategies. *Health Affairs Web Exclusive, W4*, 427–436.

Oberender, P., & Fleischmann, J. (2002). *Gesundheitspolitik in der Sozialen Marktwirtschaft [Health care policy in a social market economy].* Stuttgart: Lucius & Lucius.

Organization for Economic Cooperation and Development (OECD) (2004). *Total expenditure on health as a percentage* of GDP.

Orlowski, U., & Wasem, J. (2003). *Gesundheitsreform 2004 – GKV-Modernisierungsgesetz (GMG) [Health care reform 2004 – Health care modernization act].* Heidelberg: Economica Verlag.

Picot, A., Dietl, H., & Franck, E. (1997). *Organisation – Eine ökonomische Perspektive [Organization – An economic perspective].* Stuttgart: Schäffer-Poeschel.

Picot, A., Reichwald, R., & Wigand, R. T. (2001). *Die grenzenlose Unternehmung – Information, Organisation und Management [A company without boundaries – Information, organization and management].* Wiesbaden: Gabler.

Pitelis, C. (1991). *Market and non-market hierarchies – Theory of institutional failure.* Oxford, UK: Blackwell.

Reve, T. (1990). The firm as a nexus of internal and external contracts. In: M. Aoki, B. Gustafsson & O. E. Williamson (Eds), *The firm as a nexus of treaties* (pp. 133–161). Newbury Park, CA: Sage.

Riordan, M. H. (1990). What is vertical integration? In: M. Aoki, B. Gustafsson & O. E. Williamson (Eds), *The firm as a nexus of treaties* (pp. 94–111). Newbury Park, CA: Sage.

Robinson, J. C. (1999). *The corporate practice of medicine.* Berkeley, CA: University of California Press.

Robinson, J. C. (2001). Theory and practice in the design of physician payment incentives. *The Milbank Quarterly, 79*(2), 149–177.

Robinson, J. C., & Casalino, L. P. (1996). Vertical integration and organizational networks in healthcare. *Health Affairs, 15*(1), 7–22.

Scholz, C. (1997). *Strategische Organisation – Multiperspektivität und Virtualität [Strategic organization – Multiple perspectives and virtuality].* Landsberg/Lech.

Scott, W. R., Ruef, M., Mendel, P. J., & Caronna, C. A. (2000). *Institutional change and healthcare organizations – From professional dominance to managed care.* Chicago: The University of Chicago Press.

Shortell, S. M., Gillies, R. R., & Anderson, D. A. (1994). The new world of managed care: Creating organized delivery systems. *Health Affairs, 13*(5), 46–64.

Shortell, S. M., Gillies, R. R., Anderson, D. A., Erickson, K. M., & Mitchell, J. B. (2000). *Remaking health care in America – The evolution of organized delivery systems.* San Francisco: Jossey-Bass.

Stiles, R. A., Mick, S. S., & Wise, C. G. (2001). The logic of transaction cost economics in health care organization theory. *Health Care Management Review, 26*(2), 85–92.

The Institute for the Future (Ed.) (1999). *From hospital to health system: Taking a second look.* Menlo Park, CA: The Institute for the Future.

The Institute for the Future (Ed.) (2000). *Health & Healthcare 2010.* Menlo Park, CA: The Institute for the Future.

Thorpe, K. E., Florence, C. S., & Joski, P. (2004). Which medical conditions account for the rise in health care spending? *Health Affairs Web Exclusive, W4*, 437–445.

Wigand, R., Picot, A., & Reichwald, R. (1997). *Information, organization and management.* Chichester, UK: Wiley.

Williamson, O. E. (1975). *Markets and hierarchies: Analysis and antitrust implications – A study in the economics of internal organization.* New York: The Free Press.

Williamson, O. E. (1985). *The economic institutions of capitalism – Firms, markets, relational contracting.* New York: The Free Press.

Williamson, O. E. (1986). *Economic organization – Firms, markets and policy control.* New York: New York University Press.

Williamson, O. E. (1990). Chester Barnard and the incipient science of organization. In: O. E. Williamson (Ed.), *Organization theory: From Chester Barnard to the present and beyond* (pp. 172–206). New York: Oxford University Press.

Williamson, O. E. (1996). *The mechanisms of governance.* New York: Oxford University Press.

Williamson, O. E., & Masten, S. E. (1999). Introduction. In: O. E. Williamson & S. E. Masten (Eds), *The Economics of Transaction Costs* (pp. IX–XXII). Cheltenham UK: Edward Elgar.

Zelman, W. A. (1996). *The changing health care marketplace – Private ventures, public interests.* San Francisco: Jossey-Bass.

APPENDIX A

Assessment of Asset Specificity with Respect to Health Care Transactions

Asset specificity is considered the most important issue with respect to the determination of the mode of governance. It is defined as the specialization of assets with respect to use or users (Kay, 1993) and has reference to the degree to which an asset can be redeployed to alternative uses and by alternative users without sacrifice of productive value (Williamson, 1990, 1996; Williamson & Masten, 1999).

When asset specificity and uncertainty is low, and transactions are relatively frequent, transactions will be governed by market organizations. High asset specificity and uncertainty will produce transactional difficulties, which lead transactions to be internalized within the firm. There exists a large degree of uncertainty at each stage of health care delivery. This refers to both general uncertainty (risk) and uncertainty in the form of information asymmetry caused by principal agent relations. In addition, the frequency of health care transactions is difficult to assess as the occurrence of illness is insecure, there usually is a time lag between the financing and the provision of health care, and there typically passes some time between the actual provision of care and the effects. Finally, the following *categories* of asset specificity elucidate the degree of asset specificity of health care transactions:

Site specificity (resource immobility) with respect to health care applies to hospitals and other material assets. These assets cannot be easily redeployed and often serve as a central hub for a health system. In addition, site specificity can be caused by a fundamental transformation, which holds that a large-numbers bidding condition may be transformed into a small-numbers situation, where winners enjoy advantages over non-winners due to significant investments in durable transaction-specific assets (Williamson, 1985). This can be the case in a health network when high transaction-specific investments are made by one or some affiliates while the others have access to these investments, but have no financial stake in them. However, it has to be pointed out that the shift from inpatient to outpatient and ambulatory care settings has already and will continue to diminish this type of asset specificity. In addition, the advances in technologies, in particular telemedicine will further reduce site specificity.

Physical asset specificity (technological advantages) is high in health care in particular with respect to huge investments in medical technology.

Human asset specificity (know-how-advantages) is a critical if not the most decisive issue in health care. As the provision of health care services is people-intensive and requires highly specialized and well-trained individuals, human asset specificity can be considered to be high in health care. Know-how, experience, organizational routines, and culture play an important role in this respect (Reve, 1990).

Dedicated asset specificity (specialized investments) applies to some health systems or networks that invest in, for example, expanding their capacities for heart surgery by adding another operation room because of a high-volume (and maybe exclusive) contract with a HMO for heart surgery services.

The *specificity of brand name capital* in health care delivery is high and plays an important role because the inability of health care consumers to assess the quality of health care services due to insufficient or distorted information results in taking recourse to immaterial concepts such as reputation or brand identity. As it takes time to build a reputation or a brand identity, these assets cannot be easily redeployed.

Temporal specificity, which can be thought of as a type of site specificity in which timely responsiveness by on-site human assets is vital, is characteristic for health care provision. Emergency room services and other acute care services serve as an example.

It can be derived from the preceding that health care transactions are in general of high asset specificity. On the one hand, the emergence of new technologies and standardization of care by implementing best practices and guidelines will reduce asset specificity in the future. On the other hand, increased customization (tailoring care to the individual patient) of health care services involves increased specificity. Patient needs are idiosyncratic because no two patients are alike (Dranove, 2000). Each transaction has therefore important elements of uniqueness.

APPENDIX B

Details on the Bay Area Case Study (selected question and answers as an example for the results).

Question: Do You Apply Focal or Decentralized Coordination or Both?

Grouped answers:

Focal	Decentralized	Both
17.9%	32.1%	50%

Additional Comments (Grouped)
Referring to business strategy:

• Focal (this is important in turnaround times) ⇒ but move to decentralized structure in a couple of years.

- Centralization was important for the turnaround ⇒ decentralization is important in a growth face.
- Has become more centralized with the creation of this department ⇒ function as a hub.
- It is a decentralized organization; however, it is moving incrementally toward a more centralized one (in order to take advantage of the opportunities of the system).
- Moving from autonomy to collective action ⇒ pool talent and work together (IT facilitated this process).
- Move to integration with respect to products ⇒ make clear that standardization does not mean centralization (it just means process standardization in all organizations).

Change of focus:

- We are still centralized, but trying to decentralize.
- Power (money) is getting more centralized.
- It has been very centralized, but we are migrating ⇒ it is getting more decentralized.
- It was focal and is now decentralized.

Reasons for employing both ways of coordination:

- Think globally, act locally.
- Claims and accounting needs to be centralized; network management needs to be decentralized.
- Both (hospitals are more accountable now).
- The system sets objectives and the overall strategic direction, but leaves room for flexibility (local).
- Goals are set centrally and executed locally at individual units.
- Example: the whole IT initiative is driven regionally, but implemented locally.
- Created a situation of dynamic tension (80% decentralized; 20% centralized), because health care is local.
- Each board has obligations, but system has also obligations (two-way interaction and communication).
- "de-layer" management organization and decentralize several administrative functions ⇒ more local control.
- Objective: "tight–loose–tight" organization ⇒ the top defines the goals (tight) and passes them down to boards (loose); corporate then controls the results (tight).
- It is centrally at the one hand and therefore pretty hierarchical, but it is also very local and therefore market-orientated.

- Very market-driven from an affiliate standpoint ⇒ each affiliate can react; from system perspective ⇒ shape what the market is (e.g., every health plan has to pay the same rates, no cross-subsidizing ⇒ this is unique).
- Be a holding and an operating company.
- It is both at the same time, although it is not a mixture of the two.

POLICY

WICKED HEALTH CARE ISSUES: AN ANALYSIS OF FINNISH AND SWEDISH HEALTH CARE REFORMS

Pirkko Vartiainen

ABSTRACT

Health care organizations function in multidimensional environments, and their organizational cultures are complex and demanding. Expectations for health care services are high: patients want the most effective and newest possible treatments, politicians demand accountable service production, and health care professionals require motivating and challenging work environments. All these goals and objectives, for example, can be at the root of wicked problems in health care management. Thus, this chapter aims to explore the wickedness of health care management through an analysis of Finnish and Swedish health care reforms. The aim of these reforms is to solve the problems encountered in health care systems and organizations. The concept of a 'wicked issue' can shortly be described as a problem that is difficult to identify and solve. The reasoning behind using the concept of wicked issue as a method for analysis here is the hypothesis that the concept helps to explain and understand the social complexity involved in health care management.

International Health Care Management
Advances in Health Care Management, Volume 5, 159–182
Copyright © 2005 by Elsevier Ltd.
All rights of reproduction in any form reserved
ISSN: 1474-8231/doi:10.1016/S1474-8231(05)05006-8

Health care has been the target of management reforms in most Western European countries since the early 1980s. Most reforms have been aimed at effectiveness, enhancing quality, raising the level of management skills of health care professionals, and allowing patients greater freedom of choice. Thus, the reforms implemented in health care have been wide, many-sided and complex, and they have also overlapped each other. However, analytical discussions concerning the characteristics of the problems that these reforms aim to resolve are rare. We do know that the reforms are targeted at solving a certain problem, but it seems that the whole complexity of the problem cannot be identified.

The main objective of this study is to analyze the current status of public health care management reforms in Finland and Sweden through the lens of the concept of wicked issues. The study has two targets: to define what is meant by wicked issue, and to analyze the characteristics of health care reforms as wicked issues. The reason for choosing the concept of wicked issues as the framework for this study is the hypothesis that most serious health care management problems are wicked problems. Thus, the concept helps to describe and explain the social complexity involved in health care management. It is also assumed that the analysis of health care problems as wicked problems leads to a better understanding of health care management systems as well as to new policy making and decision-making processes. The study aims to explore how health care management deals with system-wide problems, and what kinds of solutions, or even new styles of governing, have been introduced to solve these problems in Finland and Sweden. Some of the more interesting management reform objectives discussed in this chapter are the improvement of efficiency and effectiveness, decentralization, improving access to care, quality enhancement, and patients' freedom of choice.

The main understanding of the term *wicked issue* in this study follows the definition of Clarke and Stewart (2003, p. 274), who emphasize the basic wickedness of most problems to be ones "for which there is no obvious or easily found solution." The creators of the concept, Rittel and Webber (1973, p. 160), clarify the term as follows:

> We are calling them "wicked" not because these properties are themselves deplorable. We use the term "wicked" in a meaning akin to that of "malignant" (in contrast to "benign") or "vicious" (like a circle) or "tricky" (like a leprechaun) or "aggressive" (like a lion, in contrast to the docility of a lamb).

It is necessary to separate wicked problems from tame problems. A tame problem is a problem that can be solved with straightforward and well-known problem solving. For example, suppose that you are well aware of the dosage of a certain medicine for a child, but your patient is an adult. By following the dosage requirements, you can change the dosage so that it is adequate for an adult. This is solving a tame problem. It follows, then, that an instruction or formula can always be found for tame problems.

The discussion of wicked versus tame problems leads us to the area of complexity theory. In the literature on complexity many different definitions of problem situations are found. A discussion of these situations gives the possibility for a better understanding the problem of complex systems.

Rosenhead and Mingers (2002, pp. 4–6) classify different dichotomies of problem situations by referring to the literature of complexity theory. Ackoff (1979, 1981) differentiates different kinds of problems as either 'messes' or 'problems.' A mess is a dynamic situation where system entities and their problems are changing and connected to each other. The mess creates abstract problems that can be identified; however, messes cannot be rectified by solving a single identified problem. According to Ackoff, messes need to be managed, not solved. In many ways messes share similar characteristics with wicked issues. They are problems that are parts of complex systems and their dynamics.

Schon (1987) describes these problem situations with the dichotomy of 'swamp' versus 'high ground.' According to Schon, problems that are considered high ground are very often unimportant to the system members. Still these problems inspire organization members and managers to find great technical solutions that help to solve high ground problems. On the other hand, problems that are defined as 'swamp' are often of greatest interest to the system and their members. The fact, however, is that the solving of swamp problems very often does not allow managers to find brilliant technical solutions. Instead, they have to "wade in a swamp" when managing these complex situations.

According to Ravetz (1971), problematic situations can be classified as either practical or technical. Technical problems have similar characteristics to high ground problems, and their solutions are also similar; that is, clear technical solutions. The solution of practical problems needs an intimate knowledge of the situation, which means that problems cannot be solved through a specification of optimal means, but by argumentation and discussion, which lead to alternative problem-solving methods suited to the situation.

Checkland's analysis (1981, 1985) concerning the problems of complex systems is quite similar to Ravetz. Checkland talks about soft versus hard systems thinking. According to hard systems thinking, the world consists of systems that can be objectively modeled and the problems which appear can be solved via specific and undeniable problem-solving methods. Soft systems thinking argues that a complex system cannot be modeled or optimized. Instead, complex problem-solving situations should be used as a method of learning. This means that the discussions in problematic situations have to consider the problem itself more than the potential solution.

The above discussion shows how versatile and widely deliberated the problems of complex systems are. The common denominator for all the above mentioned problem situations is the emphasis on the complexity of systems, and the dynamic situations where these problems occur. The problem-solving processes and methods of complex systems are multidimensional. All of them, however, share the idea that wicked problems or messes, for example, cannot be solved through technical solutions, but through careful discussions and argumentation.

Now that the concept of wicked issues has been defined, I shall shortly describe the Swedish and Finnish health care systems and the main reforms which have been implemented there. Then, I will go deeper into the analysis of wicked issues in health care.

HEALTH CARE IN FINLAND AND SWEDEN

Finnish Health Care

The municipalities have the main responsibility to provide health care services in *Finland*. This means that health services are financed primarily with public monies. In 2001, ~43% of total health care costs were financed by the municipalities, roughly 17% by the state, 16% by the National Health Insurance, and the remaining 24% with private sources. (Stakes, 2003).

The Ministry of Social Affairs and Health is mostly responsible for health care policy at the national level. The Ministry of Social Affairs and Health, together with several agencies and institutions, defines and prepares all health care reforms, makes proposals for legislation, evaluates their implementation, and assists the government in decision-making. In the municipalities, the municipal council, the executive board, and committees are the main decision-making bodies in the health care sector. These bodies are working in a position of trust, and are politically accountable to all members of the municipality. The decision-making process varies among municipalities. However, during recent years, there has been a significant trend toward decentralization. This means that municipal councils have allocated their power to the committees and leading officials (Järvelin, 2002).

Between national and municipal decision-making, there are also five provinces that have an official role in the Finnish health care system. The provincial state offices are administrative bodies, which promote the objectives of national and regional administration in their area. Every provincial state office has many departments, one of which is the social and health department.

Health care service provision is taken care of in the 20 hospital districts, each with several hospitals. Every hospital district provides specialized medical care and coordinates the public specialized care in its area. Primary health care is implemented through health centers. A health center is an organization that provides primary curative, preventive, and public health services in its own area. The health center system was established in 1972. At the moment, there are ~270 health centers in Finland, and all of them are owned by one or by several municipalities (Järvelin, 2002).

Swedish Health Care

The *Swedish* health care system functions at three different levels: national, regional, and local. The regional level, through the county councils, forms the basis of the health care system in Sweden, together with the central government (Hjortsberg & Ghatnekar, 2001). The Ministry of Health and Social Affairs is the leading health care organization at the national level. The Ministry, for example, plans and steers health care policy, and allocates financial assistance on special occasions. At the national level, there are eight central administrative agencies in the health care sector. One of them is the National Board of Health and Welfare, which is a supervision organization, and one of its most important tasks is to evaluate health service provision. All these agencies function under the Ministry of Health and Social Affairs.

In Sweden, the responsibility of health care service provision, from primary care to hospital care, is in the hands of the independent regional county councils. The members of the councils are selected through democratic elections. The county councils' possibility to take care of welfare service production depends on taxation. Councils have the right to levy proportional income tax in their own area. The county taxes form the biggest part of the councils' financial resources (66% in 1999), the rest of the financing comes from the state budget, fees, and other sources (Hjortsberg & Ghatnekar, 2001). All together, 21 county councils are grouped into six medical care regions. In these regions, there are nine regional hospitals, 70 county/district county hospitals, and ~950 health centers.

Municipal health care service provision is limited to school health care, environmental hygiene, care of the elderly, the disabled, and long-term psychiatric patients. However, the municipalities operate public nursing homes and provide home care for elderly and disabled people.

Comparative Analysis

When comparing the Finnish and Swedish health care systems, the main difference is the organizational level of health service provision. In Finland, the municipalities, with the right to levy income taxes, take care of both of primary and specialized care. In Sweden, health service production is implemented at the regional level through county councils. The most conspicuous similarity is the financial ground of service provision: in both countries, health care services are mainly financed via public money. The public health care system takes care of the whole population in both countries, and the private health care market is still a minor player in both Sweden and Finland.

HEALTH CARE REFORMS IN FINLAND AND SWEDEN

The Swedish health care system experienced meaningful changes during the 1980s and 1990s, both at the national and regional levels. Ideologically, the reforms have been based on different ideas. Equity was the main concern of reforms in the 1970s, while the reforms conducted in the late 1980s and 1990s mainly emphasize financial issues, effectiveness, and efficiency.

Ideologically, Finnish health care has been developed through the same principles as Swedish health care. Equality has been the main ideology, meaning that all people living in Finland have equal rights to health care regardless of their social status, wealth, or geographical place of residence. This view was strengthened through legislation, especially through the Primary Health Care Act in 1972. The health care reforms discussed in the study are briefly presented in Table 1.

Table 1. A Selective Comparison of Health Care Reforms in Finland and Sweden.

Reform Objective	Finland	Sweden
Efficiency	• Management by objectives • Changes in resource allocation • Co-operation between health care organizations	• Management by objectives • Purchaser–provider split • Contracting
Decentralization	• Changes in the state subsidy process • Reducing state regulation • Changes in coordination responsibilities	• Seven crown reform • Dagmar reform • Ädel reform
Quality	• Principles of TQM • Guidelines of quality assurance	• Principles of TQM • Patient-focused initiatives
Patients' freedom of choice	• Law for patients' status and rights • Government Resolution of the Health 2015 programme	• Different processes that strengthen patients' freedom to choose their health care provider
Improving the access to care	• These reforms are closely connected to the other mentioned reforms • Personal doctor system • "Personal responsibility" reform	• These reforms are closely connected to the other mentioned reforms • A national guarantee for Treatment

Efficiency Reforms

In both countries, the improvement of efficiency and effectiveness has been the main target of health care reforms since the 1980s. A concern for greater efficiency has mainly gone along the premise of Performance Management and Management by Objectives, even if the measures taken in the two countries are partly divergent. Efficiency measurements have often neglected the specific character of health care organizations. Available measurements, nevertheless, show that there are problems connected to organizational efficiency in health care organizations.

The discussion of high costs and low productivity in *Swedish* health care organizations was strengthened during the late 1980s and 1990s. These discussions led to management reforms in which the provider functions were separated from the purchasing functions. The management reforms also included need-based resource allocation, total cost responsibility in direct patient departments, and transfer pricing systems.

Bergman (1998) calls the development mentioned above the concept of "purchaser–provider split" and that was the main reform during the 1990s. The purchasing organizations are situated in the county councils, but the models of purchasing vary between different councils. Some of the councils prefer the large central county council purchasing organizations while others prefer district level organizations. Some of the purchaser–provider split models are also more market and competition oriented than others. However, there are two main principles that are followed in every county council. They are as follows:

• the separation between purchaser and provider, with some sort of contract between them; and
• the provider is paid by the district where the patient lives, the money follows the patient, and is related to a specific output or performance (Bergman, 1998).

Effectiveness and efficiency have also been the main development trends in the *Finnish* health care sector, partly because of the strong economical depression at the beginning of the 1990s. The economic recession affected great changes in the health care financing system. The state reduced public expenditure in all welfare sectors, and also health care resources were gradually cut. Other reasons for the lively discussion of health care effectiveness and efficiency are the comprehension that health care systems function ineffectively, and the co-operation between different health care organizations functions badly. These lacks in co-operation lead to a situation where patients are unnecessarily treated in hospitals instead of health care centers or nursing homes, for example (Järvelin, 2002).

Decentralization Reforms

Decentralization reforms are reforms that, at the macro-level, focus on reducing detailed legislation and control and simplifying the planning processes of health care systems. At the micro-level, decentralization moves authority downwards to frontline managers and even to personnel. One example of macro-level decentralization is the Finnish state subsidies reform of 1993, which increased the municipalities' authority and responsibility to reorganize and finance health care. One of the first decentralization reforms in Sweden was in the 1980s, when the county councils introduced their global budgets. This led to a situation were districts became responsible for resource allocation within their geographical area, and the central county councils managed the districts by allocating the budget among the districts (WHO, 1996). However, it is worth noticing that the wide decentralization actions carried out in the 1990s in selected countries have also created problems; for example, the structural incoherence of health care systems and coordination problems in management.

The large decentralization reform in *Sweden* in the 1970s changed the structures of health systems radically, when the responsibility was transferred from the state to the county councils. With the so-called Seven Crowns Reform of 1970, privately provided outpatient services at county council hospitals were taken over by the county councils (WHO, 1996). At the same time, county councils hired the persons working in the above mentioned outpatient service organizations. The status of county councils was further strengthened with the 1982 Health Care Act, when both financial responsibility and resource allocation were given to the county councils.

The next remarkable reform was the "Dagmar Reform" in 1985 that aimed at confirming the county councils' planning processes. The reform was intended to strengthen the county councils' authority by stabilizing their planning possibilities over ambulatory care visits to physicians and changed the financial systems of private ambulatory providers (WHO, 1996). Through this reform, the county councils' control over private establishments was strengthened, and the council's became regulators of the private health care market.

In the beginning of the 1990s, the Swedish health care system was again changed structurally. The 1992 Ädel reform moved the responsibility for long-term health care and social welfare services to the disabled and the elderly from the county council to the local municipalities (WHO, 1996). The aim of this reform was to concentrate the planning and financing of long-term care in the municipalities. In addition, the reform was aimed at increasing the efficiency of the "flow of care chain": to move elderly people that were not in need of hospital care from acute hospital care to their homes or to nursing homes.

The *Finnish* state subsidy reform in 1993 reduced state regulation of health care provision. The reform aimed at decentralization by giving more decision-making power to local authorities. It also aimed at better coordination of the functions of primary and secondary care, and gave attention to more effective health care production. However, the main changes of the reform were focused on the financing of health care. From 1993 to 1997, the state subsidies were calculated on the basis of the age structure of the population, morbidity, population density, and land area. In 1997, the subsidy system was changed, and at the moment the following criteria are used: the number of inhabitants, age structure, and morbidity. There are also additional criteria for remote areas and archipelago municipalities. The changes were remarkable, because the former state subsidy system was based on actual costs, but also on the principle that more wealthy municipalities got fewer subsidies than poor municipalities.

Quality Reforms

Quality enhancement reforms are connected to the total quality management (TQM) and continuous quality improvement (CQI) reforms implemented in the Finnish and Swedish health care systems. The general rules addressing quality systems in health care were formulated in *Sweden* in 1997. The reform continued the developments of the early 1990s by strengthening the patient-focused initiatives in health care (Hjortsberg & Ghatnekar, 2001). In *Finland*, there have been efforts concerning the quality assurance of health care. In 1995 and 1999, the Ministry of Social Affairs and Health, together with the National Research and Development Centre for Welfare and Health, as well as the Association for Finnish Local and Regional Authorities, published the guidelines on quality assurance in social welfare and health care. The guidelines concentrate on the promotion of quality as a part of daily work. They emphasize patient-orientation in service production, the use and strengthening of knowledge as a basic element of quality work, and evaluation as a part of development. On the grounds of these guidelines, quality assurance work has continued, and many separate service sectors and organizations have created their own, special quality programs.

Patients' Freedom of Choice

Patients' freedom to choose their health care service provider, hospital, doctor, etc. is an emerging theme in all Nordic health care systems. For instance, in some *Swedish* provinces, patients' rights to choose their physician are considerably larger than ever before. Patients' freedom to choose their health care provider is included in every county councils' purchaser–provider model. Patients have the freedom to choose among first-contact care providers; they can also choose between a primary health center and a hospital outpatient department. Even private physicians have a role in this, ever since the freedom of choice was introduced along with the introduction of vouchers. In Sweden, patients also have the right to choose private physicians or clinics for their first-contact care. However, in these cases the fees are subsidized only partially by the public sector (Saltman, 1998).

Finland is the first country in Europe which regulated a law for patients' status and rights in 1993. The law was mainly targeted to improve patients' possibilities to get information about their treatment and medical documents. The autonomy or the right to determine one's own affairs, also in questions of health care, was also strengthened.

The possibility to choose one's own doctor or hospital is much weaker in Finland than in Sweden. The general principle, at the moment, is that patients cannot choose the hospital or the doctor. However, the newest reform – the Government Resolution on the Health 2015 public health programme (2001) – also stresses patients' rights and possibilities to choose. The reform decreases the differences between patients' access to care by introducing criteria for access to non-urgent treatments in the country. If health care institutions maintained by the local authority or federation of municipalities cannot fulfill the criteria, treatment must be procured from another service provider at no extra charge to the patient (MSAH, 2002).

Improving Access to Care

The reforms directed to improve access to care are closely connected to the other reforms mentioned above. In Sweden, reforms aiming at improved access to care are linked to the projects dealing with effectiveness and efficiency, and in Finland to the structural changes of health care systems. The meaning of the term 'access to care' is convergent in both Nordic countries. The term refers to interventions that are taken to secure patients' possibilities to get treatment. In both countries, the reforms try to cut down existing patient queues and keep waiting times at an acceptable level. A National Guarantee of Treatment for patients was launched in *Sweden* already in 1992, with the main focus on patients' waiting times for hospital treatments—it was 3 months at the most, otherwise the hospital had to give the patient the possibility to get treatment from another hospital. The reform did not succeed very well and the guarantee was revised in 1996. The revisions made in 1997 and 1999 regulated accessibility in both primary and specialized care (Hjortsberg & Ghatnekar, 2001).

Long waiting times for care have also been a constant problem in *Finnish* health care. In the 1980s, waiting times for health center doctors, for

example, could be 2–6 weeks for non-urgent cases. Both patients and doctors were unsatisfied with the situation. The reform called the "personal
doctor system" was therefore launched during the late 1980s and early 1990s
in many municipalities. The aim of the reform was to ease patients' access to
care so that they could see their own doctor within 3 days. The results of the
project were quite good; waiting times were shortened, and patient satisfaction with the services improved. The main problem with the system was
that many small and poor municipalities could not implement the system at
all. Also, the lack of doctors in many municipalities led to the situation
where the personal doctor system could not work in practice. However, the
results of the reform led to a further development: the reform created on the
grounds of personal doctor reform is called "personal responsibility." This
concept means that doctors and nurses form a team that has the responsibility for the care of persons living in a specified area. In practice, however,
the personal responsibility system functions inconsistently in the different
parts of the country (Järvelin, 2002).

Comparative Analysis

The main characteristic of Finnish health care reforms is the fact that they are
more a chain of different incremental reforms rather than an entirety of
reforms. That is why it is difficult to form a systematic picture of the content
of these reforms. However, it can be stated that structural changes in Finnish
health care systems and organizations have been minor during recent years.
The remarkable changes in financial and decision-making levels, for example,
did not change the responsibility of the provision for health care services. The
responsibility was further shifted to local authorities. On the contrary, the
Swedish health care system has met radical structural changes in recent history. These changes have mostly been made at the organizational and production levels. Changes at the financial level have been minor, and the
Swedish health care system is still mainly financed with public money.

THE WICKEDNESS OF FINNISH AND SWEDISH
HEALTH CARE MANAGEMENT

Circularity

The elemental characteristic of wicked issues is their circularity. Circularity
has two meanings: (a) there is no definitive formulation of a wicked issue,

and (b) wicked problems have a 'no-stopping rule'. Rittel and Webber (1973, p. 161) put it as follows: "the information needed to *understand* the problem depends upon one's idea for *solving* it." Each attempt to create a solution changes the understanding of the problem. Thus, since it is quite difficult to define the problem exactly, it is also difficult to determine when it is actually resolved. To solve a wicked issue is a complicated situation: usually there are many alternative solutions. All potential alternatives may be useful, but some are better than others. The difficulty is that we never know whether the chosen solution is good enough when compared to the stakeholders' needs. Different stakeholders can even compete with one another to confirm their views as a basis of problem solving.

This circularity phenomenon links the discussion of wicked issues to complexity theory. What, then, is complexity? The definition of the complexity concept is difficult because "complexity" carries individual interpretations. For example, some situations may seem complex in the eyes of some individuals but simple in the eyes of someone else. Heylighen also (1996) stresses that the content of the complexity concept depends on the language that is used to model the system and its problems.

Heylighen (1996) searches for an explanation for complexity by going back to the original Latin word *complexus*, which signifies "entwined" or "twisted together." This signification means that some issue or situation can be defined as complex if two or more elements are combined to each other so that it is difficult to separate them. In health care reforms, both the systems that are the target of reforms, and the reforms themselves are often linked together. Thus, they both include elements that fulfill the characteristics of complexity.

The preceding definition of complexity clearly refers to the dichotomy. Phenomena that are linked together are simultaneously distinct and interconnected. Under these circumstances, it can be assumed that when a system is composed of many separate elements, the complexity of the system is greater, and more connections between these elements can be found. In practice, this means that complex systems are hard to model, and that potential models cannot easily be used as methods for problem solving.

So, distinction and connection seem to be important elements of complexity. Heylighen (1996) argues that both distinction and connection are needed in complexity. Distinction refers to heterogeneity; that is, to the fact that separate system entities behave differently. However, too powerful distinctions can lead to chaos. As an example, operations (i.e. surgical procedures) in health care have a certain order that lead to the best possible result. If this order is somehow disturbed (i.e. the different health care teams are not co-operating well enough) the whole operation can end in disaster. Connection, on the other hand, refers to the constraint that the different parts of the system are not independent. When this fact about dependency is admitted, the units of an organization can minimize the risks of chaos. Thus, connection can lead to better co-operation between the different systems or units of an organization.

When analyzing Finnish and Swedish health care reforms against the discussion in this chapter, it can be stated that the reforms fulfill many of the elements of complexity. One example of these is circularity. The reforms follow each other, and new reforms are created based on the elements of the previous reforms. Actually, the implemented reforms often do not resolve the targeted health care problems. The guarantee for care and the personal doctor system, for example, have not been able to significantly shorten the long waiting times for care. What is the reason for this? Perhaps one reason is that the reforms have been implemented without knowing the real reason for long waiting times. Another reason may be the fact that long waiting times may be a symptom of problems that have not been taken into consideration when creating the reforms. These multiple symptoms are, for example, the lack of doctors or the lack of financial resources, or even the lack of political willingness to really solve the waiting time problems. However, it is obvious that different wicked problems are linked to each other, and they have the tendency to change over time, especially when dealing with complex social systems such as health care systems.

Stakeholder Involvement

According to Clarke and Stewart (2003, p. 275) wicked issues can be resolved by "working through people." The changes cannot be made only via legislation. "The wicked issues are likely only to be resolved by a style of governing, which learns from people and works with people" (*ibid.*, p. 275). When adapted to health care management, the statements could mean that resolving wicked issues of health care depends on establishing a participatory management framework: a framework that emphasizes holistic thinking and the capacity to co-operate with other organizations, professionals, and stakeholders (Vartiainen, 2003, 2004).

Finnish and Swedish health care reforms have placed emphasis on stakeholder participation to some degree. The need for democratic decision-making, for example, stresses patients' rights to be involved in decisions about their treatment. This statement is widely known in health care systems as a patient's autonomy statement. Reforms aiming at patient participation have not been as successful as expected. The strong hierarchical and partly authoritative culture in health care organizations, for example, do not encourage stakeholders to participate in the decision-making processes very well.

The implemented reforms have also aimed at strengthening co-operation between different organizations dealing with health care questions. The results of these reforms have been variable. Co-operation among different organizations has increased, but the coordination of co-operative functions still demands improvement. It seems that the better promoter for stronger co-operation has been the lack of resources rather than all the implemented reforms. Hospital districts in Finland, for example, have created new ways of working together in recent years more than ever before. The reason for this has been the fact that hospital districts have noticed that they cannot "manage alone." This has led to a situation where some hospital districts have decided to work together by providing services for each other. This mutual co-operation is often based on the idea of specialization: hospitals that have specialized know-how over some (often very costly) treatments offer these treatments to their partners and vice versa. In practice, this means that publicly financed hospitals have started to function more and more with market-based ideas.

When thinking of the reforms as a way of solving health care problems, it can be stated that stakeholder participation in the planning and implementation of these reforms has varied. The planning process of national level reforms often considers stakeholder participation, and reforms are discussed and analyzed by different organizations both from the public and third sectors. However, the implementation of the reforms often neglects the aspect of participation. The requirement of solving wicked issues, the idea of "learning from people and working with people," is thus only partially carried out.

Problem-Solving Processes

Rittel and Webber stress that tame problems are the opposite of wicked problems. The difference between wicked and tame problems is the process of solution. Tame problems can be solved via traditional methods and processes. Conklin and Weil (2003, p. 2) call these solutions 'waterfalls.' The waterfall method "predicts that the best way to work on a problem is to follow an orderly and linear process, working from the problem to the solution." This kind of problem solving does not function in the context of wicked issues, even if the traditional methods emphasize that the following of a linear process is the best way of working with the questions of complex problems and complex organizations.

The problem-solving processes of complex organizations require nonlinear methods. Complex Adaptive Systems theory analyses nonlinear methods and the situations where this kind of problem solving is needed. According to Rihani (2002) Complex Adaptive Systems can be described with three types of behavior: order, chaos, and self-organized complexity. The literature of complexity uses several different metaphors to sketch these types, but the Kauffman (1996) illustration of water in a bathtub is probably the most well known. When the tap and plughole are closed, the water in the bathtub is in constant order. However, when the tap is opened, the water is in chaotic movement, and it is difficult to specify how the water behaves in this chaotic order. The self-organized complexity appears as the well-known vortex, when the tap is closed and the plug is removed from the plughole. In health care, this kind of metaphor can be applied to the function of a first-aid clinic. When the situation in the clinic is steady, the functions in the clinic seem to happen in an observable order, but when a big accident occurs, the functions in the clinic become chaotic. It is almost impossible to analyze how and in which order the teams in the clinic will function. However, the crisis starts a process that can be compared to the metaphor of self-organizing complexity. Both order and chaos are present in the state of emergency, but the teams in the first-aid clinic know how to function in crisis – the teams very quickly organize themselves.

When analyzing Finnish and Swedish health care reforms, it is apparent that many of the problems that the reforms aim to solve are treated as tame. This means that the health care problems are thought to be separate issues that can be solved through separate solutions. It is thought that long waiting times for treatments can be solved by increasing the number of medical students. However, the actual reason for the difficulty to get doctors to health care centers, for example, may be the high stress levels among health center personnel, busy schedules, and few possibilities to concentrate on research and further education. The example shows that the problem that on the surface seems to be tame is actually wicked, and deep analysis is needed to understand the many-sided facets behind this single problem.

It is apparent that partial and linear thinking dominates in most Finnish and Swedish health care organizations. The organizations are hierarchical and the authority of the leading professionals (especially doctors) as well as leading administrators and politicians is high. This fact complicates the resolution of wicked problems. A strong authoritative culture in an organization may effect problem solving so that wicked problems are treated as tame problems (Roberts, 2000). This means that some powerful stakeholders are chosen to conduct a linear and partial problem-solving process: to define, analyze, and solve the problem. Because of the wickedness of the problem, the implemented solution does not work very well.

Due to the complexity of health care as a professional and social system, political and professional leaders, and even researchers, do not have a clear picture concerning different wicked health care problems in Finland and Sweden. That is why the problem-solving mechanisms have remained traditional: officials and political decision makers (parliament, ministries, and communal politicians) have created improvement reforms one after another by thinking that the linear implementation of reform projects could solve potential health care problems. This custom has led to excessive reforms, which do not have any stopping rules, new improvement reforms, which overlap each other, and the result of previous projects are hardly analyzed when new and different projects are created.

The problem-solving process in the case of wicked issues should be more flexible than an orderly and linear process. Conklin and Weil (2003) prefer a process that resembles a seismograph or fountain. The "fountain model" begins with an analysis that gives an understanding of the problem, and moves to the formulation of a potential solution right after analysis. During the process it is possible, and even necessary, to move back to the stage of analysis to deepen one's understanding of the problem. Thus, the significant characteristic of problem solving in the case of wicked issues is its qualitative nature. Problems are solved through discussions, consensus, iterations, and accepting change as a normal part of the process (Article on Wicked Problem, 2003). During the formulation of potential solutions we can learn about both the problem and the solution.

Implications

Wicked issues in Finnish and Swedish health care reforms are real. Still, the consciousness of the characteristics and contents of wicked problems is quite low. Traditional thinking dominates the planning and implementation of reforms, and wicked problems are often treated as tame problems.

One reason for the uncertainty surrounding the characteristics and contents of wicked problems seems to be the lack of analysis concerning complex health care systems and their problems. However, this chapter shows quite clearly that wicked problems are a natural part of complexity although it is not always easy to recognize a problem as wicked. The recognition is difficult because health care problems are twisted together and problems that seem to be individual are seldom totally separate from the whole of the health care system. Finnish and Swedish health care systems are, however, used to solving a web of problems as if they were independent from each other and from the system. For example, the reforms analyzed in this chapter mostly deal with health care problems as separate issues. However, it would be more fruitful to plan and implement the reform targets and objectives by considering the web of health care problems in its entirety.

Another reason for the scantiness of analysis of complexity may be that decision makers, researchers, and politicians have not admitted the difficulty of modeling these complex systems. The analyses have mainly remained at the level of description. Besides abstract health care problems, for example, the lack of leadership has been treated as a tame problem.

It may also be so that the linear problem-solving method is considered as the best one from the policy-making point of view. Policy making often seeks quick solutions and quick results. That is why there may not be the possibility or time for nonlinear problem-solving processes that need much more time, discussions, and argumentation.

Therefore, it seems that some of the shortcomings in Finnish and Swedish health care reforms occur because reform planning and implementation have failed to address the obvious wickedness of the problems the reforms are aimed at eliminating.

PROPOSALS FOR IMPROVING HEALTH CARE REFORMS

What should be done to avoid the shortcomings mentioned above? The discussion below will analyze some general proposals brought forward in the literature about wicked issues in light of the Finnish and Swedish health care reforms.

Distinguish Wicked Problems from Tame Problems

It was noted earlier in this chapter that health care problems are often treated as tame problems. Thus, the problem-solving processes often lean toward simplifications, which ultimately means that the problem-solving alternatives are based on a superficial knowledge of the subject and context of the problem. This is partly because different stakeholders understand the problems differently.

One example of this is medical education and training in Finland. Different stakeholders have taken different attitudes toward the question of how many medical students Finland needs during different periods of time. Very often, for example, the decision makers in the municipalities and the Finnish Medical Association have had different views on this question. In the beginning of the 1990s there appeared to be some extent of unemployment in the medical profession. From this it followed that the Finnish Medical Association, for example, firmly worked toward a reduction in the number of medical students in universities. Discussions between different stakeholders then lead to the reduction of students in universities. However, after a few years, the Finnish health care system found itself in the situation of a lack of doctors. In many regions in Finland, there is now a huge need for qualified doctors in both primary and special health care. And this situation is becoming even more difficult due to the retirement of doctors. It is estimated that by the end of 2015, ~30% of doctors who are presently employed will be retired. Thus, the discussion to increase the number of medical students in universities has begun. Actually, the Ministry of Education decided some years ago to start a new education system for doctors by opening up a so-called "emergency education for doctors." This means that one Finnish university trains health care professionals with a polytechnic education background to become doctors. The assumption is that these persons can be qualified as doctors due to their earlier professional skills in a shorter time than students without previous education or work experience.

This example shows quite clearly how the question of the number of future doctors has been handled. At the national level, the question has been treated as a tame problem, and the solutions at a given time have been simple: increase or decrease the number of medical students in the universities. However, as it was earlier mentioned, the reason for today's lack of doctors is not only about the number of doctors. The reasons are much more multidimensional. As stated earlier, the more important reasons for the lack of doctors in health care centers may be the high stress level of the work, busy schedules, and few possibilities to concentrate on research and future education. However, many Finnish municipalities have been trying to solve the problem by raising the salaries of doctors. That is, the problem has also been treated as a tame problem at the regional level, and the measures for solving the problem have been linear and standardized. The results of the problem-solving processes have remained minor; 14% of health center doctor positions were still open in Finnish health care centers at the end of 2004, primarily due to the lack of applicants.

It is obvious that the lack of doctors cannot be treated as a tame problem. A more careful analysis of the reasons for the above mentioned problems should be done by national and regional health care administration, as well as by researchers. This analysis should include information from different stakeholder groups. The Medical Association is a powerful interest group in this case, but its information is not enough. The information from those who consume health care services, those who ultimately pay for them, and those who provide them is also needed to find better and more effective problem-solving alternatives.

Be Acquainted with the Problem at Hand

A profound understanding of health care problems could lead to a more effective planning and implementation of health care reforms. The literature on wicked issues stresses that wicked problems often arise when organizations operate in a turbulent and complex environment. Therefore, it is virtually impossible to understand the true nature of the problem if you do not understand its context. The reforms created for the improvement of health care efficiency are good examples of this.

A deep understanding of the context behind effective health care functions can lead to successful results or vice versa. For example, the introduction of purchaser–provider splits with the aim of fostering price competition among service providers via cost efficiency in Sweden has been successful in many ways. However, the evaluation system has not been able to produce a reliable enough analysis of the efficiency improvements, in spite of many reforms in the accounting and control systems. The reforms have especially failed to link the stakeholder requirements and information to the evaluation information.

The efficiency evaluations have been criticized because of their traditional input–output relationship. It has been stated that this kind of analysis ignores the non-financial dimensions of performance. This also means that the question of health care efficiency has been treated as a tame issue that can easily be solved via a linear problem-solving process by influencing the input–output relationship.

The wicked issue perspective, however, stresses a deeper understanding of the facts behind improved efficiency. From a wicked issues point of view, it can be stated that improvements in efficiency can only be achieved if the information system gathers and analyzes data from organizational, regional, and national levels. To get reliable evaluation information from health care functions, the evaluation process should include many-sided indicators and many-sided data collection. Also, in this case, the information given by different stakeholder groups becomes important. The data collected from patients gives information about the health care process from the patient's point of view. And, the data collected from clinical staff gives possibilities to evaluate medical results from the medical science point of view. The administrative staff should also be included in the evaluation process. The data collected from the administration could consist of information concerning the implementation and functions of the health care organization.

This translates to the fact that health care organizations need multidimensional performance measurement models that can help health care policy making and management to better understand the complexity of effective health care functions. In both Finland and Sweden there have been efforts toward these kinds of solutions: the adaptation of a balanced scorecard is an example of multidimensional performance measurements in health care.

Select the Applicable Problem-Solving Process

It has been stated in this chapter that wicked issues can be better solved with adaptive rather than empirical methods. The adaptive problem-solving process involves discussions with different stakeholders, many-sided analyses of data, and innovative thinking. The process introduces and rejects solutions, analyses the data again and again, and tries to find the solution that can be accepted among all stakeholders.

For example, in both Finland and Sweden there have been reforms that have aimed at improving patients' access to care and making the health care services equally available in all parts of the country. As has been stated in this chapter, the implemented reforms have only been partially successful.

In Finland, the newest reform in this area is actually starting in March 2005. The reform both strengthens patients' right to choose the doctor or hospital and introduces criteria for access to non-urgent treatments. The criteria that will be used as a priority system are still under discussion, and both municipalities and hospital districts are making plans of how to apply these criteria in their own area of health care. The critical point of view with the criteria is their practical use. It may happen that the treatments are primarily given to those patients that are better able to vocalize and emphasize their illnesses and pains.

Actually, some Finnish studies concerning equality in health care give support to the above discussion. Two newly published studies (Stakes, 2004; Heikkilä & Roos, 2004) show quite clearly that the Finnish health care system is functioning unequally. Firstly, on the grounds of these studies it can be concluded that people with high incomes use more medical care than people with low incomes. This is so even if the numbers of doctoral visits are related to the figures describing the differences in health conditions between different social groups. Secondly, the study also stresses that especially the lack of doctors in outlying areas of the country causes inequality in the possibilities to get treatment. As was earlier stated, it is quite difficult in many Finnish municipalities to get an appointment for a medical examination in health centers because many of the doctors' offices are without a full-time physician. Thirdly, a patient's social status and level of income also affect the possibilities to get hospital operations. This is partly because those with high incomes use more private doctoral services than people with low incomes, and it is via private doctors that there are better possibilities to pass the operating queues at the hospitals.

CONCLUDING REMARKS

What, then, is the reason for the fact that, in spite of many reforms and development projects, the Finnish health care system has not met the targets of equality and access to care satisfactorily? My assumption is that the reforms, which aim for the improvement to access to care and equal possibilities to get medical treatment, have been planned and implemented on the basis of traditional thinking. In other words, the national and the regional health care decision makers have not adequately analyzed the environments and contexts of the problems at hand. It seems to me that it has been especially difficult to get relevant analytical information about the linkages between different health care problems and the reforms created to solve them. Also, the efforts to illustrate and analyze potential problem-solving alternatives have remained unsatisfactory. To summarize, my assumption is that if, in the future, health care management problems are treated as wicked problems and not as tame problems, the reforms created to solve them could be more successful than they have been to this point. Especially the adoption of adaptive problem-solving processes could lead to problem-solving alternatives that can better function in complex and conflicting health care environments.

REFERENCES

Ackoff, R. L. (1979). The future of operational research is past. *Journal of the Operational Research Society, 30*, 93–104.

Ackoff, R. L. (1981). The art and science of mess management. *Interfaces, 11*, 20–26.

Article on Wicked Problem (2003). http://www.poppendieck.com/wicked.htm.

Bergman, S.-E. (1998). Swedish models of health care reform: A review and assessment. *International Journal of Health Planning and Management, 13*, 91–106.

Checkland, P. B. (1981). *Systems thinking, systems practice*. Chichester: Wiley.

Checkland, P. B. (1985). From optimizing to learning: A development of systems thinking for the 1990's. *Journal of the Operational Research Society, 36*, 757–767.

Clarke, M., & Stewart, J. (2003). Handling the wicked issues. In: J. Reynolds, J. Henderson, J. Seden, J. Charlesworth & A. Bullman (Eds), *The managing care reader* (pp. 273–280). London: Routledge.

Conklin, E. J., & Weil, W. (2003). Wicked problems: Naming the pain in organizations. http://www.3m.com/meetingnetwork/readingroom/gdss_wicked.html.

Government Resolution on the Health 2015 public health programme (2001). Helsinki: Ministry of Social Affairs and Health.

Heikkilä, M., & Roos, M. (2004). *Sosiaali- ja terveydenhuollon palvelukatsaus 2005*. Helsinki: Stakes.

Hjortsberg, C., & Ghatnekar, O. (2001). Health care systems in transition: Sweden. *European observatory on health care systems*. http://www.euro.who.int/document/e73430.pdf.

Heylighen, F. (1996). What is complexity? http://pespmc1.vub.ac.be/COMPLEXI.html.

Järvelin, J. (2002). Health care systems in transition: Finland. *European observatory on health care systems*. http://www.euro.who.int/document/e74071.pdf.

Kauffman, S. (1996). *At home in the Universe. The search for laws of complexity*. Oxford: Oxford University Press.

MSAH. (2002). *Decision in principle by the council of state on securing the future of health care. Brochures of the ministry of social affairs and health 6*. Helsinki: Ministry of Social Affairs and Health.

Ravetz, J. R. (1971). *Scientific knowledge and its social problems*. Oxford: Oxford University Press.

Rihani, S. (2002). *Complex systems theory and development practice. Understanding non-linear realities*. London & New york: Zed Books.

Rittel, H., & Webber, M. (1973). Dilemmas in a general theory of planning. *Policy Sciences, 4*, 155–169.

Roberts, N. (2000). Wicked problems and network approaches to resolution. *International Public Management Review, 1*(1), electronic Journal at http://www.ipmr.net.

Rosenhead, J., & Mingers, J. (2002). A new paradigm of analysis. In: J. Rosenhead & J. Mingers (Eds), *Rational analysis for a problematic World revisited* (pp. 1–20). New York: Wiley.

Saltman, R. (1998). Health reform in Sweden: The road beyond cost containment. In: W. Ranade (Ed.), *Markets and health care: A comparative analysis* (pp. 164–178). London: Addison-Wesley.

Schon, D. A. (1987). *Educating the reflective practitioner: Toward a new design for teaching and learning in the professions*. San Francisco: Jossey-Bass.

Stakes. (2003). Terveydenhuollon menot ja rahoitus vuonna 2001. http://www.stakes.info/files/pdf/tilastotiedotteet/tt_03_03.pdf.

Stakes. (2004). *Sosiaali- ja terveydenhuollon tilastollinen vuosikirja 2004.* SVT: Sosiaaliturva.

Vartiainen, P. (2003). The substance of stakeholder evaluation: Methodological discussion. *International Journal of Public Administration, 26*(1), 1–18.

Vartiainen, P. (2004). *The legitimacy of evaluation. A comparison of Finnish and English institutional evaluation of higher education.* Frankfurt am Main: Peter Lang.

WHO. (1996). *Health care system in transition: Finland.* Copenhagen: WHO Regional Office for Europe.

THE MANAGEMENT OF CARE FOR INTERNATIONAL REFUGEES: A COMPARATIVE ANALYSIS OF POLICIES AND OUTCOMES

Rachel Collins Wilson

ABSTRACT

Recent invasions, coups, civil wars, and ethnic crusades have caused many individuals and families around the world to flee their homelands for fear of their own safety. The exodus of refugees to foreign nations causes a strain on those nations' health care systems and resources. With the assistance of outside organizations, these countries can develop a health care management system for refugees that provides for both their immediate survival and long-term health stability, while preserving critical national resources. This chapter reviews the refugee problem and presents the short-term tactics and long-term strategies undertaken by seven very different national governments to care for the refugees that cross their borders. A model of a sound health care management system is used to incorporate the best practices of each country into a framework for approaching this multi-billion dollar issue.

As of the beginning of 2003, there were 10.4 million individuals internationally who, because of reasons of war or fear of persecution due to their

---

International Health Care Management
Advances in Health Care Management, Volume 5, 183–209
ISSN: 1474-8231/doi:10.1016/S1474-8231(05)05007-X

race, religion, gender, nationality, political views, or social group, were forced to flee their native countries and ask for asylum or refugee status from other host nations (UNHCR, 2003b). One of the main concerns of the United Nations High Commissioner for Refugees (UNHCR), the governing body that oversees the care of these transients in the hands of their host countries, is the provision of adequate health care for these individuals during their displaced state. Often, one of the most difficult tasks of providing care to these refugees has been the coordination of health care management efforts between host nations and other organizations to provide for these populations.

The field of health care management has traditionally involved the roles of professionals and organizations in providing health services in both national and international contexts (Health Care Management Division, 2002). Issues of access to care and of health care finance are foremost among several studied in this stream of research. Therefore, it is appropriate to study populations that are denied proper access to care for reasons that include financing and organization. Refugee populations are vulnerable populations for many reasons: emotional distress, contagious disease risk, and the lack of stability through shelter and sustenance. Their displacement from their home countries causes them to be at the mercy of the nations they migrate to, and because of political or fiscal reasons, those nations may be unable or unwilling to provide them with even basic care. The nature and severity of this problem varies across countries and across refugee populations. Owing to the fact that some refugee populations are cared for by national and organizational systems that appear to be of better quality than others, it is important to view this phenomenon from a comparative perspective. From comparisons across systems, a set of best practices relating to refugee health care may be accumulated.

This chapter focuses on the health care policy and systemic financial ramifications of refugee and asylum-seeker influx. First, a review will be presented of the international efforts that are in place to aid countries around the world in their assistance to refugees, focusing on the multilateral, bilateral, and non-governmental organizations outside the host countries. Next, a comparative review is conducted of seven countries experiencing varying refugee impact: Iran, the United Kingdom, Serbia and Montenegro, Germany, Guinea, the United States, and the Gaza Strip/West Bank region. This review will identify each country's issues, policies, and strategies regarding refugee health. Finally, from these nations' efforts, a list of major issues and recommended strategies is presented for moving forward effective policies for refugee care.

BACKGROUND

To set the foundation for understanding the concepts behind refugee health care provision, a number of concepts must be presented. First, the concept of a health care system is presented in this section, as it allows for a structural understanding of the phenomenon under research. Secondly, the refugee problem itself is presented – what specific challenges refugees pose for even the most developed health care systems. The last segment of background information is that of organizations that exist outside of the host countries to provide assistance to already-stressed national health care programs. This final background piece is critical to understanding how developing countries with massive refugee populations are able to provide care at all to those groups.

Refugee Care from a Health Care Systems Approach

To fully describe the refugee health care delivery process, a managerially focused framework is used. Fig. 1 illustrates a basic structure of a managerially driven health care system, wherein organization and management drives the development and attainment of resources and activities aimed at achieving certain immediate results and long-term outcomes. This model has been adapted from Filerman (1994) to include refugee-specific resources, activities, outcomes, and immediate results. Such a figure is useful because it allows for a structured process template that can be used by researchers and governments to evaluate their efforts, and determine where their strengths and weaknesses lie. In this research, it is used to evaluate the countries used as focal examples.

At the center of directed efforts is the refugee. The United Nations defines a refugee as

> A person who is outside of his/her country of nationality or habitual residence; has a well-founded fear of persecution because of his/her race, religion, nationality, membership in a particular social group or political opinion; and is unable or unwilling to avail himself/herself of the protection of that country, or to return there for fear of persecution (UNHCR, 2003a).

Also used frequently and interchangeably is the term *asylum seeker* , which is simply used to describe one who is claiming to be a refugee, or someone who is in the aforementioned condition. The refugee rights and protections

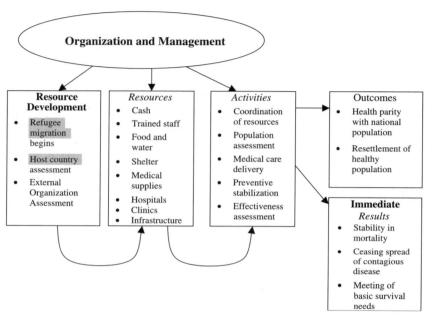

Fig. 1. A Managerially Focused Model of the Refugee Health Care System .
Modified from Filerman (1994).

agreed upon across many nations are described in the 1951 refugee
Convention, originally ratified as a way of protecting refugees from the war-
torn European countries of World War II (UNHCR 2003b). As a result of
this agreement, qualifying refugees are not to be returned to the country
from whence they are fleeing, and are to be cared for by the host governments to at least a similar level as foreign nationals living in the host country, assuming the host is one of the 145 countries originally participating in
the agreement. The United Nations acts as an overseeing body, stepping in
when host governments are not willing or able to uphold their end of the
arrangement.

   Because refugee situations usually occur by definition as a result of political or social trends, they often take a period of weeks to develop, unlike a
natural disaster, and have warning signs that can signal to nearby countries
that an influx is about to occur, such as coups, unrest, or escalating violence
(International Medical Volunteers Association, 2002). As refugees migrate

to the borders of a nation, they more often than not congregate or are encouraged to settle in camp-like establishments. The influx of refugees who are often exhausted and depleted of their natural immunity into small, overpopulated areas brings about a natural public health crisis. As a result, the crisis phase of refugee immigration begins (UNHCR, 1995). At this point, resource development to address this problem must take place, if it has not already. The host country assesses the needs of both the refugee populations and its own citizens, and external organizations affiliated with refugee causes spring into action. To address this problem, some cooperative system must be established between the host country and the external organizations.

The assessments that are made then should reveal the resources that are necessary in addressing this problem. To care for these populations, financial support is necessary to purchase medical supplies, food, potable water, and provide shelter. These must all be acquired to provide basic support. Trained staff, often volunteers, are brought into the area, and temporary clinics are constructed, often on site. Finally, hospitals are constructed in areas of major refugee impact, and a coordinated infrastructure regarding ongoing care and treatment of refugees is established.

Following through the framework in Fig. 1, once resources are obtained, activities should begin, such as the coordination of host government and external organizational efforts, ongoing needs assessments of the refugee populations, actual care delivery, stabilization of the population, and assessment of the effectiveness of these activities. The immediate goals of these activities are rapid reduction of mortality rates, ceasing the spread of contagion, and stabilizing the population by meeting their most basic needs for survival (UNCHR, 1995). Longer-term goals are to achieve a level of population health equivalent to that of the host country's population and to resettle or repatriate a healthy population. Thus completes the framework of the refugee health care management system.

As described here, this system seems to operate without a flaw, but the reality is far from flawless. Inability to fund adequate health care for their own populations, much less that for refugee populations, plagues many developing nations' efforts in meeting refugees' needs. Other developed nations turn a cold shoulder toward their increasing refugee populations, citing high taxes and low refugee productivity in the host country as reasons to shun refugees. Still other nations provide only a small improvement in stability over their neighboring countries to immigrating refugees, as civil unrest within their own borders bars them from forming a united, coordinated management effort.

HEALTH CARE MANAGEMENT CHALLENGES PRESENTED BY REFUGEE POPULATIONS

Refugee populations present specific and unique challenges to the host countries they travel to, and to external organizations whose missions drive them to care for these people. Refugees undergo two phases of health care needs that must be met. First, they go through a crisis phase during the first few days and weeks of influx (UNHCR, 1995). In the crisis phase, there are several concerns as they relate to morbidity and mortality: measles, gastro-intestinal viruses and infections, acute respiratory infections, malaria, and malnutrition. Malnutrition poses a double threat, as it can lead to starvation or death and disease from pathogens that raid compromised immune systems. Controlling death and disease in this crisis phase is challenging; however, once this is achieved, the more stable population moves toward a second phase of health care needs, in which the main concerns to be addressed include tuberculosis, vector-borne diseases (transmitted through insects), sexually transmitted diseases, and complications due to pregnancy and childbirth. Other problems come about as a result of emotional distress, primarily from torture, grief, sleep deprivation, harassment, and rape. This emotional distress works to prevent the individual's resistance to disease.

There are several inherent problems in caring for refugee populations. In the crisis phase of influx, poor nutritional status, inadequate quality and quantity of water, and inadequate shelter cause basic care to be overlooked in favor of pursuing satisfaction of basic survival needs (UNHCR, 1995). Once the refugee population stabilizes, overcrowded living conditions in refugee camps and housing areas as well as poor sanitation in these areas cause difficulties with disease control. Managing these unique population-based issues as well as the monumental task of providing financing for services is often too much for host country governments to bear themselves. Many times their countries are war-torn themselves, and thus the intervention of external multilateral and non-governmental organizations is necessary (Centers for Disease Control, 1992).

The Role of External Organizations

The role of external organizations in providing health care services to refugees is phenomenal, especially in developing or impoverished countries that bear the brunt of many refugee migrations. These organizations can be classified as multilateral, bilateral, and non-governmental in nature. The UNHCR, a United Nations body, has an extremely important role as the provider of care to refugees, and anticipates its 2004 budget to exceed $954 million in addition to the over 500 volunteer workers who help in their efforts (UN General Assembly, 2003b). Funding for UNHCR comes from private donations and contributions from many of the world's nations, as shown in Table 1. Much of the UNHCR's health care efforts are driven toward preventative measures, such as improving overcrowded living conditions, the inadequate access to food and potable water, the lack of sanitation, and the lack of shelter that exacerbate the previously mentioned threats to refugee health (UNHCR Subcommittee on Administrative and Financial Matters, 1995).

Another agency responsible for the care of a great number of the world's refugees is the United Nations Relief and Works Agency (UNRWA) for Palestine Refugees. In 2003, the agency spent $397.1 million working with refugees in the region surrounding former Palestine, including the West Bank/Gaza Strip (UN General Assembly, 2003a).

The World Health Organization (WHO) operates alongside, yet independently of the United Nations, and directs and coordinates international health activities (International Medical Volunteers Association, 2002). This organization develops standards, provides training, and monitors and evaluates public health populations around the globe. Around 190 member

Table 1. Assistance from and Contributions to the UNHCR by Countries under Study.

Nation	Assistance from UNHCR, 2004 Budget	2002 Contributions to UNHCR	Ratio – 2002 Contributions to UNHCR: GDP per Capita
U.S.	$2,702,500	$259,244,770	7202:1
U.K.	$1,308,500	$33,560,724	1280:1
Germany	$1,571,800	$30,560,090	1200:1
Iran	$20,930,700	$0	0
Serbia and Montenegro	$27,372,800	$0	0
Guinea	$24,719,100	$0	0
West Bank and Gaza Strip	$0[a]	$0	0

[a]UNRWA funded.

nations contribute to the World Health Organization. Other multilateral organizations who work in international health include the World Bank, which loans money to impoverished countries, and the UN Economic and Social Council, which includes the United Nations Children's Fund (UNICEF), the United Nations Population Fund (UNFPA), and the United Nations Development Programme (UNDP). These organizations work with vulnerable child populations, family planning, and acquired immunodeficiency syndrome (AIDS), and maternal and child health, respectively. Finally, there are non-governmental organizations, of which there are an estimated 1,500 worldwide, who contribute around 20% of external aid to developing countries (International Medical Volunteers Association, 2002). The largest of these in the international field is Oxfam International. Other organizations involved in refugee health are the International Committee of the Red Cross, and Medecins Sans Frontieres (Doctors Without Borders).

Within any refugee situation, many organizations may be working to assist the population; however, coordination between groups could almost always be improved. For example, UNHCR, Medecins du Monde, the American Refugee Committee and Medecins Sans Frontieres have collaborated to develop health posts in rural Guinea and provide these centers with cash, supplies, and administrative direction (World Health Organization, 2001). Unfortunately, in nations with more poorly developed political systems, even the aid of these external organizations is manipulated and used with varying outcome success by communities hosting refugees. Table 2 shows a summary of the various organizations involved in funding and providing health care to refugee populations.

FOCAL NATIONS' REFUGEE POLICIES AND CRITICAL ISSUES

To further illustrate the refugee issues encountered by various nations, seven countries are presented that represent socialized and privatized health care delivery systems, industrialized and developing economies, and established and preliminary health care management structures. By examining a wide variety of programs for health care management of refugee populations, a model of best practices may be derived that can serve as a template for better care across nations.

The seven focal countries include the United States, Germany, the United Kingdom, Iran, Serbia and Montenegro, Guinea, and Palestine (West Bank

Table 2. Non-Governmental Organizations Providing Assistance or Care to Refugees.

Agency Name	Provides Funding	Provides Health Care Activities
UNHCR	X	X
UNRWA	X	X
WHO	—	X
World Bank	X	—
UNICEF	X	X
UNFPA	X	—
UNDP	X	—
International Committee of the Red Cross	X	X
Medecins Sans Frontieres (Doctors Without Borders)	—	X
Medecins du Monde	—	X
American Refugee Committee	X	X
Oxfam International	—	X

and Gaza Strip). Table 3 illustrates the vast differences between these countries in terms of their gross domestic products (GDPs), populations, average health care expenditures, and severity of refugee impact, both on their populations and on their economies. Furthermore, the United Kingdom, Germany, and the United States were chosen as examples of industrialized nations due to their respective number 1, 2, and 3 positions among industrialized nations for the highest numbers of asylum applications received in 2002. Iran, Serbia and Montenegro, Guinea, and West Bank and Gaza Strip were selected from the developing nations due to their status as refugee hotbeds of activity. Each country is treated similarly throughout this section, with national refugee policies laid out, health care policies and issues delineated, and special challenges highlighted that face each individual nation.

The United States

Refugees entering the United States through proper channels are cared for through the Refugee Act of 1980, a part of the Immigration and Nationality Act (Office of Refugee Resettlement, 2002). At the end of 2002, the United States hosted 638,000 refugees, a majority of whom were awaiting decision on their asylum applications (U.S. Committee for Refugees, 2003). The U.S.

Table 3. Key Economic and Refugee Figures for Nations under Focus.

Country	GDP (Purchasing Power Parity, U.S. $)[a]	Population, 2003[a] (million)	GDP per Capita (Calculated from GDP and Population)	Health Care Expenditure per Capita, 2001[b]	Refugee Population, December 2002[c]	Refugees per 1000 Capita[d]	Refugees per $Million GDP
United States	$10.45 trillion	290.3	$35,997	$4887	638,000	2.120	0.061
Germany	$2.16 trillion	82.4	$26,214	$2412	104,000	1.262	0.048
United Kingdom	$1.53 trillion	60.1	$25,458	$1835	79,200	1.318	0.051
Iran	$458.3 billion	68.3	$6710	$363	2,208,500	32.335	4.819
Serbia and Montenegro	$23.15 billion	10.6	$2183	N/A	353,000	33.301	15.248
Guinea	$18.69 billion	9.0	$2077	$13	182,000	20.222	9.738
West Bank and Gaza Strip	$1.7 billion	2.2	$773	N/A	627,000	285	368.82

[a]Central Intelligence Agency (2004).
[b]The World Bank Group (2003).
[c]U.S. Committee on Refugees (2003).
[d]UNHCR Population Data Unit (2003).

federal government acts as a coordinating center for refugee activities and delegates to the states the responsibilities for their care. The Federal agency responsible for refugee-related issues in the U.S. is the Office of Refugee Resettlement, the U.S. Department of Health and Human Services Administration for Children and Families (U.S. Department of Health and Human Services, Office of Refugee Resettlement, 2003).

Because the United States borders neighboring countries that are stable, only about 20,000 individuals are given asylum status to stay in the U.S. as refugees each year (Office of Refugee Resettlement, 2000). Because of the small refugee impact within the U.S. relative to some other countries, resource development can be on an ongoing basis, under the direction of the Office of Refugee Resettlement. Perhaps in an effort to curb the spread of infectious disease, the Refugee Act requires that refugees are not placed in areas of high refugee concentration, a practice highly unlike the camps and tenement houses used to shelter refugees in other countries. Duplication of services is discouraged to conserve resources, and assurance that services are geographically readily available to placed refugees also helps to ensure the efficiency and effectiveness of the refugee aid system. Specialized grants and contracts are made to the States for initial medical assessment and treatment. The States are in turn responsible for upholding to their individual plans for assisting refugees, especially with medical conditions that they may bring with them that require treatment (Office of Refugee Resettlement, 2002). Infrastructure for health care within the United States is in place due to its high GDP and substantial investment in hospitals, clinics, and medical research. Through various programs, access to all of these resources is available to refugees, at least for the first eight months of their arrival.

Upon entering the United States, the 1996 Illegal Immigration Reform and Immigrant Responsibility Act (IIRIRA) dictates that asylum seekers have one year to file for refugee status (Office of Refugee Resettlement, 2000). Once granted asylum, refugees are given a small stipend of cash and medical benefits for eight months, as well as five years' access to social services to assist their integration while in the United States. Most refugee families are provided for under the Temporary Assistance for Needy Families (TANF) program; whereas money for care for single refugees and refugee couples without children are found under state-run and partially federally funded Refugee Cash Assistance (RCA) programs. Supplemental Security Income (SSI) programs can also be used for those who qualify. Finally, the Wilson/Fish program is the fourth option for receiving cash and medical benefits. This program is tailored for refugees who are not planning to ever return to their homeland and thus who must develop self-sufficiency in the States. For specific health care needs, the Refugee Medical Assistance (RMA) program is available for refugees who are not eligible for Medicaid or the Children's Health Insurance Program in their state for reasons such as employment or income status. Through these programs, refugees within the States are technically granted the same public access to care that nationals have, even though the U.S. does not have universal health care.

Current problems inherent in the U.S. system, much like other systems, include the treatment of single refugee children who have arrived in the country. These children are often detained in facilities with juvenile offenders while waiting months or years for asylum proceedings responses (U.S. Committee for Refugees, 2003). During this time, they are unduly exposed to crime, yet are not represented by legal guardians or attorneys during their process. Other concerns exist with the sometimes-arbitrary rejection of asylum seekers by Department of Homeland Security officers, who have been reported to make personal judgment calls regarding asylum seekers' claims rather than reporting them to asylum officers, as is protocol (U.S. Committee for Refugees, 2003). Also, the turning over of federal money to states to use at their discretion works against the development of a standardized approach to health care, something that could be of great concern should a population from one particular country show up in several different states with a common, previously unseen disease. Finally, recent violence and political unrest in Haiti has sent an influx of Haitian asylum seekers to the U.S. borders; however, the U.S. government usually detains individuals from this country or immediately sends them back, citing that their reasons for fleeing Haiti do not qualify them as refugees under the Refugee Convention. Such inequality of response to individuals does not portend well for the standardization, and cost reduction, of the system as a whole.

Germany

Germany housed 104,000 refugees at the end of 2002, 91,500 of which were new arrivals (U.S. Committee for Refugees, 2003). This figure actually represented a decline (−22%) from 2001. This does not include the roughly 300,000 individuals who are in the country under "toleration," or special allowance for them to stay if they face torture or capital punishment upon returning. The top five countries from which refugees fled to Germany include Turkey (13.5% of 104,000), Yugoslavia (12.5%), Iraq (10.3%), the Russian Federation (4.2%), and Iran (3.5%). The major German governmental agency responsible for the care for these refugees is the Bundesamt, which is the Federal Office for Recognition of Foreign Refugees.

More often than not, the German approach to assessing the refugee situation as it unfolds begins inland. German law prevents the acceptance of any refugee who traveled through a third country to get into Germany, unless that refugee was to be refouled, or forcibly sent back to their unsafe home country, by the country through which they passed (U.S. Committee for Refugees, 2003). Applicants who apply inland at a Bundesamt office face a much better chance that authorities will be unable to trace their journey into the country, and thus they can claim that they flew straight to German borders. Due to this barrier and given the stability of Germany's neighboring countries, it is unlikely that a large-scale refugee influx would occur in the near future.

Two types of asylum are granted in Germany (U.S. Committee for Refugees, 2003). Unlimited residence permits are granted to those who fall under the refugee definition in the Refugee Convention, and who do not travel through a third country to reach German borders. Two-year, renewable permits are granted to those who traveled through a third country to reach Germany, but were in danger of refoulement to their unsafe home countries by that third nation. This permit changes to an unlimited residence permit after eight years. Both types of refugees are allowed public assistance, including medical care, and both are allowed to work to improve their economic status. Asylum seekers in Germany are given essential medical treatment for acute diseases upon arriving, until a decision on their refugee status is made (Platform for International Cooperation on Undocumented Migrants, 2001). These individuals are also given 80% of the non-medical public assistance offered to nationals of the country, or about 40 Euros cash each month, shelter, and food. The German health care system is of similar quality to the United States, and is available to citizens through a mandated insurance program (European Observatory on Health Care Systems, 2000). The funds that comprise this program are fueled by contributions from workers and their employers alike. Hospitals, physician clinics, and medical supplies, as well as a strong health care infrastructure, are in place.

Currently, major issues that the German government struggles with include the return of Kosovars back to their country, which is arguably still unsafe for their return, and the current policy of refusing refugee status to those who are being persecuted by non-government actors (U.S. Committee for Refugees, 2003). At present, German law dictates that unless a governmental body is persecuting or threatening to persecute a group or individual, that refugee is not able to claim asylum in Germany. Pressing health care issues include the lack of medical interpreters, including those familiar with customs and medical beliefs of non-Western refugees as well as anti-foreigner sentiment on the part of citizens and some health care professionals (Platform for International Cooperation on Undocumented Migrants, 2001).

United Kingdom

The situation within the United Kingdom regarding refugees is interesting. The U.K. does not have an extraordinary refugee impact in terms of pure numbers (similar refugees per 1,000 population and refugees per $1 million GDP); however, the nation has, perhaps with the help of the media, become a hotbed of vocal anti-refugee sentiment. Perhaps for reasons of ease of entry in the past, and perhaps because of past concessions made to refugees, the number of applications for asylum filed in the U.K. increased by 20% within the past year, a trend differing that of many industrialized nations. By year-end 2002, the U.K. was home to 79,200 refugees and asylum seekers, the largest number of which arrived from Iraq, followed by Zimbabwe and Afghani refugees (U.S Committee for Refugees, 2003). Presenting oneself to the U.K. for asylum and being granted such are two very different concepts, however, and most of those actually granted asylum arrived from Somalia, then Zimbabwe and Iraq. About 15% of individuals who apply for asylum are granted refugee status.

Recent legislation in the U.K. has left refugees with little public assistance. The Nationality, Immigration, and Asylum Act of 2002 refuses public assistance to asylum seekers who do not immediately apply for asylum upon arrival, and it allows for a number of asylum seekers to be immediately refused status if they come from specified countries, including several of the former Soviet republics (U.S. Committee for Refugees, 2003). Asylum seekers are offered legal representation, and are moved through the review process, usually in a matter of weeks. Those granted refugee status are given an indefinite limit on their time to stay in the country and equal rights as citizens. Others are given four-year protections to remain in the U.K. if they fail the asylum application process, but can assert that their home countries are unsettled. This benefit will be reduced to three years as of April 2003. In response to citizen protest, the U.K. government has denied asylum applicants the right to work (U.S. Committee for Refugees, 2003).

The U.K. government has typically opted for concentration of asylum seekers and refugees into state-funded housing projects; however, they are free to move about the country as long as they periodically report. Asylum seekers are given vouchers for the equivalent of $53 per week to help sustain themselves during the period in which they may not work, and despite the provision of basic health services, asylum seekers often go hungry, cannot afford clothing or shoes, and are more often than not ill (U.S. Committee for Refugees, 2003). Both asylum seekers and refugees are offered health services through the National Health Service (NHS) as long as they apply for asylum immediately upon arrival to the U.K., although a recent law has dictated that those denied asylum must pay for non-urgent hospital care while still in the country (Refugee Council, 2004). Asylum seekers are encouraged to register with a general practitioner (GP) for their access into the NHS, and if they are denied access to care repeatedly, the NHS trust will assist the individual with finding a physician. Identity cards, while not mandatory to be shown, are one way of ensuring continuity of care throughout the asylum seeker's stay. Other benefits allotted to asylum seekers and refugees include free prescriptions, dental treatment, wigs, travel costs for treatment, sight tests, and a voucher for corrective lenses, as a part of their assistance from the National Asylum Support Service.

Iran

Iran has a unique role to play in the current international refugee phenomenon, as the country has the largest refugee caseload of any nation in the world, that of 2.21 million refugees (U.S. Committee for Refugees, 2003). The great majority of Iran's refugees have migrated from neighboring Afghanistan (90%), while others have primarily come from Iraq. Aside from the geographic proximity, Iran's extension of help to fellow Muslims brings many asylum seekers to its borders; however, refugees in Iran have few rights. The Iranian government has been trying to put an identity card system in place since 1995; however, the overwhelming influx of Afghanis into the region has rendered this effort challenging. The Iranian government coordinates resources and efforts with UNHCR; however, the magnitude of the refugee migration has caused the Iranian government to withhold cooperation on an ever-increasing scale. For example, Iran closed its borders temporarily in 2001 to Afghanis, asking that instead they congregate in camps within their own borders to wait for Iranian assistance. Furthermore, increasing incidents of forceful deportation of refugees, or refoulement, have occurred, in direct opposition to Iran's acceptance of the Refugee Convention.

Conditions for refugees in Iran are dismal. Some refugees and asylum seekers are denied the right to work, which creates problems with their ability to obtain resources legally. There exists among the Iranian nationals a xenophobic attitude, and citizens look at refugees as causes behind large unemployment rates, even though they are legally denied the right to work, and nationals view refugees in large part as criminals (Human Rights Watch, 2002). Outside the cities, due to the rapid onset of refugees, camps have been constructed at the Iranian borders. These camps have faced traditional public health crises, such as outbreaks of cholera, tuberculosis, dysentery, and malaria, as well as problems with depression and malnutrition (Iran Refugee Camps Getting Worse, 2001). Overcrowding at one border camp forced its closure to new occupants, and several outside died of the cold. Lack of security at the camps as well as nearby Taliban fighting caused safety issues to be of great concern (Human Rights Watch, 2002). Although asylum seekers and refugees are intended to be granted health care rights equivalent to that of Iranian nationals, overcrowding and overwhelming of the health care system available to care for refugees causes the intent to be lost on the reality, and refugee populations in concentrated areas experience poor health.

Even though refugee life in the camps is dismal, only some of the refugees live in the camps – most are asylum seekers (U.S. Committee on Refugees, 2003). The Iranian government does not force refugees into camps; however, refugees are restricted to movement about one Iranian province. Those living outside the camps experience healthier environments, and are afforded similar health care to Iranian nationals. As of 2002, many Afghanis were being returned voluntarily through an agreement between the Iranian government and UNHCR. The Iranian government estimates the overall cost of caring for each refugee to be $674 each year, of which $6 is shared by the international community (U.S. Committee for Refugees, 2003); therefore, the return of these refugees is in Iran's best interest.

The current state of the Iranian health care system is improving (Powell, 2003). High-quality hospitals, free primary care clinics, and a system of volunteers at the local level have improved the country's system over the past decade. Rural areas, often centers for refugee influx, are served by health houses, providing basic medical services and vaccinations.

Serbia and Montenegro

The republics of Serbia and Montenegro (the Federal Republic of Yugoslavia or FRY) declared their independence in 1992 and attempted to unite Serbs in surrounding areas into a Serbian republic over the following years (Central

Intelligence Agency, 2003). Instead, the result was an ethnic war against Albanians in the region, which provoked an international response. Fleeing persecution, Albanians outwardly migrated from Serbia and Montenegro to Kosovo, and Serbs migrated inward from Kosovo. Major problems in this region include the lack of a systematic approach to health care due to a tattered and unstable infrastructure (U.S. Committee for Refugees, 2003). Lack of border control causes an inability to assess the refugee situation accurately. Including the mainly Albanian region of Kosovo, there were 353,000 refugees in the Yugoslavian area at the end of 2002. About two-thirds of these are Croatian Serbs, and another third Bosnian Serbs. These numbers cause the FRY to be the most heavily populated area of refugees in Europe. Current efforts include repatriating those who wish to leave back to Croatia and Bosnia, and an alternative focus by the FRY government is to integrate those who wish to stay in the country permanently.

A small number of refugees live in collective centers due to financial hardship. These centers have poor living standards, inadequate water, and inadequate sanitation (U.S. Committee for Refugees, 2003). All refugees in the FRY often experience problems with documentation of their status, and many experience difficulties obtaining health care and other public services. Part of this problem exists because other refugee crises around the world, such as that in Iran, have funneled off critical resources from external organizations that were assisting the FRY. Unemployment in the region exacerbates malnutrition problems in the country as well. Finally, the lack of working medical and surgical equipment in the region, as well as the lack of information systems in clinics and hospitals, further compounds problems with access to care and public health management. Reform to the health care system is coming in the form of greater funding from tax bases, which will be used to increase by a third the current $80 per year that the government allocates per person for health care (Serbian Government, 2002).

Guinea

As of the end of 2002, Guinea was host to 180,000 total refugees, 61% of whom traveled from Liberia, and 28% of whom traveled from Sierra Leone (U.S. Committee for Refugees, 2003). Liberians and Sierra Leoneans fled their countries due to recent civil wars that have left the nations in a state of armed insurgence. Specific problems encountered that have had a lasting health care management effect include the impoverished nature of the refugees that arrive there, as many have paid all that they have to rebel soldiers to get them safely across the Guinean border (U.S. Committee for Refugees, 2003). Many refugees are malnourished from their journey, causing immunity deterioration and death. Refugees from Sierra Leone were originally fleeing civil war and human rights violations that flared in the 1990s; however, many are being helped by the UNHCR to repatriate, as conditions in that country have since improved.

The Guinean situation is compounded by a number of issues. First, the nation is relatively impoverished relative to its more industrialized counterparts. For example, the U.S. GDP per capita figure is roughly $36,000, whereas the same figure for Guinea is around $2,075 (Central Intelligence Agency, 2003). This causes a majority of the health care provision, especially during the crisis phase of refugee migration, to be borne by the UNHCR.

The Guinean UNHCR refugee shelter camps are often located in geographical regions such as rainforests, where access to quality health care is not usually available. Many refugees are only offered minimal shelter, food, water, and latrines, even after the initial time period appropriate for crisis management has passed (U.S. Committee for Refugees, 2003). As of 2001, there was only one hospital within close range of the major refugee camps, the Kissidougou Hospital, with only 12 medically well-trained people as staff (World Health Organization, 2001). Outside of the hospital, no laboratories exist at which to make diagnoses, causing some public health concern. Furthermore, primary care facilities are staffed by a non-medically trained health officer and nurses, and gaps in medicine and supply availability exist. Within refugee ranks, there are problems involving rebel-faction leaders that horde relief resources from others that are more vulnerable, and sexual exploitation of female refugees has been reported, even perpetration by the aid workers in the camps. An issue has also developed that refugees are being provided with better, free health care, whereas nationals have to pay for most of their services (Damme, DeBrouwere, Boulaert, & Lerberghe, 1998).

The continuing shortfall of basic assistance to would-be stabilized populations continues to plague Guinea, and indecision by the Guinean government regarding issues as small as printing contracts for identity cards has compounded the situation, causing refugees to be denied of the receipt of similar benefits as nationals (U.S. Committee for Refugees, 2003). As an example, the health authority for the Guinean region surrounding several major refugee camps did not have a vehicle as of 2001, nor did it have adequate office equipment (World Health Organization, 2001). The coordination between local government authorities and external organizations is minimal, with difficulty in gathering and analyzing data and low involvement in planning and oversight being the two biggest barriers to accomplishment.

There are, however, positive points about the system used in Guinea for handling refugees and their health care. Instead of forcibly keeping refugees in camps, the Guinean government has allowed refugees to settle where they want (Damme et al., 1998). This has led to the improvement in health services across the country, owing in part to UNHCR and other organizations' assistance. Roads have been improved in order to get food to dispersed refugees, and small economies have developed in rural areas due to the trade of relief items for cash. Furthermore, the dispersion of the refugee population has relieved the government from being overwhelmed with typical public health and administrative concerns; however, it is not known what the long-term effects of this freedom from concern have been. Owing to these conditions, the cost of medical care per refugee per year was estimated in 1998 at $4, as opposed to the international average of $20 per refugee per year (Damme et al., 1998).

Gaza Strip and West Bank

The Gaza Strip and West Bank is the name used to refer to the area between Israel and Jordan. Currently, the area is a source of contention between two governments who would like to settle the region and claim it: Israel and the newer Palestinian Authority. As of the end of 2002, this area hosted 1.51 million Palestinian refugees, more than 43% of the total Palestinian population (U.S. Committee for Refugees, 2003). The Gaza Strip area is organized into eight major camps, whereas the West Bank refugee population is not as concentrated and is about three-fourth the size in refugee numbers.

Problems in the West Bank and Gaza Strip are numerous, and result primarily from the violent conflict in the region, which has included suicide bombings, closures of roads that have kept refugees in critical condition from accessing hospitals, and destruction of homes (U.S. Committee for Refugees, 2003). At least 22% of refugee children suffer from acute or chronic malnutrition in the region. Part of the problem with delivery of health care in this region is the lack of an established and stable health care system on the part of the overseeing Palestine Authority and Israeli governments. The UNRWA, or the United Nations Relief and Works Agency for Palestine was developed specifically to work in this region, and is currently responsible for a great deal of the health care for refugees (World Health Organization, 2000). As of 1999, "virtually all health care providers suffer[ed] from significant budget deficits and inadequate coordination of international assistance" (World Health Organization, 2000, p. 1). Violence in the region has generated an immense need for resources. For example, in January 2002, the UNRWA budgeted $117 million for the entire year, and by July, this money had been spent. Another $140 million was needed to cover normal and emergency activities for the remainder of the year. By the end of 2002, the UNRWA cited a serious deterioration in the refugee situation in the West Bank and Gaza Strip. Major issues in this region center around the unwillingness of refugees to leave a violent area for fear that they will not be allowed to return, and the resultant casualties and mental health issues from this predicament. Likewise, the instability caused by the conflict-ridden co-occupation of this territory hinders stabilization of the populations' health.

The UNRWA has been instrumental in efforts to develop an adequate system of care, in and outside of the camps (World Health Organization, 2000). Primary health facilities, double-shift clinics, laboratories, dental clinics, maternity units, and physiotherapy clinics help to fulfill needs in both crisis and stabilization modes of refugee influx. Programs on prevention of tobacco usage and prevention of HIV/AIDS have been established as well (World Health Organization, 2000). Near the end of 2000, a public health laboratory was to be built in Ramallah to assist in rounding out the health care system there.

DISCUSSION

Upon review of the challenges and concepts surrounding refugee care in various countries, the model in Fig. 1 can be analyzed for best practice potential in some areas and for gaps that exist in current service provision across nations. Table 4 shows a summary of the strengths and weaknesses of each country as they relate to this best practice model. One of the most important issues to bear in mind is that of resources – the countries under study had widely varying access to resources, and any model that is to work across nations must take this into account, as well as the fact that what is currently working in some nations may not fit others with more urgent or widespread refugee problems.

Resources and Resource Development

As a refugee situation begins to unfold, it is critical that surrounding nations begin to immediately formulate a plan of action, if it is not already in place.

Table 4. Strengths and Weaknesses of Focal Countries' Approaches to Refugee Health Care.

Country	Strengths	Weaknesses
United States	Lack of refugee camps causes reduced likelihood of epidemic disease breakout Social services exist to assist in long-term settlement of refugees – allows for chronic disease management and improved lifestyle High-quality health care available to refugees Immediate health care for crisis intervention upon arrival	Some refugees only receive eight months of health care services Lack of national, standardized refugee health care program causes additional confusion as to how to receive health care benefits States are given discretion over use of refugee-focused financial distributions, again causing lack of a standardized approach to providing refugee care Inequality in granting of refugee status to citizens from some countries
Germany	Strict laws prevent granting of refugee status to those traveling through third countries – saves resources Same health care benefits as national population Immediate health care for crisis intervention upon arrival High quality health care system	Inequity in granting refugee status to individuals from all countries Lack of medical interpreters Reported anti-foreign sentiment among health care workers
United Kingdom	Refugee rights to health care equal to that of citizens Identity cards issued that assist in continuity of refugee's health care National health care system infrastructure in place; good quality health care available to refugees	Anti-refugee sentiment causes refugee populations to be isolated and shunned by public Refugees not allowed to work – does not assist in promotion of economic status and resultant improved health status Concentration of refugees in housing projects facilitates outbreak of disease Refugees encouraged but not mandated to register with general practitioner as means of entering national health system Identity card use not mandated

Table 4. (*Continued*)

Country	Strengths	Weaknesses
Iran	Improving quality of health care system Policies in place to grant refugees same access to health care as nationals No restrictions of refugees to camps	Increase lack of cooperation with UNHCR due to immense refugee burden Lack of security and adequate health care at camps that form Overall national xenophobic attitude causes shunning of refugee populations Denial of right to work to refugees causes inability to improve economic and health care status
Serbia/ Montenegro	Increasing funding from tax base to fund health care system improvement Commitment to offer similar health care services to refugees as national population	Lack of border control results in documentation issues and assessment problems Decrease in funding and support from external organizations Lack of strong medical infrastructure or health care system Lack of information system to track refugees
Guinea	Refugees receiving better care than nationals, for free No mandate for refugees to stay in camps Outside organizational assistance has improved national infrastructure, including health care system	Lack of resources for relatively high quality health care, even for its own citizens Rurality of refugee camps limits access to hospitals Exploitation of refugee health care system by rebel leaders and workers No identity card system in place for refugees due to political maneuvering Minimal cooperation by local governments with external authorities
West Bank/ Gaza Strip	UNRWA specifically created by the U.N. to assist in developing a response to this population Resources such as primary care and specialty clinics have been developing in region. Laboratories are to be developed soon	Lack of established health care system from lack of single overarching, accountable authority Violence causes high mortality rate Instability leads to constant crisis phase – inherent inability to stabilize population

There is no evidence from the cases studied in this research that this is not currently performed by countries that have experienced refugee influx; however, it could be done more effectively. Some nations have a geographical buffer to refugee influx as it occurs; for example, the lack of land borders with countries other than Canada or Mexico affords the United States a break in the number of asylum applicants that it might receive if it bordered a nation with a more volatile governmental situation, such as Iran, which borders Afghanistan and Iraq. For those countries bordering volatile states it is imperative that they not only assess their capability to provide shelter, food, and water to incoming refugees, but crisis intervention health care services as well. Are they well equipped with antibiotics? Are there shelters to use for quarantine and care-giving to keep initial contagion down? Do the incoming refugees have shelter and security to rest and regain their strength after their long journeys? These sorts of questions must be asked to assess the immediate needs for refugees.

Likewise, countries have to look inwardly to their own populations to ensure that their health care status is not negatively affected by the onslaught of potentially sickly individuals. Does the host government have the security in place to keep diseased asylum seekers out of the national population while they are recovering? Will providers be taken away from the current health care system to care for the refugees, and how will that impact care for nationals? Likewise, from the Guinea case, is there a way to structure the refugee system to benefit from the assistance of outside organizations, such as spreading out refugee centers to promote the improvement of the infrastructure for all involved, including refugees, without unfairly manipulating the beneficence of this help? Infrastructure improvement is not the only benefit to distributing refugees across the country. From the United States to the Gaza Strip to Iran to Guinea, nations have seen the public health advantage from allowing refugees at least limited ability to live throughout the country, as this has been documented to alleviate the spread of disease throughout overcrowded areas such as camps. Furthermore, an outcry from the public in the U.K. has developed from large housing projects being built or leased near residences, as opposed to refugees dispersing throughout the population in smaller concentrations.

Identity cards and the ability to track refugees' health-care usage is another piece to resource planning and utilization that has shown to be beneficial when adopted. The United States issues documentation for asylum seekers and refugees, as does the United Kingdom. The National Health Service for the United Kingdom goes one step further, tracking refugees' care through a general practitioner assigned to them. These two practices assist the management of health services for these individuals in several ways. First, across these individuals' lives, the documentation gives them legitimacy, whether it is for purchasing of daily goods and services or asking the government for assistance. The one downside to this legitimacy is that, for some, it could be considered a labeling instrument for stereotyping and discrimination toward these individuals. Secondly, tracking refugees' health status and care helps both in assessing that individual's healthiness and in strategic planning on a broader scale for the entire refugee system, incorporating successes and failures into care delivery in the future.

Activities and Outcomes

The final imperative piece of resource development and planning requires governments to have a plan in place for coordination between their own efforts and those of external organizations. One of the simplest ways to do this is to break down every concern for incoming refugees and nationals into resources and activities to be obtained and performed as the refugee population arrives and settles. By using such a template, governments can have a plan in place, and a brief meeting with external organizations that are assisting in that country can place them where they are most needed, and detail which activities will be the responsibility of which actor. This will also reveal where gaps exist in provision of care, so that those gaps can at least be addressed quickly.

Governments and external organizations must additionally have a plan in place for measurement and tracking of refugees' health status, progress, and utilization. Reasons for why the countries studied in this research did not have a mechanism in place for this measurement varied widely, from not having a government-run system, to not having access to adequate information systems, to the camps themselves being too unsafe for measurement, to lack of identity mechanisms for each refugee. Therefore, this critical strategic planning piece seems to be disturbingly missing from even the most sophisticated industrialized countries' systems. Without this feedback of how the population is progressing, disease management cannot thoroughly take place, and resource usage cannot be evaluated for its effectiveness. Therefore, hurdles must be overcome to develop such systems. This is easier said than done, as developing a system such as this not only takes labor, which could very well be done by volunteers, but it also requires expensive computing power to be efficient. Perhaps, soliciting the help of private organizations to donate used systems to local governments for this purpose would improve their abilities to construct these badly needed strategic tools.

CONCLUSIONS

This research attempted to address the challenges and concepts associated with the health care management of refugee populations. Organizations that assist with refugees, as well as some of the world's most refugee-inundated countries, were studied for best practices and areas of improvement to form a framework for an effective refugee health care management system. The research performed in this work could be improved and extended. First the lack of primary information for refugee conditions and care delivery systems in developing countries inhibits the analysis of practices undertaken in those countries. Without this information, it is difficult to determine the strengths and weaknesses of their systems to suggest improvements. One of the ways that this problem could be alleviated would be to perform field research in these regions to determine first, in detail, what these nations' policies are toward refugee health care activities, and secondly, what are the differences between stated policies and actual situations? Once more data are gathered in this vein, a template as suggested in the discussion could be formed and tested for improving the care to these underserved individuals.

Secondly, one of the limitations of this work lies not in the research, but in its implications. Although a framework for best practices in health care provision has been constructed, this model includes practices undertaken by countries with much greater financial resources than others. For example, the financial burden of refugee populations in Iran relative to that country's GDP is much greater than the burden placed on the U.S. relative to its GDP. Therefore, implementing the same level of medical care for Iran's refugee population may not be possible, given the resources available. However, careful coordination of activities between the host government and NGOs working with donated resources should still be implemented, regardless of financial disparities.

REFERENCES

Centers for Disease Control. (1992). Famine-affected refugees and displaced populations: Recommendations for public health issues. [Electronic version]. *41*, RR-1.

Central Intelligence Agency. (2003). *The World Factbook*. [Electronic version]. Washington, D.C.: Author.

Damme, W. V., DeBrouwere, V., Boulaert, M., & Lerberghe, W. (1998). Effects of a refugee-assistance programme on host population in Guinea as measured by obstetric interventions. *Lancet*, *351*, 1609–1613.

European Observatory on Health Care Systems. (2000). Health Care Systems in Transition. The World Health Organization Regional Office for Europe. Retrieved January 27, 2005 at http://www.who.dk/document/e68952.pdf#search = 'germany%20and%20health%20care%20system'.

Filerman, G. L. (1994). Health: The emerging context of management. In: R. M. Taylor & S. B. Taylor (Eds), *The AUPHA manual of health services management* (p. 4). Gaithersburg, MD: Aspen.

Health Care Management Division. (2002). Domain Mission. Health Care Management Division Academy of Management Home Page. Retrieved March 16, 2004, from http://divisions.aomonline.org/hcmd.

Human Rights Watch. (2002). Refugee Protection and Assistance in Iran. Human Rights Watch. Retrieved March 31, 2004 from http://www.hrw.org/reports/2002/pakistan/pakistan0202-05.htm.

International Medical Volunteers Association. (2002). The Major International Health Organizations. Retrieved February 25, 2004, from http://www.imva.org/Pages/orgfrm.htm.

Iran Refugee Camps 'Getting Worse.' (November 2, 2001). BBC News. Retrieved March 31, 2004 from http://news.bbc.co.uk/1/hi/world/middle_east/1634641.stm.

Office of Refugee Resettlement. (2000). ORR extends refugee benefits to more Asylees; issues final rule on cash and medical assistance. [Electronic version]. *Refugee Reports*, *21*(4), 12–15.

Office of Refugee Resettlement. (2002). The Refugee Act. U.S. Department of Health and Human Services, Administration for Children and Families. Retrieved March 27, 2004 from http://www.acf.hhs.gov/programs/rr/policy/refact1.htm.

Platform for International Cooperation on Undocumented Migrants. (2001). Right to Health Care for Undocumented Migrants in Germany. Retrieved March 20, 2004 from http://www.picum.org/DOCUMENTATION/Germany/BSRGermanyhc.htm.

Powell, A. (2003). *Iranian primary care produces big results*. Harvard University Gazette, January 23.

Refugee Council. (2004). Health Services for Asylum Seekers and Refugees. Retrieved March 25, 2004 from http://www.refugeecouncil.org.uk/infocentre/entit/sentit004.htm.

Serbian Government. (2002). Reform of Health Sector Will Bring a Normal System. Retrieved March 17, 2004 at http://www.serbia.sr.gov.yu/news/2002-07/03/325014.html.

The World Bank Group. (2003). World Development Indicators Database. http://devdata.worldbank.org.

UN General Assembly. (2003a). Report of the Commissioner-General of the United Nations Relief and Works Agency for Palestine Refugees in the Near East. http://domino.un.org/unispal.nsf/9a798adbf322aff38525617b006d88d7/0e236a099196750585256dbe0051251c!OpenDocument&Highlight = 2,A%2F58%2F13, accessed February 18, 2004.

UN General Assembly. (2003b). UNHCR Annual Programme Budget. http://www.unhcr.ch/cgi-bin/texis/vtx/home + NwwBmem0ABCwwwwnwwwwwwwhFqh0kgZTtFqnnLnqA-Fqh0kgZTcFqMnLpnDmoB1Gn5Dzmxwwwwwww/opendoc.pdf , accessed February 20, 2004.

UNHCR. (2003a). *Refugees by numbers, 2003 edition*. [Electronic version]. Geneva, Switzerland: UNHCR Media Relations and Public Information Service.

UNHCR. (2003b). *The 1951 refugee convention: Questions and answers*. [Electronic version]. Geneva, Switzerland: UNHCR Media Relations and Public Information Service.

UNHCR Population Data Unit. (2003). *Asylum applications lodged in industrialized countries: Levels and trends, 2000–2002*. Geneva, Switzerland: UNHCR Media Relations and Public Information Service.

UNHCR Sub-Committee on Administrative and Financial Matters. (1995). *Refugee health*. Geneva, Switzerland: Author.

U.S. Committee on Refugees. (2003). *World refugee survey 2003*. [Electronic version]. Washington, D.C.: Immigration and Refugee Services of America.

U.S. Department of Health and Human Services, Office of Refugee Resettlement. (2003). Who We Are. http://www.acf.hhs.gov/programs/orr/mission/functional.htm.

World Health Organization. (2000). Health conditions of, and assistance to, the Arab population in the occupied Arab territories, including Palestine. Fifty-third World Health Assembly, Provisional Agenda Item 16, A53/INF/DOC/4.

World Health Organization. (2001). *Rapid assessment of health system in South Eastern Guinea: Refugees, displaced, host population: February–March 2001*. Geneva, Switzerland: Author.

TAIWAN'S NATIONAL HEALTH INSURANCE: A DECADE OF CHANGE IN HEALTH CARE POLICY AND MANAGEMENT RESPONSES

James C. Romeis, Shuen-Zen Liu and Michael A. Counte

ABSTRACT

For health services researchers and health services management educators, chronicling the unfolding of a country's implementation of national health insurance (NHI) is once in a lifetime opportunity. Rarely, do researchers have the opportunity to observe the macro and micro changes associated with turning a country's health care delivery system 180 degrees. Accordingly, we report on the first decade of Taiwan's changing delivery system and selected adaptations of health care management, providers and patients.

International Health Care Management
Advances in Health Care Management, Volume 5, 211–244
Copyright © 2005 Published by Elsevier Ltd.
ISSN: 1474-8231/doi:10.1016/S1474-8231(05)05008-1

INTRODUCTION

This paper has three broad sections. First, we describe briefly Taiwan's health insurance system prior to its implementation of NHI in March 1995. We include selected general changes it has made over the decade and the structure of the current system. Second, we provide research findings from two of our studies using an NHI derived database of hospitals selected from the Taipei area. The studies describe staff-model HMO structures for hospitals (Chu, Liu, & Romeis, 2002; Chu, Liu, Romeis, & Yaung, 2003), and the implementation of outpatient prescription drug benefits for older Taiwanese citizens (Liu & Romeis, 2003, 2004). The studies are selected because they point to opportunity for comparative research. The lessons learned are:

- Major policy issues in a nation can be solved overnight.
- What may not work in one country, with cultural adjustments may work in others.
- Pitfalls in policy in one country can be assessed and avoided by other countries.

The final section discusses the unfinished business and new problems on the horizon of Taiwan's NHI and health care management. We also suggest what the U.S. and other countries can learn from Taiwan's restructuring.

This chapter is part of an ongoing program of comparative health systems research that began by taking advantage of a unique opportunity. In the summer of 1994, a management-consulting firm in Taiwan contacted us about developing a health services management education program for Taiwanese hospital executives. The goal was to train hospital executives how to manage their hospitals under a looming, not well-understood major policy shift for their delivery system. After internal and external meetings with university and Taiwan representatives, we recruited a small group of Taiwanese faculty to teach basic courses (e.g., accounting, economics, etc.) and students, we launched an executive format Master of Health Administration (MHA) and taught its first class in Taipei February 1995 – one month prior to the implementation of National Health Insurance (NHI) in Taiwan.

Based on the structural features of their (NHI) program, the training program was designed to expose students to managerial concepts and techniques developed from the U.S. post-Diagnostic-related Groups (DRG), managed care experience. We argued that the U.S. did not necessarily have *the* answers to Taiwan's delivery system problems. Rather the U.S. situation had concepts, tools and experiences that may be used to understand the intent and consequences of the proposed policy changes, and how to assess managerial decisions that would keep their hospitals competitive as the new era took shape. With experience, demands of teaching decreased permitting research collaborations to develop. The projects were of mutual interest; ones where the analysis could inform Taiwanese health policy officials and hospital executives as well as speak to the U.S., and other countries experiencing similar delivery system problems.

Accordingly, this chapter reviews and reflects on a decade of comparative health system research. We begin with a general description of the changes in Taiwan's health policy in order to provide a sense of the change and thus the behaviors that were affected. We abridge and provide two previously published studies as an indication of methods and outcomes of comparative health research. We use the studies and current experiences to discuss what the next phase of Taiwan's health policy horizon may be, and what managerial responses could be expected from the hospital executives. Finally, we reflect on what we have learned from this comparative perspective and what policy officials in other countries ought to note.

HISTORICAL CONTEXT

Prior to NHI, Taiwan's social insurance was comprised of 10 programs covering employee groups, e.g., government, labor, farmer, etc., or approximately 60% of the population, leaving approximately 8 million citizens without health insurance. This group included mostly children, older adults and the unemployed. Private health insurance did not exist and by the mid-1980s pressure was mounting for a national universal health insurance program. A Council for Economic Research and Development began planning in 1988. In 1990 the Department of Health took over remaining tasks, establishing a Preparatory Office for NHI in 1993. In August 1994, the NHI Statute was enacted and put into effect. In January 1995, the Bureau of National Health Insurance (BNHI) was established under the authority of the Department of Health, Executive Yuan and in March 1995, NHI was implemented (BNHI, 2004; Cheng, 2003).

As a single payer system, the structural framework for the NHI consists of reciprocal inter-relationships between the Insured, Providers, and BNHI. BNHI provide insurance cards establishing eligibility for services to the Insured and reimburses Providers. Providers submit claims to BNHI and deliver services to the Insured. The Insured pay co-payments to Providers and premiums to BNHI. According to BNHI (2004), most residents are required to join the program and carry a health insurance ID card. A new card, a 32 K IC, was distributed in January 2004. The new card contains medical and medication record data. In the future lab data are to be included. The intent is to improve quality and monitor utilization.

Premium revenues come from Insured (40%), Employers (33%), and Government (27%). The rates for the Insured are graduated based on income with a ceiling of 6%. Premium contributions vary by six categories, corresponding to beneficiary groups and percent contributed by the Insured, Group Insurance Applicant, and Government. Premiums for the unemployed, military, veterans are paid by the government. Benefits are extensive and cover outpatient, inpatient, Chinese medicine, dental care, rehabilitation, and preventive medical services (see www.nhi.gov.tw for inclusion and exclusion details). Co-payments are paid for both outpatient and inpatient services. Co-payment rates vary by level of care, e.g., Western academic hospitals = NT$210, Regional hospitals = 140NT$, District Hospitals and Clinics = 50NT$ (currently 1US$ = ~32NT$). Chinese Medicine and Dentistry have a flat 50NT$ co-payment that does not vary by level of care. Emergency services vary by level with academic hospitals receiving 420NT$ and District Hospitals and Clinics receiving 50NT$. Inpatient co-payments vary by acute or chronic care and number of days hospitalized with chronic stay rates lower than acute stay wards. Select groups are exempt from impatient co-payments. Currently, claims are submitted to BNHI for reimbursement and are based on a fee schedule guideline. If accepted, providers are reimbursed in a very timely fashion. Similarly, drug lists form the basis for reimbursement. Global budgets were first tested in dentistry and in July 2002 were implemented as a method of reducing medical expenses while allowing more autonomy for providers (BNHI, 2004).

Comparative total expenditure data (OECD, 2003) indicates that Taiwan has a lower percent of GDP than many European countries and the U.S. In 1997, the percent GDP for the U.S. = 13, Germany = 10.7, France = 9.4, Canada = 8.9, U.K. = 6.8, and Taiwan = 5.3. In 2001, U.S. = 13.9, Germany = 10.7, France = 9.5, Canada = 9.7, U.K. = 7.6 and Taiwan = 5.7. In 2000, per capita health expenditures for Taiwan were $1,275 and compare to $2,580 for the U.S. and 1.7 times less than OECD countries.

Current Status

In addition to providing universal access and improving the health of the society, improving quality and reducing costs have been equally important goals. One of the most heralded achievements was virtually eliminating access problems for the 40% without insurance. Between March 1995 and the end of the calendar year, enormous strides were made. By 2003, BNHI estimates that 99% of the population of 22 million is enrolled and by June 2004, universal coverage will be achieved. Further BNHI has contracts with 92% of all providers (98% hospitals and 93% of clinics) and represents 78% of beds. From 1995 to 2003, revenue has exceeded costs 3 years, fallen behind costs 3 years and equaled costs 3 years. In 2003, revenue was reported to be 338.5NT$ billion compared to 337.7NT$ billion. Financing of NHI is often heated, but this track record seems benign compared to forecasts in the U.S., e.g. the new prescription drug plan for the elderly.

A concern for Taiwan's health policy officials is utilization rates, with outpatient visits per year averaging 16.1 and hospital days per 100 persons per year 15.1 in 1994. There was an initial drop in utilization in 1995 (12.5 outpatient visits and 13.1 hospital days) but while less than 1994, there has been a gradual increase to 14.4 outpatient visits and 13.4 hospital days. Outpatient visits reflect prescription renewals, thus patients incur a visit and prescription charge. Under certain circumstances, patients with chronic illnesses receive refills for longer periods and have reduced co-payments. Our Study 2 describes this situation. Finally, the political climate surrounding NHI is debated vigorously over its implementation, but public satisfaction has increased from 33% to 78% over the course of the system (BNHI, 2004).

In summary, Cheng (2003) characterized Taiwan's National Health Insurance as a 'car that was domestically designed and produced, but with many components imported from over ten countries'. Such collaborations in manufacturing cars work well but are unique for solving health delivery problems in modern society. Taiwan's approach was bold and innovative. For other recent articles describing the Taiwanese NHI see Chiang (1997) or http://www.nhi.gov.tw. In addition, Lu and Hsiao (2003) provide a thorough complementary economic analysis of the program's first five years.

Cheng (2003) characterizes the system for U.S. and Canadian readers by suggesting that it is similar to the U.S. Medicare program for older adults and the single payer insurance programs run by Canadian provinces. What is most important about this policy change is that in a decade the system was changed dramatically and almost everyone has adapted reasonably well. Access to care was solved virtually overnight. Costs increased as expected after implementation but are currently responding to economic incentives. Utilization is becoming more appropriate. In short, there was not havoc as some forecasted.

Research Opportunity

In the next section, we provide examples of research opportunity for comparative health services management research. Our intent is to demonstrate two types of studies that can be conducted using official data. Depending on one's perspective, results can be used by either policy officials or managers. We suggest that some of the needed changes were already underway, and this helped to soften the impact of the change. Another study suggests that major corrections in program implementation can be made mid-stream and research can help further direct policy change.[1]

STUDY 1: HOSPITAL EFFICIENCY INITIATIVES

This study of Taiwan hospitals is useful to the larger health services research and management community because hospital CEOs are usually physicians, and therefore loosely resemble U.S. hospitals when physicians administratively dominated them. Another way of conceptualizing the administrative structures is a staff-model Health Maintenance Organization (HMO) that has become an increasingly important characteristic of HMOs worldwide. In Taiwan hospitals, besides central administrators, staff physicians are salaried employees of the hospital who organize and provide specialty and sub-specialty care. Based on Goes and Zhan's (1995) measurement the staff model represents the closest type of hospital–physician integration, however, agency problems may still exist when physicians are rewarded inappropriately. The staff-model management structures of Taiwan hospitals help form an organizational culture where physician-executives are actively engaged in designing various types of managerial interventions to change clinicians' behavior. Thus, Taiwan hospitals provide a good opportunity to examine simultaneously the effects of several more subtle arrangements between physicians and hospitals (e.g., the responsibility centers system and physician fee programs) within a staff-model context.

Methods

The study used Data Envelopment Analysis (DEA), which has been widely applied to the study of health care organizations (Ozcan, Luke, & Haksever, 1992; Magnussen, 1996; Ozcan, Begun, & McKinney, 1999). Efforts to measure efficiency can be divided into parametric (i.e., stochastic frontier analysis (SFA)) and non-parametric frontier approaches (i.e., DEA). The parametric frontier approach postulates a functional form with a given number of parameters to describe the production technology. In DEA, the best practice frontier is constructed from the observed inputs and outputs in the sample by linear programming techniques. The efficiency of each observation is then determined relative to the frontier. Because efficiency is measured relative to other organizations (i.e., hospitals), data errors may significantly bias the efficiency measures. Measuring allocative or cost efficiency requires data of input prices (cost data) or output prices (reimbursement rates for hospitals), which are either not available in our database or determined by governmental regulation in Taiwan. For example, the Bureau of NHI, instead of the health care market, determines the scheme of reimbursement rates. The hospital output prices contain little economic information. We focus on hospital technical efficiency, which does not require price information. As a result, the DEA is a more suitable approach in our study.

Two behavioral assumptions can be made when investigating technical efficiency in DEA. One is the input orientation model, where the focus is to evaluate the minimal use of various inputs while keeping outputs constant. The other is the output orientation model, in which the emphasis is to maximize outputs given a fixed level of inputs. The choice of either model depends on whether managers' primary priority is to reduce inputs or increase outputs in achieving efficiency (Seiford, 1996). We believe the output orientation model is more appropriate for our analysis because of the following reasons. First, our sample hospitals may have a higher proportion of fixed costs (e.g., physicians' salaries, depreciation of medical equipment, etc.) when compared with their U.S. counterparts. In Taiwan, most of physicians are traditionally hospital employees, and their salaries alone constitute a significant portion of fixed costs in hospitals. About half of the sample were government hospitals and have less control over the mix of inputs (Lo, Shih, & Chen, 1996). For example, the authority to purchase medical equipment and discharging employees is controlled mainly by the government. It is difficult for managers in government hospitals to reduce costs in the short run. Second, the reimbursement system under the NHI is mainly based on fee-for-service and influences hospital managers' attention to increase outputs instead of reducing inputs. By contrast, U.S. hospital managers tend to seek ways to trim costs instead of expanding outputs, probably because of influences of the prospective payment system.

Sample Selection and Data Sources
The sample hospitals are obtained from *The Survey of Present Status and Service Quantity of Public and Private Hospitals in Taiwan* during the

1994 – 1996 period, as compiled by the Department of Health (DOH). As the survey is important information used in hospital accreditation, the data were carefully scrutinized for both coding and measurement errors by the DOH. We only included general hospitals(i.e., those with at least Internal Medicine, Surgery, Gynecology, Obstetrics and Pediatrics departments; and no fewer than 100 beds) to reduce differences in production technology and quality of care among hospitals (Lo et al., 1996). The data set included 190 general hospitals in 1994, 170 general hospitals in 1995, and 160 general hospitals in 1996. The reduction in hospitals over the three-year period was mainly because some hospitals had closed departments essential to the qualification of general hospitals, or reduced the number of beds below the cut off point of general hospitals. It occurred to smaller hospitals or hospitals with lower accreditation status. After the implementation of NHI in 1995, access to larger hospitals with similar out-of-pocket costs had adversely affected the operation of those hospitals because they lacked resources or brand names to compete.

Because we need a complete data set for analysis, hospitals not in the file for three consecutive years are deleted. The procedure results in a sample of 130 hospitals (58 public hospitals and 72 private hospitals). In general, the deleted hospitals tended to be smaller in size (e.g., with fewer beds and personnel) and of lower accredited status. All medical centers and metropolitan hospitals were included while some local community hospitals were deleted.

Specific hospital–physician integration strategies implemented by the sample hospitals were obtained by questionnaires mailed to executives of the 130 hospitals. In total, 90 responses were received (including 43 public hospitals and 47 private hospitals), representing an overall response rate of 69.23%. Non-responding hospitals included 15 public hospitals and 25 private hospitals; the means of their inputs and outputs are significantly smaller than those of the responding hospitals. Thus, the final sample in general better represents the behavior of larger hospitals and hospitals of higher accreditation status in Taiwan. The results obtained in the study, as a result, are not readily generalized to all hospitals, but are a reasonable sample for the purposes of this study.

We merge the data for three years and calculate efficiency scores for the entire data set. Thus, we have a total of 270 observations with which relative efficiency of each observation is calculated.

Identifying Relevant Outputs and Inputs
We define inefficiencies as the differences between the actual output and the maximum feasible output. Based on prior literature (Lo et al., 1996;

Valdmanis, 1990) and suggestions from the hospital executives, we define inputs as the number of physicians (including dentists), the number of nurses, the number of other ancillary labors (e.g., pharmacist, dietitian, etc.), and the number of hospital beds. Outputs consist of total acute care inpatient days, total intensive care inpatient days (patients with severe illnesses are defined here as patients in intensive care, who receive a more complex and costly set of services), the number of admissions, the number of surgeries, the number of ambulatory visits, and the number of emergency visits.

Tobit Regression
Since efficiency scores computed from the DEA model are censored at one, an Ordinary Least Squares (OLS) regression will produce biased and inconsistent parameter estimates (Greene, 1997). Tobit analysis assumes that the dependent variable has a number of its values clustered at a limiting value. A convenient normalization in the literature is to assume a censoring point at zero.

The Effects of Hospital–Physician Integration Strategies

We mailed questionnaires to superintendents of the sample hospitals to gather information regarding specific hospital–physician integration strategies they implemented. As each strategy involves subtle organizational arrangements, we called each hospital to speak to the person who filled out the questionnaires (in many cases not the superintendent himself, but senior administrators in charge of related managerial duties) to confirm the information provided or remove any ambiguity (see Table 1). Here, RC, TQM, and PF denote the implementation of the responsibility centers , total quality management, and physician fee programs, respectively.

Responsibility Centers (RC)
The responsibility centers (RC) system holds employees of each department in the hospitals accountable for their performances; in return, it offers employees higher degree of autonomy concerning resource allocation. As a result, they may have incentives to control costs (e.g., cost centers) and enhance outputs (e.g., profit centers), and such efforts lead to higher efficiency. Although no empirical evidence exists concerning the efficiency effect of implementing the RC, Melumad, Mookherjee, and Reichelstein (1992) used an agency model to show theoretically that a RC system is better

Table 1.   The Types of Hospital–Physician Integration Strategies
Implemented by the Sample Hospitals.

Periods	Responsibility Centers		Total Quality Management		Physician Fee Program	
	Implemented	Not Implemented	Implemented	Not Implemented	Implemented	Not Implemented
1994	20	70	16	74	50	40
1995	23	67	25	65	57	33
1996	25	65	34	56	62	28

than a direct tight control over agents (physicians) when the agents cannot reveal their private information in full detail to the owner (hospitals). We believe the situation is likely to occur in the hospital setting given the medical expertise held by physicians. Thus, a RC system is expected to enhance efficiency in our analysis.

Total Quality Management (TQM) Programs

According to Deming (1986), the TQM philosophy causes a chain reaction. The prospective and continuous re-assessment of work processes and inputs yields improved quality. Improved quality results in better resource usage (lower costs) because improved processes result in less rework, fewer mistakes and delays. Although the underlying principles of TQM are generally accepted, Huq and Martin (2000) indicated high failure rates of TQM because of ineffective implementation systems. Thus, it would not be a surprise if no efficiency effects were found for hospitals identified as TQM sites. Although extant studies have not provided consistent results for the efficiency effects of TQM implementation, theoretically TQM, if done properly, is expected to enhance efficiency.

Physician Fee (PF) Programs

RC and TQM programs tend to encourage teamwork, an essential part in health care delivery. Although culture factors have been shown important in promoting teamwork (Huq & Martin, 2000; Shortell et al., 1995), hospitals may find compensation schemes which are directly associated with physician performances useful in balancing group and individual incentives. In Taiwan, many hospitals have implemented PF programs in which physicians' bonuses are computed based on medical revenues they generated. As the reimbursement scheme in Taiwan is still mainly based on fee-for-service, physicians should have incentives to expand medical services under the PF programs.

Control Variables

Besides the hospital–physician integration strategies, several relevant variables that may affect hospital efficiency based on prior literature are controlled. They are hospital size (LBED), degree of competition (COM), ownership structure (OWN), teaching status (TEA), and the effects of the implementation of NHI (Year1, Year2)

Results

The descriptive statistics of inputs and outputs used in this study are reported in Table 2. We found that differences in inputs and outputs of the sample hospitals are substantial (e.g., standard deviation of the number of hospital beds equals 545), suggesting that the sample may contain quite heterogeneous hospitals. The results indicate a need to control for

Table 2. Descriptive Statistics of the Sample Hospitals ($N = 270$).

	Mean	Standard Deviation	Minimum	Maximum
Inputs				
The number of physicians	112	161	3	970
The number of nurses	302	469	9	3,995
The number of other ancillary labors	63	76	4	436
The number of hospital beds	489	545	101	3,727
Outputs				
Total acute care inpatient days during the year	123,658	166,464	1,424	1,156,370
Total intensive care inpatient days during the year	114,499	161,725	1,419	1,132,715
The number of admissions during the year	14,808	18,631	80	136,360
The number of surgeries during the year	8,748	13,460	163	84,372
The number of ambulatory visits during the year	401,965	427,352	40,291	2,295,082
The number of emergency visits during the year	28,866	25,998	100	125,463

differences in hospital size. As discussed before, we use the number of hospital beds as proxy of hospital size in the tobit model. The measure would be useful to mitigate confounding effects resulting from variation in hospital size because the number of hospital beds has very high Pearson correlation coefficients with all input and output variables (ranging from 0.77 to 0.99). Although we require hospitals, conduct at least one hospitalwide TQM activity in the sample year to be included as TQM site; on average the TQM hospitals had 7 hospital-wide activities in 1994, 9 activities in 1995, and 10 activities in 1996. The trend suggests an increase in intensity to implement TQM over the sample period.

Tests of Effects of Implementing the Hospital–Physician Integration Strategies
We use asymptotic DEA-based tests to examine whether hospitals that implemented the specific hospital–physician integration strategies performed better than those hospitals that did not. We find hospitals that implemented RC ($F = 5.12$, $p<0.001$; $F = 16.86$, $p<0.002$), TQM ($F = 1.66$, $p<0.03$; $F = 4.16$, $p<0.001$), or PF programs ($F = 1.87$, $p<0.001$; $F = 1.81$, $p<0.001$) are more efficient than those that did not.

Tests of Tobit Regression
We find only the coefficient associated with PF programs is significant ($t = -2.88$, $p<0.001$). That is, the hospitals that implemented PF programs performed better than those hospitals that did not; in contrast, implementing RC and TQM programs are insignificant to efficiency, after controlling for other selected factors.

Concerning the results of control variables, first, the sign of LBED is negative and significant ($t = -4.32$, $p<0.001$), i.e., average efficiency in larger hospitals is significantly higher. Second, hospital efficiency increases as the COM decreases ($t = -2.99$, $p = 0.003$). Third, the OWN1 are less efficient than non-for-profit hospitals ($t = 3.70$, $p<0.001$). For-profit hospitals (OWN2) are more efficient than non-for-profit hospitals ($t = -2.42$, $p = 0.015$). Fourth, TEA are less efficient than non-teaching hospitals ($t = 2.87$, $p = 0.004$). Finally, we do not find any significant NHI effect (Year1 and Year2), indicating even a major health policy change (i.e., NHI) would not affect hospital technical efficiency automatically.

To capture the possible time-lagged effects of implementing the hospital–physician integration strategies, we conduct further tests by requiring that sample hospitals implement the strategies for at least 2 years. The requirement is particularly relevant to TQM because TQM is a cultural change and it may take a long period to observe its effect. We find hospitals that implemented PF programs ($t = -3.54$, $p < 0.001$) for at least 2 years performed better than those hospitals that did not; the effect of TQM (TM) becomes significant ($t = -2.78$, $p = 0.027$). The effect of RC, however, is still insignificant.

We also consider how the RC system is linked to performance evaluation. We redefine that RC equals one if the hospital implemented the RC system and integrated it with incentive programs in which physicians' performance was evaluated at least in part based on departmental profits for at least one year; and RC equals zero otherwise. The findings indicate that hospitals, which implemented the RC system and integrated it with formal incentive programs for physicians performed better than those hospitals that did not ($t = -3.06$, $p = 0.028$). The effect of PF programs ($t = -3.11$, $p < 0.001$) is significant, but the coefficient associated with the TQM (TM) is insignificant.

We also use asymptotic DEA-based tests to examine whether hospitals that implemented the RC and integrated it with incentive programs for physicians performed better than those hospitals that implemented the RC system, but without relating it to formal performance evaluation mechanism. The result shows that average efficiency in the former case is significantly higher than that of the later case. It suggests that when hospitals implement the RC system, to be effective, they should integrate it with formal physician incentive programs.

Discussion

In this study, we examine the effects of implementing the RC system, TQM, and PF programs on technical efficiency for Taiwan hospitals. Several interesting results are found and many possible future extensions can be pursued.

First, we find the importance of controlling for other relevant hospital–physician integration strategies that the hospitals may use. When examining each strategy individually, they are all very effective statistically. By contrast, the results look quite different when the three strategies are considered simultaneously, together with other control variables, in the tobit regression. As all prior studies investigate one hospital–physician integration strategy at a time, the study indicates the potential bias of such an approach and proposes an alternative of examining hospital–physician integration strategies as a portfolio.

Second, we find that the efficiency effect of the PF programs is very robust across different model specifications. The result may be because that the reimbursement schemes in Taiwan are mainly based on fee-for-service and the PF programs leave physicians a predictable way of maximizing income.

Third, the effect of TQM programs is significant only when they were implemented for at least two years. The result suggested TQM transition is a long time cultural change and its effect, if any, would be observed only after an extended period. Thus, persistent implementation of TQM is crucial to success. As Shortell et al.(1995) indicated that organizational culture plays a critical role in TQM implementation and subsequent effects on clinical efficiency, how Taiwan hospitals fit into organizational culture typology proposed in the literature, and what are the resulting effects would be interesting research topics to pursue.

Fourth, hospitals that implemented the RC system perform better than those hospitals that did not only in the situation when the system was integrated with formal incentive schemes (e.g., paid in part based on departmental profits). One implication of the result is that in the staff model team-based incentives can be used to motivate efficiency. Chu, Liu, and Romeis (2002) found that a RC system provides incentives for physicians to participate in correcting flaws in hospital accounting system because of the concern over performance evaluation. An improved accounting system enables hospitals to obtain accurate feedback for all managerial initiatives. The potential spill-over effect suggests the need to examine the hospital–physician integration strategies as a portfolio.

To U.S. health services researchers, Taiwan hospitals look like early stage staff-model HMOs. PF programs are shown to be effective incentives under their current NHI single payer system. As NHI adds more DRG-type constraints (case payments) and moves toward global budgets, it remains to be seen whether such incentives will continue to work as they appear now or they will change in the ways similar to U.S. hospitals. Accordingly, health services researchers, here, there, and other international settings need to monitor relationships between changes in macro policy and effective physician-integrations strategies for a given set of outcomes. The cumulative effect of such studies will significantly improve the value of the field, the systems we study and managerial decision-making.

STUDY 2: OUTPATIENT PRESCRIPTION DRUG CO-PAYMENT POLICY AND THE ELDERLY

Our second study (Liu & Romeis, 2003) examines changes in drug utilization following Taiwan's newly implemented NHI outpatient prescription drug cost-sharing program for persons over 65 years old. The study has particular relevance to the U.S. as it struggles to estimate cost and coverage for its older citizens as recently proposed by the Bush administration.

In the pre-NHI era, uninsured older Taiwanese paid for their care, including prescriptions, out-of-pocket. The NHI experienced its first operational loss in 1998, mainly because of the rapid increase in medical expenditures, especially its outpatient costs. Furthermore, drug costs have been the most important item of outpatient costs (about 33.3%), with an annual rate of increase of about 13%. We use variance analysis, a widely accepted methodology among accountants, as an attention-directing tool for policy analysis. This is coupled with regression analysis to refine the analysis.

Taiwan's Prescription Drug Co-Payment Program

To constrain the rapid increase in drug costs, the NHI implemented an outpatient prescription drug cost-sharing program beginning August 1, 1999. The program imposed no charge for outpatient prescriptions costing less than $3.125 (lower bound of the cost-sharing schedule). An additional charge of $0.625 was imposed for every increase in drug costs of $3.125 up to $15.625 (upper bound of the cost-sharing schedule) was met. All data are converted into US$ (1 US$ equals 32 NT$).

In Taiwan, prescribed medications typically are for only a few days and, thus require multiple visits for a 10–30 day supply. Refill visits also require an outpatient visit charge. Frequent outpatient visits occurred for two reasons: (1) Co-payments were low and designed to encourage patients to use clinics rather than medical centers (e.g., about $1.5 for clinics and $4.7 for medical centers). (2) The NHI reimbursement system for physicians, mainly fee-for-service, adds to physicians' incentives to increase outpatient visits.

Selected patient groups and situations were exempted from the cost-sharing program. These included: veterans, people with low incomes (earning less than 60% of average personal consumption level in the community), emergency visits, major illness (e.g., renal failure), preventive care, and people with continued prescriptions for chronic diseases. The provision to exempt continued prescriptions for chronic diseases was intended to reduce unnecessary outpatient visits for refills. Patients with chronic diseases in stable conditions can be put under this exemption provision to receive free medications for up to 30 days; the prescriptions can be refilled once. Because most patients obtain outpatient prescription drugs directly from pharmacies in hospitals after visits, Taiwan physicians strongly influence their patients' drug utilization behavior.

Sample and Method

The study hospitals for Study 2 are identical to those described in Study 1. The NHI reduced about 10,000 items of the drug reimbursement rates (49% out of total) beginning April 1, 2000. Including data after March 31st has severe confounding effects, i.e., a reduction in drug costs may come from a decrease in reimbursement rates instead of the drug cost-sharing program. Thus, our drug cost-sharing period is from August 1, 1999 to March 31, 2000 and the corresponding period of August 1, 1998 to March 31, 1999 refers to the pre-cost-sharing period. The match of sample periods reduces biases arising from monthly differences in drug utilization; it also mitigates autocorrelation in the time-series data because continuous monthly data were broken (i.e., April to July data in 1999 were excluded).

Our data were obtained from hospital outpatient claims submitted to the BNHI, and are the most reliable and valid available for this level of analysis. We focus on selected outpatient drug utilization measures instead of individual patient profiling (Tamblyn et al., 2001). Patient profiling would encounter a bias here because if patients stop appearing in our data set they may seek treatments in clinics or hospitals not in our sample (they most likely were still in the NHI system because nearly all health institutions had signed contracts with the NHI) instead of being affected by the cost-sharing program. We believe our measures better capture the drug utilization behavior of older patients given the stratified random sampling method.

Variance Analysis Method

Variance analysis has long been found useful in management control and strategic analysis. We use it as an attention-directing tool for policy analysis and health services research. Variance analysis helps managers better understand possible reasons of irregularity in costs and sales (Horngren, Foster, & Datar, 1999). Shank and Govindarajan (1993) apply variance analysis to investigate changes in market size and market share resulting from strategic positioning. Variance is generally defined as the difference between an actual result and a budgeted amount. The budgeted amount is a benchmark, a point of reference from which comparisons can be made.

Variance analysis decomposes the overall effect of a policy into the sum of variances of several specific factors important to policy-makers. The variance of each specific factor can be further decomposed into sub-levels of analyses. The process can be carried on repeatedly until the most fundamental factors are found. Thus, policy-makers can make quick diagnosis and take corrective action more effectively. The variance analysis method is a descriptive analysis and is not related to any form of statistical inferences (e.g., ANOVA).

The variance analysis method introduced here has two important characteristics. First, the total prescription drug cost variance equals the sum of lower level sub-variances. For example, the change in drug costs after the cost-sharing policy can be attributed to changes in average prescription cost and changes in volume of prescriptions. Second, the sub-variances are the factors often used as measures concerning the impact of drug policies. Thus, they should be useful to policy-makers concerning program evaluation.

Regression Analysis
An increase in drug costs per prescription and an increase in duration explain a large portion of cost variances for the cost-sharing group and non-cost-sharing group, respectively. We apply cross-sectional regression analysis to explain their increases.

We classify explanatory variables as policy effect variables and control variables. Direct policy effects are measured by a dummy variable CSP (equals 1 if the observation is from the cost-sharing period). Indirect policy effects occur because of characteristics of the cost-sharing schedule. Physicians may increase drug utilization (e.g., prescribing more expensive drugs or longer duration) if prescription costs are deemed to exceed the upper bound. When prescription costs close to the lower bound, physicians may act as the patients' economic agent (Eisenberg, 2002) by reducing drugs prescribed to avoid co-payments. Using prescriptions subject to co-payments as the base group, we let *Upper* $= 1$ if the prescription has drug costs beyond the upper bound, and *Lower* equal to one if the prescription has drug costs below the lower bound. The indirect policy effects are measured by interaction of dummy variables – *Upper*$*$*CSP* and *Lower*$*$*CSP*.

The control variables include disease types, case mix (using accreditation status as proxy; local community hospitals serve as the base group), ownership types (private hospitals serve as the base group), age, sex, and duration.

Concerning drug cost per prescription, the OLS regression for the cost-sharing group is Drug costs per prescription

$$= \alpha_0 + \alpha_1 \, CSP + \alpha_2 \, Upper * CSP + \alpha_3 \, Lower * CSP + \alpha_4 \, Chronic$$
$$+ \alpha_5 Medical + \alpha_6 Metropolitan + \alpha_7 Public + \alpha_8 Non\text{-}Profit + \alpha_9 Sex$$
$$+ \alpha_{10} Age + \alpha_{11} Duration \ldots \tag{1}$$

The OLS regression for the non-cost-sharing group is Drug costs per prescription

$$= \beta_0 + \beta_1 CSP + \beta_2 Medical + \beta_3 Metropolitan + \beta_4 Public + \beta_5 Non\text{-}profit$$
$$+ \beta_6 Sex + \beta_7 Age + \beta_8 Extended + \beta_9 Dialysis \ldots \tag{2}$$

The OLS regression for the non-cost-sharing group is Prescription duration

$$= \gamma_0 + \gamma_1 CSP + \gamma_2 Medical + \gamma_3 Metropolitan + \gamma_4 Public$$
$$+ \gamma_5 Non\text{-}profit + \gamma_6 Sex + \gamma_7 Age + \gamma_8 Extended + \gamma_9 Dialysis \ldots \tag{3}$$

The OLS regression of duration for the cost-sharing group is Prescription duration

$$= \delta_0 + \delta_1 CSP + \delta_2 Upper * CSP + \delta_3 Lower * CSP$$
$$+ \delta_4 Chronic + \delta_5 Medical + \delta_6 Metropolitan$$
$$+ \delta_7 Public + \delta_8 Non\text{-}profit + \delta_9 Sex + \delta_{10} Age \ldots \tag{4}$$

Results

Descriptive Statistics

Table 3 presents descriptive statistics. In the pre-drug cost-sharing period, 1,522,029 prescriptions were included, and 1,604,928 prescriptions were included in the drug cost-sharing period. The non-cost-sharing group was much smaller in terms of the number of prescriptions compared to the cost-sharing group and expected because of NHI policy regarding exemptions. The sample had more prescriptions from male patients than from female patients, reflecting the national demographic structure that the male elderly population was about 9.5% larger than the female elderly population. In our study, the majority (about 60%) of prescriptions came from medical centers. There was a small decrease in the number of prescriptions for local community hospitals (-3.33% in the cost-sharing group and -2.04% in the non-cost-sharing group). By contrast, there was a significant increase in the

Table 3. Sample Descriptive Statistics.

Total Sample	Pre cost-Sharing Period = 1,522,029 prescriptions; 228,444 patients; Cost-Sharing Period = 1,604,928 Prescriptions; 241,585 Patients					
	Cost-Sharing Group			Non Cost-Sharing Group		
	Pre Cost-Sharing Period (% of total)	Cost-Sharing Period (% of total)	Change in number of prescriptions (%)	Pre Cost-Sharing Period (% of total)	Cost-Sharing Period (% of total)	Change in number of Prescription (%)
Total Prescriptions	96.24	95.57	4.72	3.76	4.43	24.07
Sex						
Male	62.75	61.54	3.41	2.55	2.91	20.57
Female	33.49	34.03	7.16	1.21	1.51	31.43
Age						
65–69	28.97	25.89	−5.74	0.99	1.07	14.64
70–74	32.99	33.01	5.52	1.21	1.42	23.37
75–84	30.71	32.52	11.66	1.31	1.62	30.50
Over 85	3.57	4.15	22.44	0.25	0.31	31.17
Accreditation Status						
Medical Centers	62.40	62.83	0.69	2.54	3.12	22.83
Metropolitan Hospitals	16.44	18.93	15.15	0.74	0.83	12.16
Local Community Hospitals	17.40	16.82	−3.33	0.49	0.48	−2.04

number of prescription for metropolitan hospitals (15.15%) in the cost-sharing group and for medical centers in the non-cost-sharing group (22.83%). It suggests a possible shift of outpatient visits toward hospitals of higher accreditation status.

Average duration per prescription differed significantly across situations. For acute conditions, it was 4.9 days for the cost-sharing group, 2.3 days for the non-cost-sharing group. By contrast, average duration for chronic conditions was 22.3 days for the cost-sharing group, 29.8 days for the non-cost-sharing group. The results suggest a difference in case mix, which needs to be controlled in the analysis.

Results of Variance Analysis
In Fig. 1, we observe a significant increase in total prescription drug costs in the cost-sharing group (about 12.86%), indicating an ineffective outcome of cost containment. The main driver of drug costs is an increase in average drug price per prescription (69.20%). The second major factor influencing drug costs is an increase in the total number of patients (35.78%). Finally, average drug items per prescription decreases and results in a favorable variance of drug costs (−25.38%).

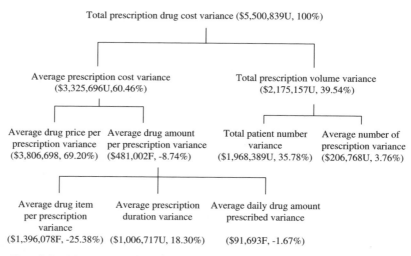

Total prescription drug cost variance ($5,500,839U, 100%)

Average prescription cost variance ($3,325,696U, 60.46%)

Total prescription volume variance ($2,175,157U, 39.54%)

Average drug price per prescription variance ($3,806,698, 69.20%)

Average drug amount per prescription variance ($481,002F, -8.74%)

Total patient number variance ($1,968,389U, 35.78%)

Average number of prescription variance ($206,768U, 3.76%)

Average drug item per prescription variance ($1,396,078F, -25.38%)

Average prescription duration variance ($1,006,717U, 18.30%)

Average daily drug amount prescribed variance ($91,693F, -1.67%)

Note: U stands for unfavorable variance, i.e., drug costs increase after the policy.
   F stands for favorable variance, i.e., drug costs decrease after the policy.

Fig. 1.   Variance Analysis for Prescription Drug Costs of the Cost-Sharing Group.

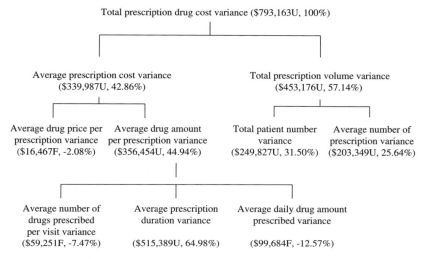

Note: U stands for unfavorable variance; i.e., drug costs increase after the policy.
F stands for favorable variance; i.e., drug costs decrease after the policy.

Fig. 2. Variance Analysis for Prescription Drug Costs of the Non Cost-Sharing Group.

The non-cost-sharing group has much higher increase rate in drug costs (51.42%) than that of the cost-sharing group. As shown in Fig. 2, the main factor contributing to the increase in drug costs is an increase in average prescription duration (64.98%), followed by an increase in the total patient number (31.50%) and average number of prescription per patient (25.64%). Average drug price per prescription, the main cost driver for the cost-sharing group, shows an opposite trend (−2.08%) in the non-cost-sharing group. The phenomenon arises from existing and continued prescriptions for older adults with chronic diseases. As these prescriptions are exempt from the cost-sharing program, more patients take advantage of the provision, resulting in longer average duration and more prescriptions per person. There were 5,621 patients under the extended prescription for chronic diseases before the cost-sharing program; the number jumped to 9,117 patients in the cost-sharing period, an increase rate of 62.2%.

Results of Regression Analysis
The regression analysis suggests that the cost-sharing program has significant effects on drug cost per prescription. In the cost-sharing period (*CSP*),

on average drug cost per prescription decreases significantly ($t = -276.72$, $p<0.0001$) compares to that in the pre-cost-sharing period. We also observe very strong interaction effects. For prescriptions with costs above the upper bound (*Upper*CSP*), drug cost per prescription is much higher in the cost-sharing period than in the pre-cost-sharing period ($t = 484.31$, $p<0.0001$). For prescriptions with costs below the lower bound (*Lower*CSP*), drug cost per prescription is slightly lower in the cost-sharing period than in the pre-cost-sharing period ($t = -7.37$, $p<0.0001$).

Concerning the control variables, patients with chronic diseases (*Chronic*) incur higher drug cost per prescription that those without chronic diseases ($t = 31.34$, $p<0.0001$). Medical centers (*Medical*) and metropolitan hospitals (*Metropolitan*) have higher drug cost per prescription than that of local community hospitals ($t = 56$, $p<0.0001$; $t = 21.3$, $p<0.0001$). Public hospitals (*Public*) have lower drug cost per prescription than private hospitals ($t = -25.01$, $p<0.0001$); non-profit hospitals (*Nonprofit*) have higher drug cost per prescription than private hospitals ($t = 17.87$, $p<0.0001$). Male patients (*Sex*) incur higher drug costs than female patients ($t = 13.97$, $p <0.0001$). Because of its small coefficient (-0.03), age (*Age*) has little influence on drug costs per prescription although it is statistically significant ($t = -9.61$, $p<0.0001$). Finally, prescriptions with longer duration (*Duration*) have higher drug cost per prescription ($t = 507.52$, $p<0.0001$).

For the non-cost-sharing group, in the cost-sharing period (*CSP*), drug cost per prescription increases significantly compares to that in the pre-cost-sharing period ($t = 12.90$, $p<0.0001$). Concerning the control variables, patients in medical centers (*Medical*) have much higher drug cost per prescription than it is in local community hospitals ($t = 26.59$, $p<0.0001$). As expected, patients with extended prescription for chronic diseases (*Extended*) are found to have much higher drug cost per prescription ($t = 48$, $p<0.0001$), so are patients under treatments for renal failures (*Dialysis*) ($t = 403.25$, $p<0.0001$).

Concerning duration for the non-cost-sharing group, *CSP* is statistically significant ($t = 11.22$, $p<0.0001$). Its coefficient is relatively small (0.10), indicating a minor effect on duration. *Extended* appears to be the most important factor for duration in terms of the size of coefficient (27.31) and level of statistical significance ($t = 2383.26$, $p<0.0001$). In addition, outpatient visits for renal failures (*Dialysis*) have significant longer duration than emergency and preventive care visits ($t = 206.58$, $p<0.0001$).

For the cost-sharing group, in the cost-sharing period, on average duration decreases significantly ($t = -374.34$, $p<0.0001$). Concerning the interaction effects, duration is longer for prescriptions above the upper bound (*Upper*∗*CSP*, $t = 614.41$, $p < 0.0001$) in the cost-sharing period than in the pre-cost-sharing period. By contrast, duration is shorter for prescriptions below the lower bound (*Lower*∗*CSP*) in the cost-sharing period ($t = -64.78$, $p < 0.0001$) than in the pre-cost-sharing period. Patients with chronic diseases (*Chronic*) have significantly longer duration than other patients ($t = 879.93$, $p < 0.0001$).

The regression equations have very large *F*-values, suggesting inclusion of relevant variables. Also, they have reasonable explanatory power with adjusted R^2 ranging from 0.29–0.98.

Discussion

The initial effects of the outpatient prescription drug cost-sharing program implemented by the NHI in Taiwan did not reverse the trend of drug cost increases among elderly Taiwanese. However, the fees collected from the program did somewhat help the financing of the NHI program. We found differential effects of the drug cost-sharing program based on the variance analysis method. The main reason of drug cost increase for the cost-sharing group is attributed to an increase in drug price per prescription; the main factor contributing to the increase in drug costs for the non-cost-sharing group is an increase in prescription duration.

Results of our regression analysis suggest that the cost-sharing program generally discourages drug utilization. The interaction effects indicate, however, that for prescriptions with drug costs above the upper bound of cost-sharing schedule drug cost per prescription and duration both increased significantly for the cost-sharing group in the cost-sharing period. This could be the main reason why we observe large unfavorable average prescription cost variance.

Did prices of prescription drug become more expensive in the cost-sharing period given the same drug mix? An increase in average drug cost per prescription in the cost-sharing period is unlikely because of drug price increases: (1) NHI generally marks down drug prices, (2) newly added drugs (usually not new drugs) were not necessarily more expensive, and (3) the percentage of changes as indicated above was very small.

Did patients become sicker and thus justify higher drug utilization? Given the short sample period and large number of prescriptions involved (results are not likely affected by extreme cases), changes in health status on the part of patients do not probably explain the observed increase in drug cost per prescription in the cost-sharing period. A more plausible explanation is that physicians prescribed more expensive drugs, and prescribe them for longer duration especially when drug costs exceeding the upper bound of co-payments.

The significant increase in average drug price per prescription indicates that many prescriptions may move above the upper bound of the cost-sharing schedule. Further examination reveals that the most significant increase in drug costs came from prescriptions over $78.125. Thus, revising the upper bound above $78.125 can be an option for policy-makers to address the cost control issue.

Our data only contain information related to outpatient drug utilization. We are unable to infer changes in health outcomes by examining consumption of other health care goods (e.g., hospitalization). A useful approximation of health outcomes is to analyze the changes in essential and non-essential drugs. We classify drugs in our database as essential drugs if they are in the WHO (1999) model list of essential medicines ("Access to essential drugs," 1999); otherwise, they are classified as non-essential drugs. We conducted similar regression analysis, and found for the cost-sharing group there was a decrease in essential drug costs per prescription in the cost-sharing period while an increase in non-essential drug costs per prescription. By contrast, for the non-cost-sharing group both essential and non-essential drug costs per prescription increased in the cost-sharing period. It suggests a potential substitution effect between essential and non-essential drugs related to the drug cost-sharing program (Chu, Liu, Romeis, Tseng, & Lin, 2005). If so, the co-payments, exerting pressure on patients regardless of their medical necessity, may threaten patients' well-being and create ethical concerns (Burton, Randel, Titlow, & Emanuel, 2001). However, a lack of detailed clinical data makes it difficult to conclude whether the changes had adverse effects on health outcomes in the elderly.

Several limitations exist in the study. First, our regression analysis is based on before–after study designs, and is weak in assessing policy outcomes causality. Second, the study focuses on outpatient drug utilization behavior for the elderly based on a sample of hospitals in Taipei. Hospitals deserve special attention because they represent about two-thirds of the total outpatient prescription drug costs incurred in Taiwan. Since outpatient drug costs in clinics were excluded from our analysis, the study cannot evaluate the overall impact of the cost-sharing program. Third, the study may overestimate the influence of medical centers and male patients. We drew observations mainly from medical centers. In Taiwan, regardless of age groups about 28.40% of outpatient prescriptions came from medical centers, 30.37% from metropolitan hospitals, and 41.23%

from local community hospitals (BNHI, 2001). In our sample, the distribution of outpatient prescriptions was about 64.94% from medical centers, 17.18% from metropolitan hospitals, and 17.88% from local community hospitals. It reflects high concentration of medical centers and older patients' strong preferences for medical centers in rich metropolitan areas like Taipei. In addition, the ratio of men to women is 1.11 in Taiwan, 1.17 in Taipei, and 1.3 in this study. Male patients appear to be over-represented.

To better control the increase in outpatient prescription drug costs, the NHI reduced about 10,000 items of the drug reimbursement rates beginning April 1, 2000, the largest such action ever. Further, research on the effect of this reduction should be very instructive for health policy researchers in Taiwan and elsewhere.

UNFINISHED BUSINESS, INNOVATIONS, AND HORIZON ISSUES

Any country's health care policy always has lengthy lists of unfinished business and issues on the horizon. Because they have essentially solved their access problems, Taiwan's unfinished business lists primarily include managing their financing and implementing quality mechanisms. In this section, we also address an issue that is on Taiwan's horizon as well as many other nations. We point to preliminary results on the economic and operational impact of Severe Acute Respiratory Syndrome (SARS) on the most prestigious academic medical center in Taiwan – one of the horizon issues we choose to highlight.

Unfinished Business

Financing the NHI Deficit
Taiwan's NHI had significant operating surpluses in its first three years of implementation partly because of favorable actuarial assumptions. In the first five years, however, the average increase in NHI expenditure was about 10%, and the average increase rate of NHI revenues was less than 4%. Thus, NHI has experienced operating deficits since 1998, and in 2002 the NHI raised the insurance premium slightly for the first time. The NHI is now close to its long-term break-even point.

To ensure the long-term financial feasibility, Taiwan's Law of National Health Insurance includes a provision that NHI should increase the premium when its accumulated surplus is smaller than one month of the average health expenditure. During 2003–2004, the NHI accumulated surplus is about 30% of the average NHI monthly expenditure, well below the mandated minimum. In the original design, the NHI premium is expected to adjust automatically to maintain financial feasibility of the program. However, the Congress scrutinized the premium increase motion proposed by the BNHI with great caution. As a compulsory policy, insurance premium increases are like tax increases – difficult to implement especially during recessionary periods. The NHI is expected to have continued difficulty implementing future compulsory premium increases.

The development has important implications for the health care market. Anticipating a tight control of NHI expenditures, health care providers are reluctant to offer new services proposed by the NHI, and have aggressively expanded their services outside the menu of NHI coverage such as comprehensive physical examinations (many similar to VIP health clubs that target wealthy executives) and cosmetic surgeries. To what degree these new out-of-pocket services moves dilutes the quality and access of regular NHI services would be important issues to assess. In addition to management initiatives such as TQM and Activity-Based Costing, many Taiwan hospitals are experimenting with Balanced Scorecard (BSC) – a strategic management approach pioneered by Kaplan and Norton (1996, 2001, 2004) to make them more strategy-focused. The impact of implementing BSC in Taiwan hospitals would be an interesting research topic.

Global Budget System
Taiwan's NHI first experimented with the global budget system for private dental clinics in 1998. With the inclusion of hospitals in 2002, the NHI has moved into the era of full global budget system. In the system, health care organization reimbursements are based on accumulated floating points calculated for the six NHI divisions, respectively. Currently, the average dollar worth of each point is approximately 0.9 for hospitals and clinics in divisions with a high intensity of medical resources (e.g., the Taipei metropolitan area). However, the dollar worth of each point is higher than 1.0 for divisions in remote areas with fewer medical resources (e.g., eastern Taiwan). The situation has differential impacts on health care providers. It created severe financial problems for health providers in more competitive markets because their net profit ratio is usually below 10%. In contrast, health providers in areas with fewer health care resources now are

financially better off. This may redirect the allocation of health care resources in different regions of Taiwan, and thus influence hospital managers to alter services in ways that may not reflect demand or be an efficient use of resources.

Many health care organizations used to use PF programs to encourage higher volume of services performed (e.g., staff model HMO example above; Chu et al., 2002, 2003). However, providing more health services may not be wise under the global budget system because the more services provided the higher the loss if the value of floating points becomes small. Furthermore, if they reduce their volume of services but competitors do not, they suffer financially because of a reduction in their market share. Moreover, if every health care organization keeps pushing for a higher volume of services, everyone is worse-off because the dollar worth for each point will be much less than one dollar. Clearly, health care organizations will benefit from better monitoring excessive providers of services and the mechanism is still pre-mature. Health executives need to consider changing the financial incentives that are mainly based upon volume of services provided. The health regulators should watch for the adverse financial effects of global budget system on hospitals as many smaller hospitals experienced financial distress and could be forced out of the market.

Since the establishment of NHI, small- and medium-size hospitals have been placed in a disadvantaged position because they are not nimble enough to react to patient needs like small clinics; and they lack the brand name and resources to compete with large hospitals and medical centers. In the first years after NHI's implementation, large hospitals, especially medical centers, expanded their scale aggressively to increase their market share. Further, large hospitals were more likely to introduce various types of hospital–physician integration strategies to improve their efficiency and effectiveness. This led to a gap between the organizational strength of smaller/ medium hospitals and large hospitals. NHI should pay special attention to those hospitals in weak competitive conditions and what are the consequences for the provision of services in their regions.

Long waiting list for patients is a complaint that often occurs for countries implementing global budget systems (e.g., Canada). The problem arises because when capitation is imposed upon individual hospitals; there are no incentives for them to continue to provide services once the level of capitation is achieved. However, in the initial stage of the global budget system the concern over long waiting lists appears insignificant in Taiwan; hospitals have to compete for market share because the budget is set for each NHI division that has many hospitals. In 2004, the NHI experimented with a

Canadian type of capitation for selected academic medical centers and created long waiting lists immediately. Because of severe negative responses from the public, NHI decided to stop the experiment in 2005. The incident suggests that health care organizations worldwide respond to financial incentives in a very predictable way.

Control of Drug Costs

Although drug costs are included as a part of the global budget system, drugs are reimbursed based on a fixed reimbursement rate schedule (one dollar for one point) instead of floating points for other health services. Thus, significant increases in drug expenditures will reduce the amount left for other health services. To mitigate the moral hazard problem in drug utilization, the NHI further expanded the scale of outpatient prescription drug co-payment schedule. The upper ceiling of the co-payment is now 1,000 NT\$ (with co-payments = 200 NT\$) instead of 500 NT\$ (with co-payment = 100 NT\$) in 2000.

Further, the NHI is aggressively reducing the reimbursement rates for prescription drugs. Preliminary data by Chu et al. (submitted) investigates the initial effects of Taiwan's prescription drug reimbursement rate reduction policy in the elderly with hypertension based on outpatient treatment data. About 477,000 outpatient prescriptions or about 137,000 patients aged 65 and older with hypertension were drawn from 21 hospitals in the Taipei area for the study using a stratified random sampling method.

The study indicated that about 8,900 items of drugs (roughly 45% of the total) experienced rate reductions in the NHI formulary. Those drugs, however, appeared only in about 3% of prescriptions. Thus, the policy had limited impact on total outpatient drug expenditures. The study found evidence that physicians substituted drugs experiencing rate reductions with drug experiencing no rate reductions. However, physicians appeared to be reluctant in reducing the use of essential drugs even when facing rate reductions, possibly attempting to avoid an adverse health outcome. The results may suggest less concern over the quality of health service because of the policy. Overall, the NHI reimbursement rate reduction policy offers a mechanism to change prescribing behavior of physicians by reducing excessive profits on certain drug items based upon reliable database of reported drug transaction prices. The NHI implemented further drug rate reduction policy, which targeted drug of higher utilization in 2002 and 2003. Future studies are needed to examine the effects of the follow-up policies because they would have larger impact on drug cost control.

Enhancing Quality Control

Controlling health expenditures is anticipated, and thus the NHI directs increased attention to quality of health services. The Department of Health has systematically and consistently fostered the continued import, internal development and diffusion of a variety of quality assessment, and improvement methodologies. These have included:

* continued refinement and monitoring of profession-specific and hospital quality assurance programs (Huang, 1996);
* application of new external peer review techniques in hospital accreditation processes (Huang, Hsu, Kai-Yuan, & Hsueh, 2000);
* implementation of hospital quality management/process improvement initiatives such as TQM/ Continuous Quality Improvement (Counte & Meurer, 2001);
* a comprehensive hospital outcome-based quality performance indicator project that created a tool, which can be used to systematically compare Taiwanese hospitals referred to as the Taiwan Quality Indicator Project (TQIP) (Liao, 2000) and
* continued assessment of consumer satisfaction with NHI (Lu & Hsiao, 2003).
* payment for quality proposals are being evaluated, e.g., five diseases (cervical cancer, breast cancer, TB, diabetes, and asthma are being studied as pilot projects. Data from the pilot projects will inform further research and include cancer, hypertension, chronic B and C-type hepatitis, and schizophrenia.

The simultaneous presence of a large number of highly trained health services researchers, productive professional linkages in and outside Taiwan, comprehensive and accessible data bases, and consistent governmental research funding have resulted in numerous research projects addressing different facets and outcomes of NHI. These investigators and health care policy-makers as well also appear to be clearly attuned to external developments and health care issues that arise in other developed societies.

Thus, at this stage, the health services research community in Taiwan is now in a position to address "second generation issues (G2)" regarding quality monitoring and improvements in its health care system. Illustrative concerns include:

1. Compared to external best practices, how successful have Taiwanese hospitals been in implementing comprehensive, hospital-wide process improvement systems based on TQM or CQI principles and methods?

2. What are the major barriers to quality improvement in Taiwanese hospitals that have been identified? How can they be effectively managed?
3. What specifically do senior managers in Taiwanese health care organizations need to do to assist quality improvement efforts in their organizations (Bradley et al., 2003)?
4. What is the comparative utility of the wide array of alternative methods of improving health care quality processes and outcomes including new approaches such as physician incentive systems (Epstein, Lee, & Hamel, 2004)?
5. How do measurable improvements in health care processes affect subsequent clinical and financial performance outcomes?
6. How can BSC methods (Kaplan & Norton, 1996) be used to help hospital executive managers develop optimally effective organizational strategies and better understand their current levels of performance in different domains and major opportunities for improvement?

Horizon

SARS illustrates a challenge that Taiwan's NHI and the rest of the world has to face in the years to come. In addition to being a rising economic power, China is notorious for being the source of new emerging infectious diseases to its neighboring countries. SARS first emerged in China in November 2002, and spread to Hong Kong, Vietnam, Canada, Singapore, Taiwan, and more than 20 other countries at unprecedented speed. The new disease caused worldwide panic because of its threat to human life (8,422 cases and 916 deaths as of August 7, 2003) as well as the social and economic disruption (economic losses estimated at US$30 billion in the Far East alone).

While the epidemiology is well known, Chen, Chen, Liu, Romeis, and Lee (2004) assess resource consumption of fighting SARS and operational impact on health care organizations based upon experiences of the National Taiwan University Hospital (NTUH), which treated more SARS patients than any other hospital in Taiwan. The NTUH's experiences with 158 SARS patients indicated that SARS has severe externality (spillover effects) on hospital management. The treatment costs of SARS, after controlling for sex, age, and average length of hospitalization, were not significantly higher than that of pneumonia. Only expired SARS patients had much higher treatment costs than pneumonia control patients.

As SARS patients were only a small group in terms of their prevalence, the total SARS treatment costs are relatively small in importance to hospital management and health policy. However, because of the novelty of the virus and its rapidly progressive infectious nature, SARS had a tremendous impact on hospital operational and financial conditions. For instance, in the peak of SARS crisis, NTUH's number of surgeries dropped from 3,576 in May 2002 to 519 in May 2003, an astonishing decrease rate of 85%. The situation improved slightly as the number of surgeries dropped form 2,950 in June 2002 to 1,525 in June 2003, a decrease rate of 48%. Thus, designing appropriate health polices (e.g., financial assistance programs to infected hospitals and health care workers) are important to NHI for possible future emerging infectious diseases and will have important implications for other countries. China's obstruction of WHO into Taiwan's epidemic confounded the situation and may be solved with Taiwan recognized with Observership status (www.doh.gov.tw).

Other horizon directions are bold steps for the culture and its politics. Taiwan has eschewed primary care providers such as family physicians and general practioners or gatekeepers. Some physicians provide these services but do not identify as these specialties. Since March 2003, the NHI has planned a "Family Doctor Integrated Delivery System". The concept has two goals. One is to enlarge the routine scope of medical services to include diagnosis, treatment, health education, and prevention. The second goal is to reduce inappropriate utilization in general, and to encourage use of district hospitals and clinics instead of more costly regional and medical center hospitals. Taiwan's family physician program is proposed to be a network of medical care for communities that patients' will consult for appropriate care and follow-up.

Much of Taiwan's successes with developing and implementing NHI can be attributed to leaving physicians to use a fee schedule and reimbursing them promptly. In 2001, BNHI began to propose revisions to the fee schedule, and explore adapting the concepts and methods associated with the U.S. resource-based relative value scale (RBRVS) mechanism; medical service reimbursement based on a formula of value of resources provided. In March 2003, the first edition was completed. Next steps will be review and revision and pilot testing. The plans are to have RBRVS become a foundation for payment reform (BNHI, 2004).

Finally, Taiwan's long-term success is in the hands of its citizens. NHI may be seen as an historical accident – where public demand overlapped with political circumstances and political leadership provided some policy makers with the wish of their careers. After implementation, the goal has been to develop a system that provides for the needs of the population within fiscal constraints. Cheng (2003) cautions that Taiwan's experience could be a

Tragedy of the Commons – where commonly owned property face risks of depletion from overuse by some selfish individuals who have little regard for the common good. Here he speaks of patients who overutilize services at a level that threatens the larger system. In turn, he proposes a serious education program coupled with economic incentives. We can easily imagine the economic message, but the G2 reform is considering how to avoid the tragedy of the common by educating the citizenry to understand their behavior with their physicians'. A working proposal is to freeze annual contributions toward the NHI by employers and government out of general funds, and to let increases in health spending by the NHI to the insured's premium rate based on assessed income. This may stem overutilization, but may have an equally onerous effect of increasing delay in seeking care.

CONCLUSION

Our overall objectives for this chapter were to demonstrate the value of comparative research through our experiences over the last decade chronicling the implementation of Taiwan's NHI system. A teaching opportunity led to research, which sheds light on our own policies. We provide two examples of studies to indicate conceptual and analytical strategies. Our results indicate that similar to health services research in the U.S. and other countries, comparative research is never complete; the target keeps moving, and thus keeps challenging researchers. Finally, comparative research in Taiwan has demonstrated that a country can overhaul its delivery system in a short period of time, achieve dramatic results, and leave consumers highly satisfied. It is possible to virtually eliminate lack of access to care overnight. It is often heard that to accomplish this in the U.S. would be a long and cumbersome process. It might but need not be. We are struck by the idea that when universal access is achieved in societies, financing and quality problems may be easier to resolve. In this regard, Taiwan remains instructive. Another instructive situation is NHI's response to SARS. If such a situation occurred in the U.S., the financial loss would probably be born by the treating institution. We may be reasonably well prepared to respond to the clinical aspects of the epidemic, but may be inadequately prepared for the economic and operational impact. Finally, comparative research leads to questions of reform for any society's policy officials. Following Cheng's (2003) observation about Taiwan, it would seem quite possible to for the U.S. to redesign, and produce a delivery system that borrows heavily from the experience of other countries' best practices.

NOTES

1. Permission to quote extensively from these two previously published studies has been obtained from *Medical Care* and its publisher, Lippencott Williams & Wilkens. The reader is encouraged to review the original if our editing lacks clarity.

REFERENCES

Access to essential drugs. (1999). *WHO Drug Information, 13*(4), 218–224.

Bradley, E. H., Holmboe, E. S., Mattera, J. A., Roumanis, S. A., Radford, M. J., & Krumholz, H. M. (2003). The roles of senior management in quality improvement efforts: What are the key components? *Journal of Healthcare Management, 48*(1), 15–28; discussion 29.

Bureau of National Health Insurance. (2001). *National health insurance annual statistical report.* Taipei: Taiwan, Republic of China.

Bureau of National Health Insurance. (2004). *National health insurance annual statistical report.* Taipei: Taiwan, Republic of China.

Burton, S. L., Randel, L., Titlow, K., & Emanuel, E. J. (2001). The ethics of pharmaceutical benefit management. *Health Affairs, 20*(5), 150–163.

Chen, Y. C., Chen, M. F., Liu, S. Z., Romeis, J. C., & Lee, Y. T. (2004). SARS in teaching hospital, Taiwan. *Emerging Infectious Disease, 10*(10), 1886–1887.

Cheng, T. M. (2003). Taiwan's new national health insurance program: Genesis and experience so far. *Health Affairs, 22*(3), 61–76.

Chiang, T. L. (1997). Taiwan's 1995 health care reform. *Health Policy, 39*(3), 225–239.

Chu, H. L., Liu, S. Z., & Romeis, J. C. (2002). Does the implementation of responsibility centers, total quality management, and physician fee programs improve hospital efficiency? Evidence from Taiwan hospitals. *Medical Care, 40*(12), 1223–1237.

Chu, H. L., Liu, S. Z., Romeis, J. C., & Yaung, C. L. (2003). The initial effects of physician compensation programs in Taiwan hospitals: Implications for staff model HMOs. *Health Care Management Science, 6*(1), 17–26.

Chu, H. L., Liu, S. Z., Romeis, J. C., Tseng, Y. F., & Lin, L. J. (2005). *Do drug reimbursement rate reductions work? Evidence from Taiwan's outpatient hypertension treatments in the elderly.* Unpublished manuscript. Saint Louis: Saint Louis University.

Counte, M. A., & Meurer, S. (2001). Issues in the assessment of continuous quality improvement implementation in health care organizations. *International Journal for Quality in Health Care, 13*(3), 197–207.

Deming, W. E. (1986). *Out of the crisis.* Cambridge: Cambridge University Press.

Eisenberg, J. M. (2002). Physician utilization: The state of research about physicians' practice patterns. *Medical Care, 40*(11), 1016–1035.

Epstein, A. M., Lee, T. H., & Hamel, M. B. (2004). Paying physicians for high-quality care. *New England Journal of Medicine, 350*(4), 406–410.

Goes, J. B., & Zhan, C. (1995). The effects of hospital-physician integration strategies on hospital financial performance. *Health Services Research, 30*(4), 507–530.

Greene, W. H. (1997). *Econometric analysis.* New York: Macmillan Publishing Company.

Horngren, C. T., Foster, G., & Datar, S. M. (1999). *Cost accounting: A managerial emphasis* (10th ed.). Upper Saddle River, New Jersey: Prentice Hall.

Huang, P. (1996). Quality assurance in Taiwan, the Republic of China. *International Journal for Quality in Health Care, 8*(1), 75–82.

Huang, P., Hsu, Y. H., Kai-Yuan, T., & Hsueh, Y. S. (2000). Can European external peer review techniques be introduced and adopted into Taiwan's hospital accreditation system? *International Journal for Quality in Health Care, 12*(3), 251–254.

Huq, Z., & Martin, T. N. (2000). Workforce cultural factors in TQM/CQI implementation in hospitals. *Health Care Management Review, 25*(3), 80–93.

Kaplan, R. S., & Norton, D. P. (1996). *The balanced scorecard: Translating strategy into action.* Boston: Harvard Business School Press.

Kaplan, R. S., & Norton, D. P. (2001). *The strategy-focused organization: How balanced scorecard companies thrive in the new business environment.* Boston: Harvard Business School Press.

Kaplan, R. S., & Norton, D. P. (2004). *Strategy maps: Converting intangible assets into tangible outcomes.* Boston: Harvard Business School Press.

Liao, S. (2000). Taiwan launches QI project. *Target: Quality.* Elkridge, MD: Quality Indicator Project, Maryland Hospital Association.

Liu, S. Z., & Romeis, J. C. (2003). Assessing the effect of Taiwan's outpatient prescription drug copayment policy in the elderly. *Medical Care, 41*(12), 1331–1342.

Liu, S. Z., & Romeis, J. C. (2004). A variance analysis approach for assessing the effect of Taiwan's outpatient prescription drug cost-sharing policy. *Health Policy, 68*(3), 277–287.

Lo, J. C., Shih, K. S., & Chen, K. L. (1996). Technical efficiency of the general hospitals in Taiwan: An application of DEA. *Academia Economic Papers, 24*(3), 375–396.

Lu, J. F., & Hsiao, W. C. (2003). Does universal health insurance make health care unaffordable? Lessons from Taiwan. *Health Affairs, 22*(3), 77–88.

Magnussen, J. (1996). Efficiency measurement and the operationalization of hospital production. *Health Services Research, 31*(1), 21–35.

Melumad, N., Mookherjee, D., & Reichelstein, S. (1992). A theory of responsibility centers. *Journal of Accounting and Economics, 15,* 445–484.

OECD (2003). *Health data 2003.* Washington, DC: Organization for Economic Cooperation and Development.

Ozcan, Y. A., Begun, J. W., & McKinney, M. M. (1999). Benchmarking organ procurement organizations: A national study. *Health Services Research, 34*(4), 855–874.

Ozcan, Y. A., Luke, R. D., & Haksever, C. (1992). Ownership and organizational performance: A comparison of technical efficiency across hospital types. *Medical Care, 30*(9), 781–794.

Seiford, L. M. (1996). Data envelopment analysis: The evolution of the state of the art (1978–1995). *The Journal of Productivity Analysis, 7,* 99–137.

Shank, J. K., & Govindarajan, V. (1993). *Strategic cost management: The new tool for competitive advantage.* New York: The Free Press.

Shortell, S. M., O'Brien, J. L., Carman, J. M., Foster, R. W., Hughes, E. F., Boerstler, H., et al. (1995). Assessing the impact of continuous quality improvement/total quality management: Concept versus implementation. *Health Services Research, 30*(2), 377–401.

Tamblyn, R., Laprise, R., Hanley, J. A., Abrahamowicz, M., Scott, S., Mayo, N., et al. (2001). Adverse events associated with prescription drug cost-sharing among poor and elderly persons. *Journal of the American Medical Association, 285*(4), 421–429.

Valdmanis, V. G. (1990). Ownership and technical efficiency of hospitals. *Medical Care, 28*(6), 552–561.

WHO. (1999). Essential drugs. *Drug Information. 13,* 249–262.

PERFORMANCE

MEASURING AND MANAGING QUALITY IN HOSPITALS: LESSONS FROM A FRENCH EXPERIMENT

Etienne Minvielle and John R. Kimberly

ABSTRACT

We present a description and analysis of the current reforms in the French system of "assurance maladie", or its health insurance system, particularly as they bear on quality at the hospital level. The measurement and management of quality play a significant role in the reform, thus providing a particularly timely example for health care policy makers, researchers, and managers. We discovered several lessons from the French experience. First, the issue of workload influenced thinking about how best to build a given indicator, and led to careful evaluation of the added value of additional data collection. In some cases the indicators are actually more of a screen or filter than an actual assessment of quality, with particularly high or low values signaling the need for further investigation rather than serving as assessments per se. Second, the development and implementation of quality indicators (QIs) demand the involvement of professionals in the process. Third, process indicators seemed to be more useful than outcome indicators. Fourth, expectations for quality management should be aligned with feasibility and with the reality of measurement system. For example, the workload is closely tied to the state of the hospital data collection systems (indicators selection). Lastly, the

International Health Care Management
Advances in Health Care Management, Volume 5, 247–272
Copyright © 2005 by Elsevier Ltd.
All rights of reproduction in any form reserved
ISSN: 1474-8231/doi:10.1016/S1474-8231(05)05009-3

*twin objectives of quality improvement and accountability do not neces-
sarily mesh easily or well.*

As the costs of providing health care have continued to escalate in virtually
every country around the globe, a variety of cost control initiatives has been
undertaken, from government-mandated price controls on products and
services to market-oriented reforms designed to introduce competition into
the production and delivery of health services to increasing the out-of-
pocket contributions by individual consumers. At the same time, a number
of reports from such influential organizations as the Institute of Medicine
and the World Health Organization point to huge problems in quality of
care, suggesting that both large numbers of lives and large amounts of
money could be saved by improving quality.

Are costs and quality in health care inextricably intertwined in such a way
that cutting costs necessarily leads to compromises in quality? Although
rhetoric abounds on both sides of this question, few would argue that the
performance of health systems, as well as the performance of the organizational entities that comprise those systems, does not encompass elements
of both costs and quality. We believe that the fundamental issue in assessing
performance at both the system and organizational levels is *value*, and value
is a judgment, incorporating both quantitative and qualitative dimensions,
about whether the quality of the service provided justifies its cost. The
calculus for determining value can be extremely complex, and there is no
widely shared "gold standard" of measurement. Indeed, much of the current
focus on "outcomes" and "evidence-based" medicine represents efforts to
bring more sophistication to the measurement of the quality component of
the value equation.

Concern with quality has been a central issue for the profession of medicine
for decades. It became more visible with the publication of Donabedian's
classic article on evaluating quality in 1966 (Donabedian, 1966), and increasingly politicized as research on quality expanded and attention was
drawn to the topic through articles in leading journals (e.g., Donabedian,
1988; Chassin, 1996; Blumenthal, 1996; Chassin & Galvin, 1998; Thomson,
1998; Berwick & Nolan, 1998). And while it is certainly the case that momentum for assessing quality developed initially in the United States, the
questions and concerns raised there quickly spread to other parts of the
world. And also just as other countries can learn much – both positive and
negative – from various experiments with measuring and managing quality in
the United States, much can be learned from experiments undertaken abroad.

It is with this latter point in mind that we present in this chapter a description and analysis of the current reforms in the French system of "assurance maladie", or its health insurance system, particularly as they bear on quality at the hospital level. As you will see, the measurement and management of quality play a significant role in the reform, thus providing a particularly timely example for policy makers, researchers, and managers in health care to consider.

The chapter begins with some background on the international context, then describes the French context and Coordination for Measuring Performance and Assuring Quality in Hospitals (COMPAQH) (Minivielle, Michel, Grenier-Sennelier, Daucourt, & Corriol, 2003), the initiative in measuring and managing quality that is currently underway. It continues with the lessons learned thus far, and concludes with some observations about future directions in the management and measurement of quality in health care globally.

QUALITY AND THE "IRON TRIANGLE" IN HEALTH CARE

Around the globe, the search is on for new approaches to managing the contradictions emerging from the "iron triangle" in health care, the relationships among cost, quality, and access (Kissick, 1998). In the ideal system, the citizenry of every country would have access to high-quality care at a cost that was reasonable both to the individual and to the collectivity. The reality, however, seems to be that trade-offs must be made among the three. Different countries have made different choices about what to provide and what trade-offs to make, but there is a common set of factors that all countries are facing and that stress their health systems, no matter what choices have been made.

Increasing Expectations

Citizens expect more from their systems, and are increasingly unhappy with the *status quo*. International surveys by Blendon, Schoen, DesRoches, Osborn, and Zapert (2003) at Harvard point to some of the specifics. The promise offered by new technologies and new medicines no doubt fuels these expectations, and tends to focus attention on the medical component of systems at the expense of the preventive component. Scientific advance

coupled with commercialization of the fruits of research leads to an ava-
lanche of new treatment possibilities, possibilities whose potential is rapidly
and widely disseminated. As awareness of these possibilities spreads, expectations escalate.

Reluctance to Pay More

Citizens expect more from their health care systems, but are reluctant to pay
more, whether the payment is direct, in the form of increasing co-pays or
increased premiums, or indirect, in the form of increased taxes. Efforts to
expand access and/or services or to improve quality that require increased
financial outlays are met with resistance, even when it appears that expanded
access or improved quality may actually reduce costs in the long run.

Concerns about Safety and Quality

Recent research documenting widespread problems with patient safety and
quality has raised public concern and led to calls for improvement. How
such improvements can be made without increased spending, however, is
not obvious.

Concerns about Equity

Around the globe, there is increasing awareness of the fact that health resources – be they hospitals, nurses and physicians, technology, medicines,
and/or public health initiatives – are not equally available to all citizens.
Every country faces problems of underserved populations, and some countries are facing devastating health crises that they are unable to deal with on
their own. Recognition of the gap between what we know about improving
health status and what is available leads to mounting pressure which reduces
its magnitude.

Each of the factors noted above, increasing expectations, reluctance to
pay more, concerns about safety and quality, concerns about equity, puts
pressure on health systems to respond. Together, they keep health care as a
political agenda item in the spotlight in most countries. In the case of
France, the "iron triangle" is further complicated by the way in which
health policy has evolved over the past two decades. This evolution has left
the country facing severe labor shortages in the health sector, has tended to

have a near-exclusive focus on cost control, has resulted in waiting lists for elective procedures, and has significant quality and safety problems. Furthermore, as it moves toward a financing scheme based on Diagnosis Related Groups (DRGs), it has not addressed prevention in a significant and sustained fashion, and has tended to separate cure, care, social care, public health, and health policy (Moisdon, 2000; de Kervasdoué, 2004).

Our focus in this chapter is restricted to the measurement and management of quality in the hospital sector. Clearly, France is buffeted by the same set of pressures that other countries face in this regard, as well as some that are perhaps somewhat idiosyncratic. But the end result has been a proliferation of initiatives for assessing hospital performance in more and more countries, with corresponding opportunities to learn from the experiences in specific cases.

It is fair to say that important strides have been made in the measurement of hospital performance and quality, and that the United States has played a leading role in this work. Both public agencies and private payers have been involved in a variety of initiatives, sometimes separately, sometimes collaboratively, to better define, measure and manage quality. The National Committee for Quality Assurance, for example, has promulgated a set of performance indicators for health plans that have become widely used. The National Quality Forum has brought public and private payers together with consumers, researchers, and clinicians to broaden consensus on performance measures and best practices for a growing portfolio of health care settings, conditions, and treatments. The Agency for Healthcare Research and Quality (AHRQ) has developed a variety of performance indicators, including Patient Safety Indicators. The Leapfrog Group, a coalition of major employers, has moved boldly to tie provider payment to selected performance indicators. And perhaps most important, the Centers for Medicare and Medicaid Services (CMS) has taken significant steps toward a quality strategy based on quality measurement and incentives. Even if the available indicators are less than perfect, the CMS, National Quality Forum, and Leapfrog initiatives, all advocate that developing financial incentives to motivate improvements in performance should become a top national priority for hospital care.

Other English-speaking countries have developed similar initiatives. In Canada, for example, the province of Ontario has developed a "report card" that publishes performance data from 95 provincial health care institutions. In the United Kingdom, a series of reforms has resulted in the development of league tables with the Performance Assessment Framework and of professional practice guidelines under the auspices of the recently established

National Institute for Clinical Excellence (NICE). The commercial website named Dr. Foster has begun posting comparative data on public and private hospitals. And similar initiatives are taking place in Australia and New Zealand.

The burgeoning interest in performance and quality is not limited to English-speaking countries. Recently, national initiatives have been launched in several European countries, including the Netherlands, the Nordic countries, Spain, and Germany. And both the OECD and the WHO have focused attention on performance at the hospital level. A summary of the principal initiatives undertaken in Western Europe in the past 10 years is presented in the appendix.

Key Questions about Hospital Quality and Performance

Each of these initiatives has to address and resolve a common set of questions in some way. The following eight questions address definitional, contextual, statistical, teleological, and ontological concerns, as well as issues of accountability, performance, and incentives.

How are Performance and Quality Defined?

Many definitions of these two terms are used, both in the literature and in practice. Furthermore, they are tied to multiple levels; individual, organizational, regional, and national levels. These levels are, of course, linked, but they involve different units of analysis and different metrics. While in this chapter we are focusing primarily on performance and quality at the organizational level (the hospital), we need to consider how issues at this level shape and are shaped by performance and quality at other levels. For example, the performance of an individual surgeon is affected by the way in which work in the hospital in general, and the surgical suite in particular, is organized and managed. The performance of a hospital is affected by the characteristics of the labor pool from which it can hire. Although historically definitions of the two abound, we see an emerging consensus around the definition of hospital performance. This consensus includes *effectiveness* (provision of services based on scientific knowledge to all who could benefit and not providing services to those not likely to benefit), *finance/productivity, equity, responsiveness, appropriateness, safety* and *quality*. The latter consists of four components: patient safety, effectiveness, responsiveness, and appropriateness. This consensus puts finance/productivity, equity, and quality as the cornerstones of performance (the iron triangle once more) and clinical effectiveness, responsiveness, accessibility, and safety as the cornerstones of quality (Hurtado, Swift, & Corrigan, 2001). Some boundary issues remain (e.g., that between appropriateness and equity), but considerable progress is being made in separating the three components of the iron triangle. Each is a specific domain of performance, not an overall goal in and of itself.

Under what Conditions is Change Possible?

The introduction of new initiatives is challenging under the best of circumstances. The health sector, being highly institutionalized and highly professionalized, is also characterized by substantial inertia. The measurement of quality raises the visibility of the work of everyone in the system, and particularly of physicians. It would not be surprising, therefore, to encounter a certain lack of enthusiasm on their part for the implementation of efforts to monitor and evaluate their work more systematically. And as we have argued elsewhere, quality in hospitals is an organizational problem (Minvielle & Kimberly, 2000; Kimberly & Minvielle, 2003). So it is reasonable to ask whether hospitals have the resources (and the resolve) to change the way they work, given that such change requires not only tangible resources but also skill in managing substantial changes in culture as well. Attention needs to be paid to system and organizational readiness for change, and, as a practical matter, to the question of how best to introduce change when readiness is low.

How Should Statistical Controversies be Resolved?

The development of quality indicators (QI) is inevitably accompanied by statistical controversies. The use of mortality rate illustrates the problem vividly. This statistic is a negative final outcome indicator; it is the first indicator to be widely and publicly reported in the United States, and because of its ready availability, it is very attractive to the media. But a number of reasonable objections have been raised about its use (Iezonni, Shwartz, Ash, Hughes, Daley, & Mackiernan, 1995; Iezzoni, 1997; Landon, et al., 1996; McKee & Hunter, 1995; Leyland & Boddy, 1998; Ansari, Ackland, Jolley, Carson, & McDonald, 1999; Thomas & Hofer, 1999). It is a rare event, and requires a large database to insure sufficient precision; it is very sensitive to the characteristics of patients prior to admission to the hospital and thus requires sophisticated risk adjustment; and its relationship to quality of care, no matter how defined, is open to question. Similar questions can be raised about virtually any indicator of quality, thus highlighting the necessity of insuring stakeholder consensus insofar as appropriateness is concerned.

What is the Objective being Sought?

The measurement of quality is not and should not become an end in itself. Rather it is part of a process, the objective of which can be improvement in quality, increased accountability for quality, and/or control of quality through payment for quality outcomes.

What is the Evidence Base Underlying the Construction and Choice of Indicators?

It may seem obvious that validity should be clearly and compellingly demonstrated. However, in the interplay among politics, science, and the media, this obvious point can get lost (McGlynn, 2003a). In the case of France, for example, the media frequently used length of stay as a QI, with the underlying hypothesis that a shorter length of stay is correlated with quality improvement.

How Should Quality Improvement be Linked to Accountability?

Providing information to citizens/consumers about hospital performance is a two-edged sword. We have seen that National Quality Reports, "report cards", League Tables, and provider profiles have become more widely used, and that hospital rankings sell magazines. In France, issues of popular magazines that contain hospital rankings are among the most popular in any given year. Armed with information, consumers are theoretically in a position to take more responsibility for managing their own health, and this is something to be applauded. However, if quality improvement and accountability are closely linked, it will be in the hospital's interest to score well on whatever quality measures are used, thus incentivizing gaming of those measures. Paradoxically, by linking performance with accountability, tension will almost inevitably be generated with quality-improvement goals.

What Level of Performance is Sufficient?

This question is both extremely sensitive and at the heart of any measurement system. And it generates a series of additional questions. What, for example, do above- and below-average scores tell us? And what should be the consequences of being one or the other? What do benchmarks tell us? And given the current fascination with benchmarking, to what extent do benchmarks actually mislead rather than inform? These questions all inevitably arise as soon as policies tying consequences to the measurement process are articulated.

How might Incentives be Better Aligned with Policy Objectives?
There should be tight coupling between objectives and incentives; otherwise we will be in the position of "rewarding A while expecting B". Behind this question, of course, is the issue of paying for quality. If we are to move in this direction, it will be extremely important to insure that the incentives deriving from the terms of payment will actually help promote and improve quality rather than diminishing it.

These questions were all considered as the French project was conceived and launched, and their articulation early in the process helped shape the scope and direction of the project substantially. It should be noted, however, that by comparison, France has lagged behind other developed nations in attention to quality. In fact, it was not until 1998, after a popular magazine *Science et Avenir* published a quality ranking of hospitals, that the issue of hospital performance began to emerge as socially and politically significant ("Le Palmarès des Hôpitaux," 1998). This initial effort was quickly picked up by other magazines, and the rankings proliferated. Since then, the French Ministry of Health in collaboration with the National Agency for Accreditation has developed a national project, and this project is the focus of our chapter. But before describing the French project, which focuses on hospitals, we should locate it in the context of the French health care system as a whole.

THE FRENCH HEALTH CARE SYSTEM

The health care system in France is complex, but its most significant features are the way it is funded and the way citizens can access it. With respect to funding, in 1945, France adopted a universal insurance system (called Social Security) that covers health insurance, income supplements based on family size and income, and retirement. Everyone in France who has a paid job contributes to the universal insurance system fund in an amount proportional to his or her income. For salaried workers, the contribution is paid in part by the employer and in part by the employee. The system is under governmental control but is managed by independent agencies that have a specific status: elected trade-union representatives and appointed representatives of corporations sit on the boards of these agencies. The largest group of agencies manages Social Security for salaried workers and is organized in a pyramid of local, regional, and national Health Insurance Agencies. The universal health insurance system paid for 71.6% of all health care costs in France during 1995, whereas the government paid for 3.6%. The rest was paid for either out-of-pocket or by private insurance that employed individuals who can obtain if they want to, at modest cost. The system does not, in principle, receive income tax money but must balance its budget. This financial autonomy is relative, however: the government defines both the scale of contributions from employed individuals and the proportion and type of health care costs that are covered.

The Access System

With respect to access, all levels of the health care system are accessible to everyone. There is no gatekeeper system, and patients with minor problems can go to the office of a primary care practitioner or to specialist of their choice, to a hospital outpatient clinic, or to a hospital emergency room. Since 2004, however, patients are required to consult a GP before seeing a specialist. Direct access to a specialist is still possible, but patients must pay a larger portion of the cost out of pocket.

The Hospital System

In 2001, France had 3,836 hospitals with approximately 480 000 beds. Of these, approximately 50% were acute care beds. Although the public sector is dominant, a dynamic private for-profit and not-for-profit sector delivered 50% of all surgical and obstetrical services that year. Public hospitals fall into three categories: large regional teaching hospitals with strong links to medical schools; smaller general hospitals with 100–600 acute care beds; and small community hospitals whose main role is to offer beds with limited technological resources. All public hospitals are local public organizations and each has its own board of trustees, usually chaired by the mayor of the town.

In the for-profit private sector, hospitals are considerably smaller than most public hospitals, and in the past, most were physician-owned. Since the mid-1980s, however, there has been a trend towards consolidation into larger groups, although on a smaller scale than in the United States. A summary of the main features of the French hospital system is presented in Table 1.

Table 1. France: Key Health Care Figures.

General Data		
Country area	547,027 sq. km.	
Population	58,891,913	
Percent of population < 20 years	31.8	
Percent of population aged 21–64 years	49.9	
Percent of population > 64 years	16.3	
Life expectancy at birth, women	82.4	
Life expectancy at birth, men	74.9	
Health Expenditures	1985	2001
National health expenditures (2001 Euros)	64 613 millions	123 330 millions
Percent of National Domestic Product	9	8,8
Percent of Hospital health expenditures	44.1	43
Health Professionals	1985	2000
Number of physicians	120,929	194,000
Number per 100,000	218.7	330.21
Percent of General Practitioners	56.3	50.1
Percent of Specialists	43.7	49.9
Other health professionals:	358,851	445,789
Hospital Sector	Public and private (non for profit sector)	Private (for-profit sector)
Number of hospitals (2001)	2460	1376
Total number of beds (2001)	383,274	94,924
Number of beds per 1000 pop.	1985	2000
	12.7	10

Source: French Ministry of Health (2001).

How Hospitals are Paid

The operating costs of both public sector and private not-for-profit hospitals are covered by a budget allocated prospectively each year. Annual discussions are held at the national level to define the rate at which hospital expenditures increase nationally. At the time, this national rate was marginally adjusted at the regional level using funds earmarked for specific health programs by government outreach agencies called the Regional and District Offices of Health and Social Affairs (Directions Régionales et Départementales des Affaires Sanitaires et Sociales, DRASS and DDASS, respectively), which were under the authority of the prefects, administrative officers of each district. For public hospitals, this adjusted rate is applied to past expenditures in each hospital to determine the amount of money that will be allocated to the hospital for the year to come. Since 1980, a case-mix-adjusted budgeting method, using a French adaptation of the DRG system has been used (Programme de Médicalisation du Système d'Information, PMSI).

In 1992, a cap was also placed on total expenditures of the private-for-profit sector, excluding physician fees. Hospitals in this sector are paid on the basis of a per-diem amount for the hospital room and nursing care based on the complexity of the surgical procedure for which the operating room was used, and on a lump sum for medications, except particularly expensive ones. This global expenditure cap is managed through a price–volume mechanism, i.e., the proportion paid is decreased if volumes are high and vice versa. And a new initiative launched in 2005, Tarification à l'Activité, introduces a common mode of payment private–public, based on a generalization of the DRG system.

The Need for Improved Efficiency and Quality

A review of the functional and political dynamics of the French health care system over the last 20 years has led most observers to agree that substantial improvement in both efficiency and quality should be priorities for the government. Total hospital care expenditures increased from 40 billion Euros in 1975 to about 123 billion in 2001. Although one might argue that the structure of the system created favorable conditions for the development of high-quality hospital care, macroeconomic data indicate that a similar result could probably have been obtained at a lower cost during the last 20 years. France spent 8.8% of its GNP on health in 2000, of which slightly less than half was for hospital care, as shown in Table 1. This places France just behind the United States, the leading health care spender in the world, generating considerable pressure to rein in the rate of growth in expenditures.

The World Health Organisation comparative analysis of health care systems around the globe completed in 2000 suggests good overall performance of the French system. However, critics of the WHO report question the extent to which results in terms of health are related to the availability of hospital care. Furthermore, in the 1980s, serious safety concerns arose regarding AIDS and about the equity of the health care system. More recently, concerns about nosocomial infections (NI) have been raised by the French media, and well-organized consumer groups have denounced the lack of transparency of the hospital system regarding information about quality of hospital care. Public awareness of quality as an issue in hospitals has thus been raised considerably, and has provided a strong impetus for change.

MADE IN FRANCE: THE COMPAQH PROJECT

In response to many of the forces described above, the French Ministry of Health and the French National Evaluation and Accreditation Agency (ANAES) decided in 2003 to develop a national project for hospital quality, the COMPAQH (Coordination for Measuring Performance and Assuring Quality in Hospitals) project.[1] The general objective of this project is to identify a set of QIs that could be generalized to all French hospitals (acute care, rehabilitation, or psychiatric hospitals) by the end of 2005. The project takes a pragmatic view of the notion of performance, one in which quality is an important dimension to consider, equal to those of cost and equity.

Stakeholders

The project is coordinated by the French National Institute for Medical Research (INSERM), in collaboration with an academic regional structure (the Aquitaine Committee for Quality Evaluation, CCECQA). It is supported by the French Ministry of Health and the French National Evaluation and Accreditation Agency (ANAES). The different hospital federations (public and private) as well as three important health consumers associations are also partners of this project. Other groups interested in its development are the Regional Hospital Agencies, the main national health insurance agency of the French Social Security system, and some important health professional associations. They all are in agreement that consensual definition of a set of indicators would facilitate development of a common framework for measuring and managing quality in French hospitals.

A Steering Committee of 14 members representing the principal stakeholders was formed and represents the following institutions:

- Ministry of Health (Hospital Division), 2 members
- National Evaluation and Accreditation Agency (ANAES), 2 members
- Sickness Fund, 1 member

- Federation of Consumer Groups, 1 member
- Federation of Public Hospitals, 1 member
- Federation of Private for-Profit Hospitals, 1 member
- Federation of Private non-Profit Hospitals, 1 member
- Federation of Cancer Centers, 1 member
- Federation of French Supplemental Health Insurers, 1 member
- Panel of 36 participating hospitals, 3 members

The 36 French hospitals that agreed to participate in the initial work of COMPAQH include 16 public, 7 private non-for-profit, and 13 private for-profit institutions. Twenty-four are acute care facilities involved in Medicine, Surgery, and Obstetrics, four are centers specialized in Cancer, four are Rehabilitation and Long-Term Care facilities, and four are Psychiatric hospitals. The project coordination team is composed of four physicians, one statistician, one project manager, one secretary, and seven data mining experts (their mission is to help hospitals for collecting data required by the indicators).

Dissemination Strategies

In order to disseminate the results, a strategy composed of three steps was developed. In the first step, eight National Priorities were defined by the French Ministry of Health: pain management, continuity of care, nutritional disorders management, iatrogenic risks (including NI), patient satisfaction, follow-up of practice guidelines, management of human resources, and accessibility.

As a second step, given these eight National Priorities, a set of 42 QIs was selected: a set of 6 core QIs and 8–18 specific QIs depending on the hospital type. To illustrate, the QI for acute care hospitals include the following:

CORE SET: Medical/anaesthesic record conformity, time to discharge letters, nutritional disorder screening, score on patient satisfaction questionnaire (overall, care, information, welcoming, staff availability and behavior, feeding, respect for privacy, comfort, and discharge preparation), staff turnover, and score on prevention and control of NI.

SPECIFIC SET: Pain treatment, traceability of pain assessment, therapeutic education, short term absenteeism, request forms for medical test appropriately filled in, cancelled one-day surgical procedures, follow-up of practice guidelines for breast surgery, prostatic cancer, myocardial infarction, and stroke, and caesarean section rate, surgical NI, emergency waiting time, and in-patient mortality in low-death DRGs.

The third step is a test period (2004–2005) designed to allow for feedback on routine use of these indicators (mainly based on feasibility and metrological aspects). It also requires recommendations regarding a benchmark process in which these indicators can be used. These early results will be relevant not only at the physician and the hospital level, but also at the national level, where there is interest in creating a system of payment based, in part, on performance on QIs.

Process for Selecting National Priorities and Quality Indicators

A four-step process guided the selection of QIs: (1) establishing a list of national priorities for QI; (2) assembling a potential list of QIs related to these priorities; (3) evaluating the preliminary list; and (4) developing consensus on the final list.

Step 1: Establish a List of National Priorities for QI
This first list was based on a review of the literature on the different national initiatives developed in industrialized countries, in consultation with the Ministry of Health. Four criteria were considered for selecting these priorities:

- the importance of the topic (number of citations in the different national initiatives,[2] scientific evidence about the epidemiological impact of the disease or event on population health)
- potential variation in quality across the hospitals
- feasibility (ability to develop QIs, evidence-based which supports the development of these indicators)
- the potential gain in quality in relation to previous results (e.g. for the main clinical conditions, QIs show results from 40 to 65% of adherence to the practices guidelines; the gap can be interpreted as potential gain from improving these practices).

Additionally, compatibility between the findings of this review and features of the French context were taken into account (e.g., in the United States, pain management now appears to be a less important issue than 10 years ago, suggesting that more improvements have been made during the last decade, when it became a crucial issue in the French context).

Once completed, this list was submitted to different stakeholder groups in the hospital field (physicians, hospital directors, sickness fund, Regional Agencies in charge of hospital management, the Regional Hospital

Agencies, and consumer groups) and was modified based on their feedback, resulting in the eight national priorities presented above.

Step 2: Assemble a Potential List of QIs Related to these Priorities
The COMPAQH staff made a preliminary selection of 81 QIs, based on literature analysis and evidence about the scientific soundness of quality measures and the effectiveness of methods for improving quality. For each priority, a second literature review was conducted in order to identify related QIs. In other words, each selected QI had to be linked to one specific national priority. Again, the selection process was guided by the four criteria, criteria similar to the four described by McGlynn (2003b):

- Importance (including, the fact that the measure capture key aspects of the process for accomplishing the priority or represent an important outcome; variation in quality, and potential improvements in terms of performance).
- Feasibility (including, the workload required for the data collection, the acceptability by the professionals).
- Scientific soundness (considering the reliability and validity aspects as well as the adequacy of risk adjustment).
- Usability (i.e., utility in decision-making; clarity of the results; ease in connecting to quality improvement actions).

Following these steps, a first list of 81 QIs was created (which corresponds to 8–12 QIs per national priority).

Step 3: Evaluate the Preliminary List
Each QI was presented in a pamphlet describing operational definition, rationale, methodology, workload, and responsibility for data collection Then, representatives from the 36 hospitals in the panel ranked the 81 QIs with a validated evaluation tool that contained the four dimensions described above: importance, feasibility, scientific soundness, and usability (that means the hospital panel did a second round of evaluation). More specifically, the hospital panel rated the criteria of importance, feasibility, and usability on a scale of 1–10 in which 1 represents a poor evaluation, and an expert panel of statisticians rated the criterion of scientific soundness on the same scale. A global score was then created by summing the scores obtained on each scale.

Step 4: Develop Consensus on the Final List

Based on a structured voting process (Delphi method, two rounds), the hospital panel selected a comprehensive set of QIs from among the 81 QIs. The global score of each QI gave a first rank submitted to each member of the hospital panel (a list by sector was been produced which represents a total of four lists). In addition, scores obtained on each scale and variation between them and the global score were diffused. This first list served as a basis for the search for consensus. To guide the process, two categories were created, the "top 20" and the non-selected group of QIs. The "top 20" corresponds to the QIs that had the best scores compared to the others. Each member of the panel could modify the "top 20" list by replacing one of these QIs with one coming from the other group. In addition, each of the 8 National Priorities had to be represented by at least one QI. Voters returned their results to the COMPAQH staff running the voting exercise.

After the results of the initial vote had been compiled, the staff presented a second list in which any changes made had to have been advocated by more than 20% of the respondents. Using the same principles as in the first round, a second round of voting then took place. Eighty-two percent of those voting in the first round voted in the second round. Finally, in a face-to-face meeting the results from the two round-voting process were discussed, and the pilot committee validating the final list, which included 42 QIs, from four lists (Medicine–Surgery–Obstetrics, Cancer, Psychiatric and Rehabilitation).

Lessons From the French Experience

A set of carefully chosen QIs is a necessary but not sufficient condition for developing a quality measurement system for French hospitals. Coincidentally, collection of data on indicators is also a key element in the new accreditation initiative under the auspices of the ANAES. Thus, there are good reasons for hospitals to participate fully in the effort, and the next two years of the COMPAQH project will be devoted to data collection and provision of feedback on the managerial implications of implementing the indicators.

After a little more than one year's experience with the project, there are some lessons that we have learned. Perhaps most important, both professional and institutional stakeholders agree on the importance of developing reliable and valid QIs. This consensus is somewhat surprising given the conventional wisdom about the difficulty of introducing change into health care systems around the globe, and suggests reexamining some of our basic assumptions about the intransigence of professional behavior. As one physician noted during one of the many roundtables held during the first year "We are entering a new cycle in the development of measures. Even if there will be serious negative effects, it is better than the current situation where we know next to nothing about the quality of care delivered in hospitals." When compelling evidence can be marshaled that a problem exists, professionals, like most others, will be motivated to take remedial action.

If there was consensus regarding the desirability of developing QIs, there were also challenges during this first phase of the project regarding feasibility and utility in the areas of both quality improvement and accountability. With respect to feasibility, the initial activities of the project were very time consuming for both the project coordination team and for the participating hospitals. For many hospitals, the initial enthusiasm that was generated by their involvement in many roundtables and conferences waned somewhat – and in one case, evaporated entirely – as they experienced the amount of work that was required to develop each indicator. As a consequence, the amount of additional work required became implicitly a criterion for selection of indicators, and irrespective of their importance, some indicators were not selected for this reason. An example is the number of falls among elderly patients. The definition of falls was not consensual, and the process of data collection about falls suffered from a lack of reliability.

The issue of workload also influenced thinking about how best to build a given indicator, and led to careful evaluation of the added value of additional data collection. To illustrate, the utility of developing an adjusted rate for comprehensiveness was intensively debated because of the additional workload that would be generated by collection of data on each variable that was to be part of the adjustment. Ultimately, it was decided that the unadjusted rate was preferable because the marginal benefit of an adjusted rate was more than offset by the cost of additional data collection. For this reason, in some cases the indicators are actually more of a screen or filter than an actual assessment of quality, with particularly high or low values signaling the need for further investigation rather than serving as assessments per se.

Another lesson we draw from the experience is that process indicators are more useful than outcome indicators, for at least two reasons. First, they permit the accumulation of a large sample of cases, thereby permitting statistical differences to be demonstrated more easily (Eddy, 1998). And second, they result in findings that are easier to translate into corrective actions for improving quality. It is easier, for example, to do something about non-conformity to practice guidelines than about poor results in terms of mortality for a given clinical condition such as acute myocardial infarction.

A further lesson, unsurprisingly, is that the workload is closely tied to the state of the hospital data collection systems. A particularly vivid example is the patient record: each indicator that requires collection of data from this record (e.g. the date required for assuring that a letter has been sent in a short time (less than 8 days) to the physician who follows the patient) is dependent on its own quality (degree of informatization, information shared, relevant, and accurate data). This inevitably shapes the strategy for selecting indicators, because one always starts with available data. Indicators based on existing data are thus preferred, although this does not exclude the possibility of developing better indicators in the future. AHRQ in the United States, for example, has developed 20 patient safety indicators exclusively based on data coming from the DRG system (AHRQ, 2005). The use of available data also puts pressure on to improve the quality of existing systems. To the extent that the scientific credibility of measures is determined by the quality of existing information systems, this pressure is a positive constraint.

The additional work created by the development and implementation of QIs attenuates the need for involvement of professionals in the process. If they are to be assessed by such indicators, the indicators themselves must be acceptable to them. In the French experiment, professional associations were involved from the beginning in the selection, design and monitoring of the indicators, and every indicator has the official approval of the relevant professional association or organization. The French Society of Cardiology, for example, approved the measure for respect of practice guidelines for AMI.

At this early point, we can also draw some lessons from the COMPAQH project regarding objectives. With respect to the objective of quality management we would note two potential problems. First, there is often a time lag between the initiation of corrective action and the reflection of the consequences of this action in the measurement system. For example, the SAE system, a national database in France, gives results on a variety of performance indicators but with a lag of between one and a half and two years. Care must be taken to insure that expectations are aligned with the reality of the measurement system. And second, there is the risk of developing and implementing indicators for which no corrective actions are feasible in the short run. For example, in the French project, providing access for the handicapped can require revisiting the overall architecture of the hospital, something that simply cannot happen in the short run. So once again, expectations must be aligned with a clear sense of feasibility.

A final lesson is that the twin objectives of quality improvement and accountability do not necessarily mesh easily or well. The French experiment provides a particularly good illustration of this general point with the case of NI. A public debate about the number of deaths due to NI, fueled by extensive coverage in the media, revealed the complexity of the scientific issues involved. From an expert point of view, it was estimated that roughly one-third of the 4,000 deaths attributed to NI could have been avoided. However, leaders of an association of consumers, with the support of the media, took the position that no deaths from NI are acceptable, and were thus unable or unwilling to make a distinction between avoidable and unavoidable deaths. This debate underlines the importance of effective communication strategies. Complex issues often underlie statistical reports, and, if they are not understood, indicators can be misinterpreted, leading to unproductive conflict.

Future Considerations

The French experiment with measuring and managing quality has faced a number of challenges early in its development, and it will most certainly face new challenges as it develops further. Some of these new challenges can be deduced from what has already occurred: professionals need to continue to be involved in all aspects of the experiment from the design of indicators to the comparative assessment of performance; information, IT, and analytic capabilities must be expanded; information systems in hospitals must meet a common set of requirements including a high degree of standardization across providers, high regularity of data collection, high accuracy of data collected, and relevant statistical analysis of data. In addition to these relatively obvious issues, three newer questions have emerged:

From Measurement to Quality Management?
As an indicator is being designed, it is important to consider how the construct it measures will be used subsequently. As noted earlier, process indicators can generally be tied more closely to corrective action than outcome indicators. It is also important to pay attention to the temporal relationship between the management period and the evaluation period. Some information systems require one or more years to register data and provide measures, thereby creating a problem for taking corrective action. In the same

vein, there can be a significant lag between the time-corrective action is taken and the time the consequences of that action are reflected in the measurement system (Naylor, Iron, & Hnada, 2002). In either case, the possibility of lags needs to be taken into account in order to insure alignment between expectations and the realities of measurement procedures.

How Should Measurement be Linked to Accountability and Quality?
As noted in the previous section, the connection between quality and accountability is not straightforward. To draw the two closer, it might be useful to pay closer attention to communication in the direction of patients and to the simplification and contextualization of information. There is a real need for individuals or organizations that can act as translators, that can explain and adjust information provision to demand and that can act as go-betweens between patients and providers (Hibbard & Jewett, 1997).

Second, more needs to be known about the real impact of accountability (through public reporting) on quality. Does increased accountability lead to quality improvement? There is some evidence in the literature that public reporting of performance data improves quality (Berwick, James, & Coye, 2003). Provider organizations are sensitive to public image even in the absence of market pressure emanating from consumer choice. But there is also some question about how much impact public reporting has and whether the impact is positive or negative. It has been argued, for example, that report cards for cardiac surgeons have resulted in some surgeons referring complex cases elsewhere. The clear implication of this controversy is that we need to understand more clearly the impact of accountability measures on provider behavior and hence on quality.

Can We (or Should We) Pay for Quality?
Provision of appropriate incentives for quality, as noted earlier in this chapter, is the current Holy Grail being pursued in health care. And we must remember that both financial and non-financial incentives can be used to motivate quality improvement. In the U.K., for example, hospitals can "earn autonomy". Hospitals that score well on the measures used are subject to less frequent assessment and less bureaucratic control. In France, as in the U.K., the U.S., and many other countries, the general idea that quality can be "purchased" is a new avenue of reform, and we can expect a number of new initiatives based on this idea to be implemented in the not-too-distant future.

As various possibilities are contemplated, there appear to be some common themes; consumers should be able to choose providers on the basis of performance on a cost/quality ratio; payers should be able to reward or penalize providers on the basis of demonstrated performance on quality measures; and selective contracting should be encouraged, as any given provider may perform better in some areas than in others (Rosenthal, Fernandopulle, Song, & Landon, 2004).

It is interesting to note that this approach represents a significant departure from more traditional approaches to the allocation of financial resources for health services, approaches that focused on type rather than quality of service provided as the basis for payment to hospitals and physicians. By focusing on type of service and paying differentially by type, payment systems rewarded volume. The advent of DRGs introduced the notion of efficiency into the provision of services; those who could provide services efficiently were rewarded, while those who could not were not. The idea of rewarding providers on the basis of quality is still largely an aspiration, however, not a reality (Maynard, 1998).

CONCLUDING REMARKS: MOTIVATING IMPROVEMENT IN QUALITY

The actual introduction of new modes of competition based on quality would thus mark a substantial break with past practice, practice based on classical micro-economic principles of price competition that hold quality constant. While this break is in many ways appealing, some caution needs to be used, particularly in the context of the French system (de Pouvourville & Minvielle, 2002).

- One of the basic principles of the French social insurance system is that quality should be the same from one establishment to the next. This principle effectively orients the system not toward discriminating among providers on the basis of quality but rather toward assuring that they provide similar levels of quality.
- It must also be noted that those managing the system have imperfect knowledge of the quality of service provided from one establishment to the next. At best, they can make approximate categorical judgments such as "good", "average", or "poor". This imprecision is amplified depending on the level of system management; it is stronger at the national level than at the regional or ARH level.
- Finally, those managing the system necessarily have selective knowledge about quality in a given establishment, knowledge that varies with respect

to domains of activity. Because of this selective knowledge, they have to make a choice: either they assume that if quality in the domains they know is high, quality in the establishment as a whole is high; or they have to limit themselves to a selective form of reasoning.

These cautions suggest that competition on quality can only be partial, and that concerns about reducing observable inequalities with respect to quality will dominate. It thus appears to be more reasonable to focus attention on the kinds of incentives that might be introduced to improve quality.

In this regard, one important incentive might operate through public dissemination of information on hospital performance in areas of particular concern such as, in the French context, risk or equality of access. This incentive might also be linked to new ways of allocating hospital resources or to planning or accrediting activities – low levels of quality in certain areas or in the establishment as a whole could result in the extreme in revocation of an operating license or more likely in the specification of certain remedial actions. Incentives might also link the three. It is thus possible to imagine ways in which incentives could be constructed so as to help create a true system focused on quality improvement rather than isolated, fragmented initiatives.

While construction of such a system might be highly desirable in the abstract, this vision raises a number of important questions concerning the nature of the incentives (redistribution, bonus, sanction), the type of measure used (the incentives may be more or less selective depending on the domains of activity of concern), and finally the kind of mechanism put in operation. (What part of the allocation might be redistributed without leading to discrimination on the basis of quality? What form of contracting might be employed?) As the experiment matures, these questions will have to be addressed and answers, no matter how problematic and imperfect they may be, will have to be found. In our view, while the French are rather late in moving in this direction, the scope of their involvement is such that the rest of the world will learn much from the way the experiment unfolds, particularly regarding the relationships between cost and quality. These insights in themselves will go a long way to helping other countries wrestle with the complex questions about the provision of health services they all face.

NOTES

1. Since January 2005, the ANAES has been included in a new structure called the Haute Authorité de Santé (the High Authority of Health).

2. National Health System (UK), Australian Council on Healthcare Standards (Aus), JCAHO(US), Agency for Health care Research and Quality (US), Quality Indicators Project Maryland (US), Medicare Quality Improvement Organization (QIO), National Quality Forum (US), Victorian Government Health Information (Aus), Cleveland Health Quality Choice (US), FOQUAL (Suisse), Hospital report project Ontario (Canada), CRAG(Ecosse), Institut canadien d'information sur la santé, FAACT(Foundation for Accountability).

ACKNOWLEDGEMENT

Funding for this chapter is based was provided by the French Ministry of Health and the National Agency for Accreditation and Evaluation. We thank Catherine Grenier-Sennelier, Clément Coriol, Valentin Daucourt, and Philippe Michel, members of the coordination staff of the COMPAQH project. Although the analysis and conclusions presented are our own and do not necessarily reflect the views of our colleagues, we are deeply indebted to them for their support and assistance.

REFERENCES

AHRQ. (2005). *Guide to patient safety indicators* (No. 03-R203). Washington, DC: Agency for Healthcare Research and Quality, Department of Health and Human Services.

Ansari, M. Z., Ackland, M. J., Jolley, D. J., Carson, N., & McDonald, I. G. (1999). Inter-hospital comparison of mortality rates. *International Journal for Quality in Health Care, 11*(1), 29–35.

Berwick, D. M., James, B., & Coye, M. J. (2003). Connections between quality measurement and improvement. *Medical Care, 41*(1 Suppl.), I30–38.

Berwick, D. M., & Nolan, T. W. (1998). Physicians as leaders in improving health care. *Annals of Internal Medicine, 128*(4), 289–292.

Blendon, R. J., Schoen, C., DesRoches, C., Osborn, R., & Zapert, K. (2003). Common concerns amid diverse systems: Health Care experiences in five countries. *Health Affairs, 22*, 106–121.

Blumenthal, D. (1996). Part 1: Quality of care – what is it? *New England Journal of Medicine, 335*(12), 891–894.

Chassin, M. R. (1996). Improving the quality of care. *New England Journal of Medicine, 335*, 1060–1063.

Chassin, M. R., & Galvin, R. W. (1998). The urgent need to improve health care quality. *Journal of the American Medical Association, 280*, 1000–1005.

Donabedian, A. (1966). Evaluating the quality of medical care. *Milbank Memorial Fund Quarterly: Health and Society, 44*(3), 166–203.

Donabedian, A. (1988). The quality of care: How can it be assessed? *Journal of the American Medical Association, 260*, 1743–1748.

Eddy, D. M. (1998). Performance measurement: Problems and solutions. *Health Affairs, 17*(4), 7–25.

Hibbard, J. H., & Jewett, J. J. (1997). Will quality report cards help consumers? *Health Affairs*, *16*(3), 218–228.

Hurtado, M. P., Swift, E. K., & Corrigan, J. M. (Eds) (2001). *Envisioning the national health care quality report*. Washington, DC: National Academy Press.

Iezzoni, L. I. (1997). The risks of risk adjustment. *Journal of the American Medical Association*, *278*(19), 1600–1607.

Iezzoni, L. I., Shwartz, M., Ash, A. S., Hughes, J. S., Daley, J., & Mackiernan, Y. D. (1995). Using severity-adjusted stroke mortality rates to judge hospitals. *International Journal for Quality in Health Care*, *7*(2), 81–94.

de Kervasdoué, J. (2004). *L'hôpital. Que sais-je?* Paris: Presses Universitaires de France.

Kimberly, J. R., & Minvielle, E. (2003). Quality as an organizational problem. In: S. S. Mick & M. Wytenbach (Eds), *Organizational innovation and health care*. San Francisco: Jossey-Bass.

Kissick, W. (1998). *Medicine's dilemma*. New Haven: Yale University Press.

Landon, B., Iezzoni, L., Hughes, J. S., & Mackiernan, Y. (1996). Judging hospitals by severity-adjusted mortality rates: the case of CABG surgery. *Inquiry*, *33*(2), 155–166.

Le Palmarès des Hôpitaux. (1998, October). *Science et Avenir*, 32–71.

Leyland, A. H., & Boddy, F. A. (1998). League tables and acute myocardial infarction. *Lancet*, *351*(9102), 555–558.

Maynard, A. (1998). Competition and quality: rhetoric and reality. *International Journal for Quality in Health Care*, *10*(5), 379–384.

McGlynn, E. A. (2003a). An evidence-based national quality measurement and reporting system. *Medical Care*, *41*(1 Suppl.), I8–15.

McGlynn, E. A. (2003b). Selecting common measures of quality and system performance. *Medical Care*, *41*(1 Suppl.), I39–47.

McKee, M., & Hunter, D. (1995). Mortality league tables: do they inform or mislead? *Quality in Health Care*, *4*(1), 5–12.

Minvielle, E., & Kimberly, J. R. (2000). Conclusion. In: J. R. Kimberly & E. Minvielle (Eds), *The quality imperative: Measurement and management of quality in health care* (pp. 185–204). London: Imperial College Press.

Minvielle, E., Michel, P., Grenier-Sennelier, C., Daucourt, V., & Corriol, C. (2003). *COMPAQH: Rapport D'Etape 2003*. Paris: INSERM,

Moisdon, J. C. (2000). What is the value of your DRG's? New management tools in the French hospital sector. *Sociologie du Travail*, *42*(1), 31–51.

Naylor, D., Iron, K., & Hnada, K. (2002). Measuring health system performance: Problems and opportunities in the era of assessment and accountability. In: P. C. Smith (Ed.), *Measuring up: Improving health system performance in OECD countries* (pp. 13–34). Paris: Organisation for Economic Co-operation and Development.

de Pouvourville, G., & Minvielle, E. (2002). Measuring the quality of hospital care: The state of the art. In: P. C. Smith (Ed.), *Measuring up: Improving health system performance in OECD countries* (p. 380). Paris: Organisation for Economic Co-operation and Development.

Rosenthal, M. B., Fernandopulle, R., Song, H. R., & Landon, B. (2004). Paying for quality: providers' incentives for quality improvement. *Health Affairs*, *23*(2), 127–141.

Thomas, J. W., & Hofer, T. P. (1999). Accuracy of risk-adjusted mortality rate as a measure of hospital quality of care. *Medical Care*, *37*(1), 83–92.

Thomson, R. G. (1998). Quality to the fore at last. *British Medical Journal*, *17*, 95–96.

APPENDIX

Comparisons of Quality Initiatives in Selected Countries

The main national initiatives in the development of QIs in the last 10 years are presented in the table below. This overview is not exhaustive. National quality initiatives are underway in countries such as Spain, Portugal, Italy, and Norway. Moreover, a number of East European countries are currently launching similar initiatives.

Country	Target level in health system	Type of System (external, internal)	Context
U.K.	National, regional, local	External: league tables	Quality as main national priority Coordinated by NHS (NSF, NICE, CHI, NPSA, NPF)
U.K. Scotland	Local	External: benchmarking, site web	Commercial, Dr. Foster
	National	External: clinical outcome report	National Health System –Scotland
Denmark	National, Regional	External: public disclosure Internal: audit process	Danish national project (Government)
Germany	National	External: clinical performance measures	Federal Consortium for Quality, the Coordinating Committee (a joint committee of both the physicians and the hospitals committee)
Netherlands	National	External: integrated in a four dimensions model (consumer orientation, finance, quality, ability to learn)	Ministry of Health, Welfare and Sport
Sweden	National	Internal and external: clinical outcomes (based on National Quality Registers)	Federation of Swedish country councils and National Board oh health and Welfare (independent from the MOH)

NSF, National Service Frameworks; NICE, National Institute for Clinical Excellence; CHI, Commission for health improvement; NPSA, National Patient Safety Agency; NPF, National Performance Frameworks; MOH, Ministry of Health.

A DIAGNOSTIC TOOL FOR HRM BENCHMARKING WITHIN A HEALTH CARE SYSTEM

Tim Mazzarol, Geoffrey N. Soutar and Douglas Adam

ABSTRACT

We outline the design and development of a diagnostic tool for use in health care organisations to assist in benchmarking the management of human resources. Key areas of focus were the way in which employees perceived their work roles, work loads, satisfaction with their work life and their views of clients, peers, front line supervisors and senior management. Using a cross-section of metropolitan and regional health services, the study used focus groups and large-scale survey research to capture data on these employee perceptions. Principal component analysis identified a series of 'factors' associated with the key elements found within human resource management (HRM) frameworks. The diagnostic tool we developed offers a way of measuring employees' perceptions of their work environment and offers managers within large health care service organisations a potentially useful tool for benchmarking human resources.

International Health Care Management
Advances in Health Care Management, Volume 5, 273–295
ISSN: 1474-8231/doi:10.1016/S1474-8231(05)05010-X

Health care, particularly as it applies to a hospital system, occurs in a complex management environment. Contemporary health care requires the application of sophisticated technology, as well as highly skilled staff who are usually employed in small teams that operate within large organisations. As a service industry, the quality of health care is contingent on the overall skill and performance of the people employed within the system. While there are many management tools for monitoring and benchmarking the efficiency and effectiveness of technology and other tangible assets in health care systems, this is often not the case for people.

Benchmarking has been defined as "a structured approach for looking outside an organisation to study and adapt the best outside practices to complement internal operations with creative, new ideas" (Schuler, 1998, p. 40). It has been used to guide organisational performance by identifying best practice and comparing current behaviour to such "benchmarks" (Fong, Cheng, & Ho, 1998). However, benchmarking can also have an internal focus as, for example, when it is used to examine changes in an organisation's practices and performance over time (Glanz & Dailey, 1992). Internal benchmarking comparing employee satisfaction and performance against ideal performance standards, or comparing one subunit within an organisation with another is recognised as a legitimate approach and has been followed in this study.

One area where benchmarking has been used successfully is in the management of human resources. A number of studies have found links between a range of HRM practices e.g., training and skills development, the use of teams, and employee participation and empowerment and organisational outcomes, such as increased productivity, quality and sales (Osterman, 1994; Pfeffer, 1994; Fitz-enz, 1997). Within the health care services field the primary focus for HRM benchmarking has been on financial measures such as hourly labour costs, recruitment and separation rates and how these relate to an overall human capital return on investment (ROI) measure (Kocakulah & Harris, 2002). Also measured have been absenteeism and staff turnover (Rodwell, Lam, & Fastenau, 2000; Runy, 2003; Stack, 2003), and expenditure on training and development with a focus on how different parts of an organisation compare against common criteria (Howes & Foley, 1993).

While these studies have examined the link between HRM practices and performance at an organisational level, it has been suggested that there is also a need to study outcomes at an individual employee level. For example, Browne (2000, p. 55) argued, "HRM practices are only progressive if the concern for organisational-level outcomes is matched by a concern for the well-being of employees who are directly affected by these practices." It also seems reasonable to suggest that individual employee outcomes (e.g. employee satisfaction and morale) will have an impact on the performance of the organisation as a whole. This is particularly true in a service context, where customers often look for tangible indicators (such as the quality of their interaction with employees during service delivery) to assist in their evaluation of a largely intangible service (Lovelock, 1996). In situations such as this, customers are exposed to the consequences of HRM practices, whether they are good or bad. HRM benchmarking can be undertaken using both internal and external measures; however, it is important to link any performance measures to the organisation's strategic goals and to have clear outcomes (Becker & Huselid, 2003). Consequently, it is important to understand HRM practices and the present paper discusses the development of a diagnostic tool for use in benchmarking HRM practices in a health care context.

AN HRM FRAMEWORK FOR THE EFFECTIVE MANAGEMENT OF PEOPLE

The Health Workforce Reform Task Force of the Health Department of the Government of Western Australia originally commissioned the research underlying this study to develop a questionnaire to assist health care organisations benchmark their HRM practice. Two years prior to this study commencing a separate study was undertaken by a commercial consulting team to identify a set of HRM indicators that might be used by the WA Health Department to benchmark the performance of their human resources. Using a qualitative methodology that employed a series of workshops and focus groups in which facilitators from the consultancy working in conjunction with members from the Health Service identified a list of 33 potentially measurable performance indicators was identified. These were grouped into a five-part framework: namely work organisation, leadership, availability for work, utilisation of people and performance development. These elements are discussed in turn in subsequent sections.

The Work Organisation

The first of these elements was Work Organisation, which is the way in which work is identified and structured to achieve organisational, enterprise and customer outputs. This element can be measured through four indicators: (i) the number of 'reporting' levels of management from the CEO/GM to the last manager in the reporting chain inclusive of both; (ii) the average span of control or number of direct reports that managers have; (iii) the percentage of people who consistently work in workplace teams; and (iv) how effectively the work group/department/organisation worked as a team to meet the needs of the business/organisation.

The first two were not included in the HRM diagnostic tool as existing reports were thought to be a better way of collecting such data. The organisational structure and managerial span of control are more accurately captured via internal records than via a self-administered questionnaire of this kind. These two items may be important within larger health care systems, particularly where management is concerned. However, an analysis of the other two indicators was undertaken. The majority of employees who work within large health service organisations operate in team environments. Further, management's commitment to the team concept is vital in the success or failure of teams (Drew & Coulson-Thoms, 1996) and teamwork contributes to the enhancement of work quality, customer satisfaction and productivity (Montaque & Pitman, 1995).

Leadership

The second element (Leadership) was defined as creating an environment in which people:

1. know what is expected of them individually and as a group;
2. understand organisational issues and the need for change;
3. are motivated and enthusiastic to achieve;
4. make necessary changes happen.

The initial research comprising a series of facilitated workshops held with HRM staff and other health service managers suggested 10 indicators, namely: external customer/client satisfaction; employee perceptions of internal customer satisfaction; employee involvement in improvement initiatives; employee perception of management performance; employee understanding of business issues; absenteeism per employee; employee identification with organisation's vision and goals; employee involvement in business planning and decision making; employee satisfaction with work life and the number of formal grievances per employee.

In the present study, external customer or client satisfaction and absenteeism were not measured. The former was beyond the study's scope and had been addressed by other research, while the latter was measured through the payroll system. The other indicators were measured using approaches suggested in similar organisational contexts. For example, other service industries have found that asking one question about internal customer satisfaction is inadequate as satisfaction is a multidimensional construct (Turner & Pol, 1995; Hajjat, 2002). Customer service is also thought to be multidimensional and has often been measured through the SERVQUAL scale, which has reliability, tangibles, assurance, empathy and responsiveness dimensions (Parasuraman, Zeithaml, & Berry, 1988; "Strategies for service quality," 1994).

The other key indicators within the Leadership dimension examined employees understanding of their role within the organisation and how well they aligned their own goals with those of the organisation. The importance of an organisation having a clear vision and mission that gives focus and direction to employees is a characteristic of companies that have successfully introduced quality management ("Customer service," 1994). Employee involvement in strategic planning is beneficial to the implementation of an organisation's new vision and mission (Allen, 1995) and has been successfully used in large health service organisations to secure employee buy-in and commitment to the organisation's goals (Hillebrand, 1994).

Employee satisfaction with their work life is recognised as an important element in the development of a successful organisation although, in the past, many organisations did not measure such indicators well, due to the difficulties involved (Louise, 1996). The use of quantifiable measures of employee satisfaction offers managers a means of benchmarking such 'soft systems' and strategically monitoring trends in people's performance (Yeung & Berman, 1997).

Availability for Work

The third element within the HRM framework was employees' availability for work to ensure appropriately skilled people are available to achieve organisational goals. Five indicators measured this element: (i) the available hours (the prime indictor); (ii) absenteeism per employee; (iii) planned and non-productive hours per employee; (iv) standard paid hours per employee; and (v) additional work hours as a percentage of the total standard paid hours. None of these indicators was measured in the current study as they were already captured in existing HRM systems.

Utilisation of People

The fourth element within the HRM framework was the utilisation of people, which is the degree to which people effectively spend time contributing to the achievement of organisational goals. Four indicators measured this element: (i) income-revenue per employee per annum; (ii) profit per employee; (iii) staff to client/customer ratio; and (iv) average employee hours per patient or diagnostic-related grouping (DRG). As with the last element, these indicators were not included in the present study as they were measured in existing systems within the health service.

Performance Development

This final element in the HRM framework was associated with the way jobs and people are developed to achieve organisational goals. Ten indicators were identified as potential measures of this element, namely: the percentage of employees formally appraised; annual training and development hours per employee; the percentage of customer satisfaction change over time; the percentage of training that matches training needs analysis; the percentage of employees who receive specific follow up action or review after poor evaluations; the percentage of improvement in employee performance after training; employee satisfaction with performance management processes; the percentage of performance management actions implemented annually; the percentage of employees who feel equipped to do their job and the equity of access to training.

The requirement to measure employee competence and the benefits from training and ongoing performance appraisal has been recognised as important to the health services sector (Waddell, 2001). However, such measures can be difficult to obtain. Of the 10 indicators, only employee satisfaction with performance management processes and the equity of access to training were included as the other indicators are either measured elsewhere or cannot be assessed through individual responses to a survey, which was the approach chosen, as outlined in the next section.

THE PRESENT STUDY

The study was undertaken in three stages. The first stage led to the identification of the framework discussed in the previous section. As already mentioned, this stage involved discussions with senior HR managers in the health service sector who represented a cross-section of health service organisations (e.g., a hospital and its allied health services) in the metropolitan and regional areas of Western Australia. During the second stage, pilot studies were undertaken in a large metropolitan, two small metropolitan, and a regional health service organisation. Focus groups were held with a cross-section of staff at each of these health service organisations during this stage. The pilot studies were followed by a large-scale survey of all employees at these sites.

Prior to the commencement of the second stage the research team held meetings with senior managers from across the WA Health Service including representatives from the hospitals and HR management area. These agreed that the primary focus of the survey should be on the employees or staff operating within the Health Service. The need for a single survey instrument or multiple instruments for each centre was also discussed. It was agreed that there may not be a need for multiple instruments. Centres which may seek to know how their performance on the HRM indicators was rated would be able to be separately identified from a single common instrument. Demographic items within the survey would enable individual centres and employee groups to be identified. Should individual centres wish to add specific questions to the survey at a later stage this would be possible once a common core of question items had been developed. Several key observations were made. The first of these was that the rapid pace of change in the Health Service had affected many employees and it was uncertain whether all employees would feel that they are involved in improvement initiatives or what that involvement would mean. Second, employee perception of management performance was likely to be a function of outcomes and process. It was considered desirable for consultations to take place with managers themselves about this issue. Third, employee understanding of business issues was not felt to be uniform across the system but something that would vary from centre to centre depending upon its size and culture. Finally, a key measure of employee satisfaction with their jobs was considered to be how well they were "liked" within their communities. This was thought to be particularly so for regional centres. It was decided to follow up many of these issues during the focus group discussions.

Sampling and Data Collection

Four focus groups were undertaken with a cross-section of staff members from the participating health centres. The sessions helped in refining the identified performance indicators and examining how employees understood the indicators. The focus groups were designed to provide a representation of opinions and they included between 8 and 12 people in each session, with nurses, administrative staff, allied health and technical support staff being represented. Doctors were not represented in any of the focus groups due to the difficulties in securing their participation. The research team, which was experienced in such a research method, facilitated all of the focus groups using a common discussion protocol based on the HRM Framework. Each session was taped and subsequently transcribed for later analysis.

Following the focus groups and the development of the questionnaire, a survey was prepared and distributed through the HR managers of each of the participating health service organisations. Each questionnaire contained a covering letter from the HR mangers that explained the purpose of the study and an envelope into which completed questionnaires could be placed and sealed for return to the research team. This was important, as some of the findings were considered potentially sensitive. The sample was drawn from the four health care services (e.g. large metropolitan, two small metropolitan and one regional centre) that had participated in the focus groups. All employees in these four health service organisations were sent a questionnaire via the internal mail. Participation in the survey was voluntary and all responses were anonymous. After the distribution of 1,700 surveys a total of 403 completed questionnaire were returned, providing a response rate of approximately 24%. While a higher response rate would have been desirable, the level of response was good when it is considered that the survey was voluntary and relatively complex.

Responses to questions that asked about years of work, job categories, full and part-time employment, management levels, education and training levels, age, gender, ethnicity and disability were compared to known figures for the sector. The analysis suggested that the sample was a good representation of the nursing, administrative, technical, general and allied health staff working within the WA Health Service, although participation in the study by doctors was low (4.2%). Despite this limitation, the final sample compared favourably with the true population in terms of demographics with a good cross-section of management levels represented (33.5% of sample).

Measures

As already discussed, the questionnaire contained a series of items that was designed to measure the Work Organisation, Leadership, and Performance

Development elements of the HRM framework. Items were asked as statements to which respondents indicated their agreement using a seven-point Likert-type scale that ranged from strongly disagree (1) to strongly agree (7).

Eight items asked about the need to work in teams, with respondents being asked to indicate whether this was a requirement of their jobs and, if so, the percentage of their working time that was spent in a team environment; while another eight items asked about internal customer satisfaction. Nineteen items asked about management performance and six items asked about the respondent's identification with the organisation's vision and goals. Workplace satisfaction was measured using a 39-item scale, while four items asked about grievance handling procedures within the organisation. Satisfaction with the performance measurement process was measured using 15 items, while two items asked about the respondent's satisfaction with their access to training and development.

ANALYSIS

Following the collection of data, a series of principal components analyses were undertaken to assess the underlying structure of the data and to refine the scales that were used to measure the various factors. Scale refinement was obtained by examining item-to-total correlation scores (Churchill, 1979) that provided an indication of the contribution each item made to the reliability of the scale, measured by Cronbach's (1951) coefficient alpha and, as such, suggested which items might be removed.

Each group of items was evaluated using Kaiser's (1974) measures of sampling adequacy (MSA), which is one of the best measures for determining the suitability of a set of data for factor analysis (Stewart, 1981). An MSA below 0.50 is unacceptable, while those below 0.60 are of doubtful value (Kaiser, 1974). In each case, a principal components factor analysis procedure with varimax rotation was used to provide a "simple structure". In keeping with the usual principal components approach, only factors with eigenvalues greater than one were retained (Hair, Anderson, Tatham, & Black, 1992). The variance explained for each factor, which is determined by summing the eigenvalues of the retained factors and dividing by the number of items (Hair et al., 1992), analysis is also reported. It is generally hoped that the retained factors should explain at least 60% of the variance in the data, which was the case in the present study.

RESULTS

Each of the principal component analyses is shown in Tables 1–5, which display the items, the factor loadings for each item, and coefficient alpha.

Work Organisational Teamwork

Employees' perceptions of teamwork effectiveness were examined in the first analysis. Respondents were asked to indicate whether their duties required them "to work within a team environment" and the average proportion of their time spent working in a team environment as part of their working week. It was found that around 75% of a respondent's time was spent working as part of a team and that 95% of respondents were required to work in teams. The focus groups had highlighted the importance of communication between team members, team leadership, participation of team members, team esprit de corps, success of team goal achievements and goal congruence among team members and employee satisfaction with their place in the team.

The MSA for the teamwork items was 0.92, suggesting they were suitable for factor analysis. Six of the items loaded onto a single factor with an eigenvalue of 5.14 that explained 64% of variance. Following the removal of two items with low item-to-total correlations, a four-item scale shown in Table 1 emerged that was extremely reliable (alpha = 0.91) (Nunnally,

Table 1. Teamwork Effectiveness Questions to be used in the Final Survey.

Question Items	Factor Loadings
Esprit de corps	
• My work team enjoys a high degree of team spirit and esprit de corps	0.77
• My work team is successful in achieving its objectives	0.74
• All members of my work team fully participate in decision making and achieving our goals	0.72
• All members of my work team fully understand the team's goals	0.69
Eigenvalue	5.14
Percent of variance explained	64.3
Alpha	0.90

Note: Mean score based on a scale where 1 = strongly disagree, 7 = strongly agree.

Table 2. Customer Satisfaction Questions to be Used in the Survey.

Question Items	Factor	1	2
Service Quality			
• Most of our customers are satisfied with our organisation		0.82	
• Not many of our customers complain about this organisation		0.79	
• Customers are well looked after in this organisation		0.74	
• The quality of service we provide is very good		0.69	
Feedback			
• I frequently receive formal feedback as to how well we satisfy our patients			0.86
• I frequently receive formal feedback as to how well I satisfy those within my centre whom I serve			0.86
	Eigenvalues	3.47	1.49
	Percentage of variance explained	56.2	67.3
	Alpha	0.80	0.78

Note: Mean score based on a scale where 1 = strongly disagree, 7 = strongly agree.

1967). Given the nature of the items in the scale, the factor was named "esprit de corps".

Internal Customer Focus

During the focus groups an important issue was whether the employee provided services to a specific set of clients or to a broad range across the system. Nursing staff were particularly sensitive to the level of support they felt the organisation provided them to fulfil their duties. Their ability to service their patients was frequently measured in terms of the nurse/patient ratio found within the wards. As one nurse commented:

> To me it means if I'm a typical nurse on the ward, it means I've got enough staff to service the number of patients that I've got at that time, so I expect management to have rostered adequate staff to do the job in hand at the level of activity that we've got.

Those in non-clinical areas, who did not have regular contact with customers, found it more difficult to identify how well they were being served or were serving. The formal measurement of the satisfaction of internal clients was usually measured through how many complaints were received. For those in areas such as engineering, client satisfaction was measured by

Table 3. Management Performance Questions.

Question Items	Factor	1	2
Management equity			
• I feel confident that this organisation's senior managers will treat employees fairly		0.80	
• Senior management does not show favours among the different functional areas at this organisation		0.78	
• Senior management at this organisation are willing to defend the resources and rights of the employees		0.78	
• Senior management at this organisation are able to acquire additional resources for their employees		0.74	
• I trust senior management to do what is in the best interest of this organisation's employees		0.73	
Leadership			
• Senior management at this organisation have the courage to achieve the objectives they set			0.56
• Current senior management have the knowledge and skills to effectively lead this organisation			0.47
• Senior management has a clear idea of where this organisation is going			0.46
	Eigenvalues	10.72	1.06
	Percentage of variance	56.4	62.0
	Alpha	0.94	0.83

Note: Mean score based on a scale where 1 = strongly disagree, 7 = strongly agree.

whether equipment functioned. It was generally felt desirable to have better feedback on satisfaction from internal and external clients.

Employees' perceptions of internal satisfaction were examined in the second analysis, as can be seen in Table 2. The MSA in this case was 0.78; suggesting factor analysis was likely to be useful. Two factors with eigenvalues of 3.47 and 1.49 that explained 67% of variance were found. Four items that asked about the quality provided to internal customers loaded onto the first factor, which was termed "service quality", while two items that asked about satisfaction with feedback received loaded onto the second factor, which was named "feedback". The reliability for both scales were acceptable (alphas were 0.80 and 0.78, respectively). Results are shown in Table 2.

Table 4. Employee Identification with Visions and Goals Questions.

Question Items	Factor Loadings
Identify with Vision & Goals	
• Staff are aware of this organisation's goals	0.85
• This organisation is successful in achieving its objectives	0.84
• Staff are aware of this organisation's objectives	0.83
• Staff are aware of this organisation's vision	0.82
• This organisation is successful in achieving its goals	0.72
Eigenvalues	3.60
Proportion of variance	60.0
Alpha	0.86

Note: Mean score based on a scale where 1 = strongly disagree or 7 = strongly agree.

Management Performance

The focus groups identified key measures of management performance. The first of these was how supportive the manager was towards employees. The second was the level of communication or consultation provided by the manager and the extent to which the manager informed employees about what was expected of them and the things they needed to know. A third element was the extent to which the manager was viewed as approachable, accessible and whether the manager was trusted. A fourth element was whether the manager's decisions resulted in effective outcomes and the manager's flexibility when an outcome was different from that which had been anticipated. Further elements were the willingness and ability of the manager to defend the resources and rights of the employees within the system against other groups and the ability of the manager to acquire additional resources to assist employees successfully complete their work. Finally, the focus groups identified as important issues, whether the manager was viewed as knowledgeable or expert and whether the manager was fair in dealing with employees and equitable in allocation of work tasks to employees. As noted by one employee:

> What I was going to say is that you can have two different people on in the same situation and one is total confusion and a complete stuff up, and the next one everything runs smoothly, and it' is basically the manager's ability to allocate the resources to the right point where it's required at the right time.

In the third analysis, items that asked about managers' performance were examined. The MSA was 0.95; suggesting factor analysis was likely to be

Table 5. Employee Satisfaction Index Workplace Satisfaction.

Question Items Factor	1	2	3	4	5
Co-Workers					
• Satisfied with the people you work with in your job	0.76				
• Satisfied with the quality of the people in your unit	0.74				
• Satisfied with the people you talk to in your job	0.67				
Job interest					
• Opportunities for interesting work in your job		0.82			
• Opportunities for challenging work in your job		0.81			
• Your choice to learn new things in your job		0.77			
• The chance to learn different jobs		0.74			
Resources					
• The resources available to your unit			0.69		
• The information provided to you			0.58		
• The way top management runs this organization			0.56		
Work Load					
• The time to do your job properly				0.83	
• The amount of overtime you do				0.75	
• The amount of pressure in your job				0.70	
Performance Review					
• Feedback about your performance review					0.90
• Results of your performance review					0.90
• Your area or work team's performance review					0.82
• The performance management process					0.73
• Feedback provided to you					0.62
• This organisation's disciplinary system					0.42
Eigenvalues	9.40	2.27	2.02	1.58	1.09
Percentage of variance	37.6	46.7	54.6	61.1	65.5
Alpha	0.77	0.89	0.72	0.75	0.91

extremely useful. As can be seen in Table 3, the items loaded onto two factors with eigenvalues of 10.72 and 1.06 respectively that, together, explained 62% of the variance. Five items relating to perceptions of management's fairness and supportiveness loaded onto the first factor, which was named "management equity" and three items relating to leadership skills loaded onto the second factor, which was named "leadership". The scales were very reliable (with alphas of 0.94 and 0.83).

Employee Identification with Organisational Vision and Goals

It was felt that employees would identify with organisational vision and goals on at least two levels. The first level was their work unit or professional group, while the second level was the centre to which they were attached. All of the focus groups suggested a low level of employee identification with the vision and goals of their organisation but most felt that they understood and identified with the vision and goals of their individual subunits. Some identified with the common vision and goals of their professional body, which spanned more than one organisation. This is common in health services, where nurses and doctors orient more towards their respective professional bodies than they do toward their own organisation. Mintzberg (1999) describes this phenomenon as the *"pull to professionalise"*.

For some centres, the level of employee identification with the overall vision and goals of their organisation was viewed as a function of senior management. In organisations where management had devoted time and energy to building and communicating a common vision and goals, employees were more likely to identify with the organisation's common vision.

The MSA for the items that measured employees' identification with the organisation's vision and goals was 0.82. As can be seen from Table 4, five of the items loaded onto a single factor with an eigenvalue of 3.60 that explained 60% of the variance, which was labelled "identify with vision and goals." The scale was reliable (alpha = 0.86).

EMPLOYEES' WORKPLACE SATISFACTION

The focus group discussions on job satisfaction centred on developing an understanding of the factors that made participants "satisfied" with their work. As a result of this process a common set of criteria emerged. The first was the need for acknowledgement, recognition and feedback for good work or effort. Such acknowledgement was desired from management, co-workers and clients. The second criterion was the need for satisfactory financial compensation, although the focus groups suggested that, while financial remuneration was important, it was not sufficient for most employees to feel fully satisfied with their work. This is consistent with the two-factor theory of motivation in which salary and work conditions are satisfiers or "hygiene factors", while achievement, educational enhancement and professional recognition are true motivators (Herzberg, Mausner, & Snyderman, 1959;

Herzberg, 1968). Further, both are important in the management of health service employees (Gunnar-Vaughn, 2003).

A more important influence was the ability of the worker to see the successful outcome of their work effort. This might involve seeing the product of work effort used successfully by other colleagues or elsewhere in the system. Employee satisfaction was also influenced by their autonomy and responsibility. Many employees were specialists and took pride in their professionalism. Being able to use their discretion in problem solving and decision making while completing their work was a source of satisfaction. The focus groups suggested that employee satisfaction was likely to be impacted by the level of time and resources provided. A lack of time or resources to effectively complete work tasks was considered to be a common source of frustration and dissatisfaction. The education and training received to enable people to perform their work was also important. Much of the work in the health service sector requires specialist training and skills as; if employees are not adequately trained they cannot perform effectively and therefore, are dissatisfied.

When asked what factors were likely to be sources of dissatisfaction, four factors were identified. The first was isolation as being isolated from colleagues and not being able to obtain feedback on performance or information was a major source of dissatisfaction. Isolation was not necessarily a function of geography, but more a function of communication. The second was a lack of the resources needed to enable employees to successfully achieve objectives. The third was poor management and incompetent co-workers. Because many employees worked in teams with different professional backgrounds, friction can arise if one group does not complete its work. Alternatively, those taking over shifts might find the previous shift was poorly organised or did not complete its tasks, impacting negatively on the subsequent shift and leading to dissatisfaction.

Workplace Satisfaction

Thirty-nine questions were used to measure satisfaction with work on three key subcategories [employee satisfaction with their workplace; employee attitudes toward their work;and employee satisfaction with supervision and fellow workers]. Twenty-five items asked about workplace satisfaction. The factor analysis found an MSA 0.88, which suggests that the analysis was likely to be very useful. An initial analysis found six factors with eigenvalues ranging from 9.41 to 1.03 that explained 70% of the variance.

Some items were excluded, however, due to low item-to-total correlations, leaving 19 question items that loaded onto five satisfaction factors, as can be seen in Table 5. Three items loaded onto the first factor that related to satisfaction with "co-workers", while four items loaded onto the second factor that was related to the intrinsic interest employees had with their job; which was termed a "job interest" factor. Three items loaded onto the third factor that was related to satisfaction with resources, information and how well management runs the organisation, leading to its label as a "resources" factor. Three items loaded onto the fourth factor that was related to satisfaction with the time available to complete work and work pressure, leading to its being labelled a "work load" factor. Six items that were related to individual and team performance review and feedback loaded onto the fifth factor, which was labelled as a "performance review" factor.

Employee Attitudes Toward Work

A further principal component analysis was undertaken on 24 items that asked about respondents' attitudes toward work, supervisors and fellow workers, as can be seen in Table 6. The MSA in this case was 0.82 and an initial solution found seven factors with eigenvalues ranging from 5.84 to 1.077 that explained 62% of the variance. Thirteen items loaded onto five factors. Two items loaded onto the first factor that related to willingness to remain in their current occupation and was labelled "loyalty". Two items loaded onto the second factor that was related to pride in being associated with the organisation and was labelled "organisational pride". Three items loaded onto the third factor that related to concerns over depression, unhappiness or worries arising from work and was labelled "work pressure". Three items loaded onto the fourth factor that was related to job enjoyment and pleasure and was labelled "work enjoyment". Three items loaded onto the fifth factor that was related to feelings that the job had meaning and that others understood what they did in this job and was termed "job identification". Three items loaded onto the sixth factor that was related to interactions between employees and staff and external clients and was labelled "interaction". Two items loaded onto the seventh factor that was related to "supervision".

Table 6.   Employee Attitudes to Work, Supervisors, Fellow Workers.

Question Items Factor	1	2	3	4	5	6	7
Loyalty							
There is not much to be gained by sticking with this organisation indefinitely	0.65						
It would take very little change in my present circumstances to cause me to leave this organization	0.64						
Organisational pride							
I told my friends that this organisation is a great organisation to work for		0.67					
I am proud to tell others that I am part of this organisation		0.66					
Work pressure							
I'm often worried because of my work			0.79				
I'm often depressed because of my work			0.79				
I often feel miserable because of my work			0.73				
Work enjoyment							
I'm often cheerful about my work				0.81			
For me my work really flies by				0.80			
I'm often enthusiastic about my work				0.76			
Job identification							
Very few people in this organisation know what I do					0.70		
Very few people in this organisation understand what our unit does					0.70		
Very few people in this organisation understand how everything fits together					0.70		
Interaction							
Clinical and non-clinical staff in this organisation enjoy interacting with each other						0.80	
Non-clinical staff in this organisation enjoy interacting with patients						0.80	
Staff in this organisation are focused on patient needs, desires and attitudes						0.65	

Table 6. (*Continued*)

Question Items	Factor	1	2	3	4	5	6	7
Supervision								
Your immediate supervisor								0.88
The way your supervisor is carrying out his/her job								0.86
	Eigenvalues	5.84	2.23	1.88	1.47	1.29	1.17	1.08
	Percentage of variance	24.3	33.6	41.5	47.6	52.9	57.8	62.3
	Alpha	0.82	0.82	0.79	0.76	0.63	0.71	0.96

Note: Mean score based on a scale where 1 = strongly disagree and 7 = strongly agree.

DISCUSSION

The importance of benchmarking human resources (HR) has become a focus of research and analysis within large organisations in recent years, providing strategic guidance to HR departments as to ways to enhance worker satisfaction and organisational productivity (Glanz & Dailey, 1992). Most efforts to benchmark HR performance have been limited to such readily measured indicators as payroll cost, absenteeism and turnover, with a tendency for HR managers to avoid more sophisticated measures and to, therefore, make decisions more through intuition than evidence (Hilltrop & Despres, 1994). Nevertheless, benchmarking HR indicators is a desirable objective that offers benefits to organisations (Ulrich, Brockbank, & Yeung, 1989). This is particularly the case for many public health service organisations that have faced major pressures for work place reform and enhanced productivity in recent years at a time when public-sector health budgets have been under strain (Bach, 2000). Successful health care service HRM requires a strategic approach within which HR processes are regularly monitored and reviewed, with substantial input and participation from employees who then are able better to align their own goals with those of the organisation, and receive suitable rewards and recognition for effort (Zairi, 1998).

The present study supports Hackman, Oldham, Janson, and Purdy's (1975) research, which outlined a framework for the strategic redesign of work to achieve enhanced job-enrichment and performance. The framework recognised the importance of offering employees variety in the skills and tasks they undertook in their work, while allowing them to understand the significance of these tasks in a wider employment context. Also of importance was allowing employees autonomy within their decision-making and adequate feedback on their performance. This combination has a positive influence on employees' psychological states, leading to improved motivation, greater satisfaction, enhanced performance and lower absenteeism and turnover. The focus groups and the structure of the key elements within the employee satisfaction index that was outlined in Tables 5 and 6 reinforce the relevance of this framework.

Hackman et al.'s (1975) research has been used in measuring the relationship between job-structure and employee motivation among hospital staff in service support functions (Lee-Ross, 1999, 2002), focussing on the inter-relationships between the core dimensions of the job, employees' psychological states and affective outcomes (measured by satisfaction, enhanced performance and employee commitment). It recognises the need to look beneath the superficial level of hours worked, absenteeism and staff turnover when benchmarking HRM performance (Stack, 2003).

The constructs identified in the study provide a means of measuring employees' views on:

• their workplace's organisation (e.g. teamwork effectiveness) and customer orientation;
• employees' understanding and satisfaction with their leadership;
• employees' identification with organisational goals; and
• employees' satisfaction with their work, workplace, supervision and co-workers.

They provided measures of most, if not all, of the criteria identified in the HR framework for the effective management of people that was initially developed by the Health Workforce Reform Task Force within the Government of Western Australia. The scales offer a diagnostic tool that can assist in benchmarking HRM processes and could be used in a periodic survey of employees, with the mean scores being compared across periods. HR managers within geographically dispersed health service organisations, such as in Western Australia, can also use the tool to compare employee responses from different health service organisations and using such data, can better understand existing HR performance measures, such as absenteeism, sickness or turnover statistics.

Similar scales have been used by large service organisations to benchmark customer satisfaction (Parasuraman, Berry, & Zeithaml, 1991), allowing managers an opportunity to collect comparable and quantifiable attitudes data to assist strategic HRM planning. The tool is a means of measuring some of the less tangible issues associated with human resources that have been recognised as being important to productivity and performance. From a policy perspective, the ability of a health care management system to regularly measure the attitudes and perceptions of its human resources and to observe statistical changes in these views is highly important. Health care is a complex service industry and quality is determined in large part by the way people are managed, organised and motivated. Regular use of a bench-marking survey allows managers to monitor the way in which employees respond to different variables over time and to use this to measure the likely impact of different HRM policies. Comparisons between centres or regions can also be made if the tool is used across an entire health care system.

CONCLUSIONS, LIMITATIONS AND FUTURE RESEARCH

Benchmarking HRM performance is internationally recognised as an important goal (Drost, Franye, Lowe, & Geringer, 2002). International comparisons of HRM practices provide useful guidance to organisations seeking best practice (Rodwell et al., 2000). However, there has been limited research into health service organisations, many of which are public sector entities (Bach, 2000).

The diagnostic tool developed in the present study provides a potentially useful way to measure employee perceptions and attitudes that can supplement existing HR performance indicators. As a benchmarking tool, the scale is focused internally rather than externally. While offering an enhancement over many existing quantitative measures that address such factors as hours worked and absenteeism, it remains limited in its application. The scale items used in the diagnostic tool are only indicators of employee perceptions and attitudes and provide only broad indicators of satisfaction. Such measures must be used in concert with other HR indicators and must be gathered on a regular basis that enables statistical comparisons from one period to the next.

While these measures were developed using a sample of Western Australian hospitals, employees who participated in the study included a wide range of occupational types, including doctors, nurses, allied health professionals, administrators, technical support personnel, and hotel services and maintenance staff. The generic nature of the indicators makes them suitable for many applications within the health services sector, although they are likely to be of greater value in clinical environments.

REFERENCES

Allen, R. (1995). On a clear day you can have a vision: A visioning model for everyone. *Leadership & Organisational Development Journal, 16*(5), 36–41.

Bach, S. (2000). Health sector reform and human resource management: Britain in comparative perspective. *International Journal of Human Resource Management, 11*(5), 925–942.

Becker, B., & Huselid, M. (2003). Measuring HR? *HR Magazine, 48*(12), 56–62.

Browne, J. H. (2000). Benchmarking HRM practices in healthy work organizations. *American Business Review, 18*(2), 54–61.

Churchill, G. A. (1979). A paradigm for developing better measures of marketing constructs. *Journal of Marketing Research, 16*(1), 64–73.

Cronbach, L. J. (1951). Coefficient alpha and the internal structure of tests. *Psychometrica, 16*, 297–334.

Customer service. (1994). Customer service can reap rich rewards. *Health Manpower Management, 20*(4), 7–8.

Drew, S., & Coulson-Thoms, C. (1996). Transformation through teamwork: The path to the new organization? *Management Decision, 34*(1), 7–17.

Drost, E. A., Frayne, C. A., Lowe, K. B., & Geringer, J. M. (2002). Benchmarking training and development practices: A multi-country comparative analysis. *Human Resource Management, 41*(1), 67–86.

Fitz-enz, J. (1997). Highly effective HR practices. *HR Focus, 74*, 11–12.

Fong, S. W., Cheng, E., & Ho, D. C. K. (1998). Benchmarking: A general reading for management practitioners. *Management Decision, 36*(6), 407–418.

Glanz, E. F., & Dailey, L. K. (1992). Benchmarking. *Human Resource Management, 31*(1–2), 9–20.

Gunnar-Vaughn, R. M. (2003). Motivators get creative. *Nursing Management, 34*(4), 12–13.

Hackman, R. J., Oldham, G., Janson, R., & Purdy, K. (1975). A new strategy for job-enrichment. *California Management Review, 17*(4), 57–71.

Hair, J. F., Anderson, R. E., Tatham, R. L., & Black, W. C. (1992). *Multivariate data analysis with readings*. New York: Macmillan.

Hajjat, M. (2002). Customer orientation: Construction and validation of the CUSTOR scale. *Marketing Intelligence & Planning, 20*(7), 428–441.

Herzberg, F., Mausner, B., & Snyderman, B. (1959). *The motivation to work*. New York: Wiley.

Herzberg, F. (1968). One more time: How do you motivate employees? *Harvard Business Review, 46*(1), 53–62.

Hillebrand, P. L. (1994). Strategic planning: A road map to the future. *Nursing Management, 25*(1), 30–32.

Hilltrop, J. M., & Despres, C. (1994). Benchmarking the performance of human resource management. *Long Range Planning, 27*(6), 43–57.

Howes, P., & Foley, P. (1993). Strategic human resource management: An Australian case study. *HR Human Resource Planning, 16*(3), 53–65.

Kaiser, H. F. (1974). An index of factorial simplicity. *Psychometrika, 39*, 31–36.

Kocakulah, M. C., & Harris, D. (2002). Measuring human capital cost through benchmarking in health care environment. *Journal of Health Care Finance, 29*(2), 27–38.

Lee-Ross, D. (1999). A comparative survey of job characteristics among chefs using large and small-scale hospital systems in the UK. *The Journal of Management Development, 18*(4), 342–350.

Lee-Ross, D. (2002). An exploratory study of work motivation among private and public sector hospital chefs in Australia. *The Journal of Management Development, 21*(7/8), 576–589.

Louise, C. (1996). Analysing business performance: Counting the 'soft' issues. *Leadership & Organisation Development Journal, 17*(4), 21–25.

Lovelock, C. H. (1996). *Services marketing.* London: Prentice-Hall.

Mintzberg, H. (1999). The structuring of organizations. In: G. Lewis, A. Morkel, G. Hubbard, S. Davenport & G. Stockport (Eds), *Australian and New Zealand strategic management: Concepts and cases,* (2nd ed.). Sydney: Prentice Hall.

Montaque, J., & Pitman, H. (1995). Currents: Human resources. *Hospital & Health Networks, 69*(24), 20.

Nunnally, J. C. (1967). *Psychometric theory.* New York: McGraw-Hill.

Osterman, P. (1994). How common is workplace transformation and who adopts it? *Industrial and Labour Relations Review, 47*(2), 173–189.

Parasuraman, A., Zeithaml, V. A., & Berry, L. L. (1988). SERVQUAL: A multiple-item scale for measuring consumer perceptions of service quality. *Journal of Retailing, 64*(1), 12–40.

Parasuraman, A., Berry, L. L., & Zeithaml, V. A. (1991). Refinement and reassessment of the SERVQUAL scale. *Journal of Retailing, 67*(4), 420–450.

Pfeffer, J. (1994). *Competitive advantage through people.* Boston: Harvard Business School Press.

Rodwell, J. J., Lam, J., & Fastenau, M. (2000). Benchmarking HRM and the benchmarking of benchmarking. *Employee Relations, 22*(4/5), 356–374.

Runy, L.-A. (2003). Staffing effectiveness: A toolkit for JCAHO's new standards. *Hospitals & Health Networks, 77*(3), 57–63.

Schuler, R. S. (1998). *Managing human resources* (6th ed.). Cincinnati: Southwestern College Publishing.

Stack, S. (2003). Beyond performance indicators: A case study in aged care. *Australian Bulletin of Labour, 29*(2), 143.

Stewart, D. W. (1981). The application and misapplication of factor analysis in marketing research. *Journal of Marketing Research, 18,* 51–62.

Strategies for service quality (1994). Addressing the issues of management and quality. *International Journal of Health Care Quality Assurance, 7*(4), 3–40.

Turner, P. D., & Pol, L. G. (1995). Beyond patient satisfaction. *Marketing Health Services, 15*(3), 45–53.

Ulrich, D., Brockbank, W., & Yeung, A. (1989). Beyond belief: A benchmark for human resources. *Human Resource Management, 28*(3), 311–335.

Waddell, D. (2001). Measurement issues in promoting continued competence. *Journal of Continuing Education in Nursing, 32*(3), 102–106.

Yeung, A. K., & Berman, B. (1997). Adding value through human resources: Reorienting human resource measurement to drive business performance. *Human Resource Management, 36*(3), 321–335.

Zairi, M. (1998). Building human resources capability in health care: A global analysis of best practice – Part 1. *Health Manpower Management, 24*(3), 88–96.

IMPLEMENTING A REGIONAL HEALTH INFORMATION NETWORK: IMPACT ON HEALTH CARE PERFORMANCE AND THE MANAGEMENT OF CHANGE

Manolis Tsiknakis, Angelina Kouroubali, Dimitris Vourvahakis and Stelios C. Orphanoudakis

ABSTRACT

The rising of chronic illness and the continuous aging of the global population requires a re-organization of health care systems based on relations and exchange of information to address patient needs in the community. The re-organization of health care systems involves interconnected changes and the development of integrated health care information systems and novel eHealth services. In Crete, the Foundation for Research and Technology-Hellas has developed HYGEIAnet, a Regional Health Information Network (RHIN) to contribute to the re-organization of health care systems and information sharing. We present HYGEIAnet, some of the most critical and novel eHealth services developed and deployed, discuss the impact of an RHIN on health care processes, and explore innovative models and services for health delivery

International Health Care Management
Advances in Health Care Management, Volume 5, 297–329
ISSN: 1474-8231/doi:10.1016/S1474-8231(05)05011-1

and the coordination of care. We then critically discuss lessons learned regarding the effective management of change to overcome organizational and cultural issues in such large-scale initiatives. The paper concludes with policy and practice recommendations for managing change processes in health care organizations.

Health care is a sector that currently experiences a number of pressures, both from inside and outside. The continuing innovation in medicine and health care technologies results in new methods and tools in health care. The demographic changes of an aging European population, combined with citizen empowerment, stretch the limits of what countries can offer as services of their national health systems. Governments are confronted by the urgent need to limit the rise in health care costs and achieve cost containment without compromising quality, euity and access. Consequently, new ways to organize and deliver health services are being investigated and experimented with. Public–private partnerships in care delivery are emerging. Citizens and patients are given more responsibility in the management of their own health and chronic illnesses. In today's challenging, dynamic, information and knowledge-intensive environment, it is not surprising that Information and Communication Technologies (ICT) are increasingly viewed as central to any strategy aimed at increasing productivity, controlling costs and improving care.

Health consumes a significant portion of national budgets in developed countries. Between 1960 and 1996, the percentage of GDP spent on health care by the OECD countries nearly doubled, rising from an average of 3.9–7%. There is no sign of any slowing down, and countries such as the U.S. are predicting increases of over 15% per annum (PriceWaterhouseCoopers, 1999). The expenditure on health in Europe was over 700 billion euros in 1999, of which an estimated 14 billion of 2% was spent on ICT. The prediction is that this market is set to double over the next 5 years (Deloitte & Touche, 2000). This growth is due to many factors including the maturing of the market, i.e., health catching up with other information-intensive market segments, and the rapid developments in medical science itself resulting in new treatments and therapies. The gap between the demand for health care from an increasingly well-informed and expectant public, and the ability of the state and health care organizations to meet this demand is widening all the time. Efficiency and cost-effectiveness are the key drivers in health care today, with the twin aims of delivering enhanced quality of care at the same or reduced cost. There is documented evidence from a number of trials that patients who are encouraged to take responsibility and assume an active role in their own health care management do better, enjoy a better quality of life, have fewer complications and cost less (Grimson, 2001). Paternalism is giving way to partnership; process centered health care is giving way to patient centric care; and consumer health care is emerging as a significant driver in the sector.

Citizens in developed countries are already spending an increasing percentage of their disposable income on health care and are making more decisions about their own treatment (PriceWaterhouseCoopers, 1999). Other important trends in health care include the movement towards shared or integrated care in which the single doctor–patient relationship is giving way to one in which an individual's health care is the responsibility of a team of professionals across all sectors of the health care system. This is being accompanied by a very significant growth in home care, which is increasingly viable even for seriously ill patients through sophisticated eHealth services facilitated by intelligent sensors, monitoring devices, hand-held technologies and the Internet. It is seen as better for patients by providing a more comfortable and familiar environment, and better for the health care system as a whole by reducing costs.

The shareable, ubiquitous and integrated electronic health record (I-EHR) is a fundamental requirement for integrated care (Katehakis, Tsiknakis, & Orphanoudakis, 2002). The I-EHR will be a lifelong, cradle to grave, record of an individual not necessarily stored in one place. The informed, knowledgeable and increasingly demanding patients will be at the heart of the health care system. Preventive medicine, which, at least in democratic countries, fundamentally requires the active engagement, understanding and involvement of the citizen or consumer, will no longer be the least of the concerns in health systems. The emphasis will shift to systems concerned with promoting wellness rather than treating illness. At the same time, medical errors are a growing cause for concern and a number of countries and health care organizations are mounting major campaigns to significantly reduce the number of errors. Approximately 100,000 Americans die each year from preventable errors in hospitals (Corrigan, Kohn, & Donaldson, 1999), which is more than the combined number of deaths from breast cancer, AIDS and motor vehicles (NCH, 2000). Medical errors generally result from a complex interplay of multiple factors, and reducing their frequency requires a combination of technical, social and organizational approaches. However, one single solution, which has been proven to significantly reduce medication errors, is the replacement of manual ordering systems by reliable automated ones (Bates, 2000).

The U.S. Institute of Medicine (IOM) (2001) in its report, "Crossing the Quality Chasm: A New Health System for the 21st Century" acknowledges the need of an integrated health system based on self-organizing subsystems to achieve a shared purpose. Local adaptation, innovation and initiative are essential ingredients for successful health systems. Subsystems need to follow a few simple rules adapted to local circumstances while examining performance. The current approach to health care is contrasted with the new approach proposed by the IOM (2001, p. 71) in Table 1. The new rules set forth are representative of the future developments in health care. Information and relationships form its core and patients are its main focus.

Given the complexity and diversity of health systems moving towards the new approach, improvements in health care systems must develop from within, from people who have the ability to change their behavior based upon experience and reflection. Dawson (1999) argues that the first step in achieving change is for those involved to realize that change is possible:

> Work in health cannot be subject to mass standardization and detailed hierarchical control. It needs to be customized to the context. Unless there is local ownership and commitment to solve the inevitable problems which arise, to train and motivate the people in the front line of action, to assemble appropriate resources and support, then [...] health indices are unlikely to improve.

Despite the facts that health systems undergo constant changes and improvements must develop from within, most health organizations are largely

Table 1.   Simple Rules for the 21st Century Health Care System.

Current Approach	New Rule
Care is based primarily on visits	Care is based on continuous healing relationships
Professional autonomy drives variability	Care is customized according to patient needs and values
Professionals control care	The patient is the source of control
Information is a record	Knowledge is shared and information flows freely
Decision-making is based on training and experience	Decision-making is evidence-based
Do no harm is an individual responsibility	Safety is a system property
Secrecy is necessary	Transparency is necessary
The system reacts to needs	Needs are anticipated
Cost reduction is sought	Waste is continuously decreased
Preference is given to professional roles over the system	Cooperation among clinicians is a priority

dominated by highly structured, hierarchical and historically determined norms and assumptions. Administrative changes are often taken as attempts to limit the freedom and quality of medical practice for the convenience or benefit of managers, corporations, insurers or government. Medical practitioners have a professional culture that is resistant to top-down management approaches (Contandriopoulos, Lauristin, & Leibovich, 1999).

In practice, regardless of careful management plans, hierarchies emerge, relationships and technologies develop and specialties become established (Anderson & McDaniel, 2000). The need for continuous transformation applies especially to patient-centered health care. The nature of the medical profession has an inherent component of uncertainty and transformation. According to its philosophical foundations set in ancient Greece, it is a profession in flux, where continuous education and improvement occurs to face the spectrum of human condition (Pellegrino, 2001). Hence, if health care providers view their profession as a vocation, the assumption of 'reluctance to change' is a mere paradox. Change is no longer a problem to resolve but an opportunity to improve health care delivery and customer care. With the current global increase of chronic conditions (WHO, 2002), health care providers are called to be particularly flexible, to work in teams and incorporate activities geared towards long-term care. The collaboration of the primary care sector and home care with the emergency and hospital sectors is a fundamental principle for continuity of care and patient-centered care. In-depth understanding of change mechanisms allows health care organization and staff to embrace and manage it effectively. Policies need to be translated into meaningful actions at a local level. To sustain region-wide efforts, it is important to account for ongoing maintenance and financial support.

A 'high-performing health sector' needs to have the following critical features (Coye & Detmer, 1998):

- Information technology (IT) to support patient care
- Transfer of knowledge about best practices and generation of new knowledge without 'reinventing the wheel'
- Aligned incentives for improved performance
- Encouragement of innovation
- Willingness to collaborate with academic enterprises
- Community-based interventions to alter fundamental determinants of health
- Purchaser and consumer education
- Accountability.

Successful systems are most likely to be the ones that offer opportunities for "ongoing professional involvement, relative stability and security, and the capacity to support improvements in practice with useful and timely information" (Coye & Detmer, 1998, p. 765).

In Crete, the Foundation for Research and Technology has developed HYGEIAnet, an Integrated RHIN. HYGEIAnet was set up to respond to the challenges arising from three global factors:

- A changing operating environment comprising a number of issues like informed citizens demanding personalized health services and the legislation and guidelines on privacy and security of personal information.
- Changes in health care delivery comprising the move towards evidence-based care and provision of integrated health services (citizen-centered services, continuity of care or seamless care) across organizational boundaries. In addition, extending care to the outside of the walls of care organizations and making the patient a member of the care team, especially in the case of chronic diseases, moving from care to health or wellness management.
- Technology push stemming from the rapid advancement in Internet and wireless technologies combined with the emergence of content providers and new business models for IT services (e.g. application service providers, ASP, Internet Service Providers, ISP, internet-portals, eHealth and eCommerce).

The fundamental objective for developing HYGEIAnet was to enable information sharing and medical collaboration among all stakeholders of the regional health economy and assist in the re-organization of the health care system based on innovative technological solutions and eHealth services (Katehakis et al., 2002).

The implementation of the RHIN in Crete observed several of the critical features of 'a high-performing health sector' and had an impact on the provision of health care services. The rest of the paper discusses a range of novel eHealth services deployed in HYGEIAnet and presents diverse service delivery models having the potential to enhance continuity of care and improve access and quality of care through the use of integrated services. The paper also presents the evaluation experiences from the deployment of such services and provides a critical review of factors related to organizational and social issues acting as impediments to successful implementation. The paper concludes with implications for policy and practice.

REGION OF CRETE AND HYGEIANET

The island of Crete is the southernmost point in Europe. It is Greece's biggest island and the fifth largest in the Mediterranean. It is about 260 km long and 12–60 km wide. North and south are separated by a mountainous range that spans the length of the island. The unique morphology of its terrain combines isolated and scarcely populated areas on the high mountains, with densely populated areas along the northern and southern coast. Crete has a population of ~ 600,000 people. As an island, Crete is isolated from the mainland, rendering access to mainland health care services difficult. The size, population and location of Crete render necessary the autonomy of health care services to minimize use of medical services in Athens and abroad. The improvement of health care services through IT is particularly important for Crete for two main reasons. First, the population more than doubles during the summer because of tourism, increasing the demand for health care services and information needs; second, the number of accidents doubles or triples in the summer. Tourists are involved in more than 40% of these accidents. ICT can contribute to strengthening self-sufficiency in providing adequate health care to the island's own population and to visitors.

The Institute of Computer Science at the Foundation for Research and Technology (ICS-FORTH) in Crete undertook the development of HYGEIAnet, the integrated RHIN on the island of Crete, as a pilot and a model for similar initiatives at a national and European level (Fig. 1). An RHIN is fundamentally designed to bring timely health information to, and to facilitate communication among, those wishing to make informed health decisions for themselves, their families, their patients and their communities.

HYGEIAnet represents a conscious and systematic effort towards the design, development and deployment of advanced eHealth and mobile Health (mHealth) services at various levels of the health care hierarchy, including home care, primary care, pre-hospital health emergency management and hospital care. Specifically, eHealth services for timely and effective patient management are routinely used in (a) pre-hospital emergency management, supporting patient tele-monitoring and management during transportation from the scene of an accident to the appropriate health care facility, (b) home care, supporting the remote management of asthmatic patients, (c) primary care and hospital care, supporting synchronous and asynchronous collaboration of medical professionals in the domains of Cardiology and Radiology, and (d) an eHealth service providing access to

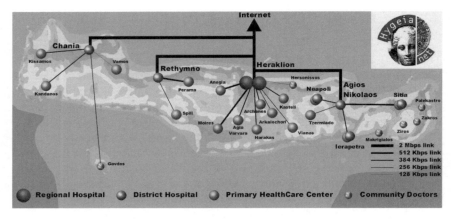

Fig. 1. HYGEIAnet, the Regional Health Information Network in Crete.

an integrated, lifelong electronic health record (I-EHR) is being used to support continuity of care across organizational boundaries.

HYGEIAnet has been established as a scalable RHIN and is based on an open architecture. It provides the tools for the integration of specialized autonomous applications, a Health Information Infrastructure (HII) to support these applications and relevant services for health care. The creation of a HII requires the successful resolution of many medico-legal issues related to privacy, security, encryption and authentication, issues that are fully reported in (Tsiknakis, Katehakis, & Orphanoudakis, 2002). It also requires the definition of a reference architecture to provide the framework for the gradual integration of heterogeneous, autonomous, networked information systems. Addressing such issues and requirements successfully has been a major and rather unique achievement of HYGEIAnet.

In the course of designing HYGEIAnet, special effort was made to address the requirements of the user groups involved and to use state of the art technology compliant with world standards. Real-life operations started in December 2001 and are currently implemented in the Region of Crete, Greece, South and Eastern Belfast HSS Trust, Ireland and a cluster of islands belonging to the Regional Health Authority of South Aegean, Greece. HYGEIAnet users include health professionals in remote and isolated primary care facilities, medical as well as paramedical staff of the pre-hospital health emergency services, various medical specialists (e.g. cardiologists, radiologists, pediatricians and pathologists) and asthmatic patients and their families.

Some of the core services offered in HYGEIAnet will be briefly discussed in the sections to follow, together with qualitative and quantitative results regarding their cost–benefits, impact on the quality and access to care, as well as their impact on performance.

Pre-Hospital Emergency Services

Health emergency care relies heavily on the effective and timely intervention of 'on-the-field' operators not only to save the lives of accident victims, but also greatly reduce the harmful effects of injury. In a number of cases, these injuries can be severe and can sometimes turn into permanent disabilities, which inevitably result in a great increase in both direct and indirect social costs. The resulting high direct social costs stem from expenditure for medical treatment, subsequent rehabilitation and, in many cases, the need for extra assistance; whereas, the high indirect social costs can range from a simple absence from work to the more permanent loss of employment due to the possible inability of the victim to perform his or her previous duties.

Taking into consideration the characteristics of the Region of Crete, the fact that the population more than doubles during the tourist period, the number of accidents doubles during that period and tourists are involved in more than 40% of these accidents, it becomes imperative to meet the challenge for effective and timely response management. Consequently, the systems and services developed in the domain of pre-hospital health emergency management services address two inter-related issues: (a) supporting the operators of the emergency services coordination center for optimal decision-making regarding the type and severity of each case and the dispatching of appropriate resources for the management of the emergency and (b) supporting the medical or paramedical staff of mobile units for effective patient management during transportation from the emergency scene to the appropriate hospital organization. The pre-hospital emergency system address these issues providing (a) decision-support and protocol-based dispatching, (b) continuous patient tele-monitoring through the acquisition, transmission, analysis and storage of vital signs and collaboration between the personnel of the emergency units and the doctors in duty on the Co-ordination Center, and (c) continuous tracking of ambulances and other mobile units, through the use of Global Positioning System (GPS) and Geographic Information Systems (GIS) technologies, required for the optimal use of the available resources and optimal response management. The system is able to monitor not only incoming vital signs and continuous

12-lead ECGs from mobile units, but also, resource-related decisions of the operator/dispatcher such as the feedback to its proposed actions, in addition to providing decision-support in the form of suggestions with a focus on resource management issues (e.g. which mobile unit should be sent? which hospital should be used? and other similar issues).

Given that the first 60 min, also known as the Golden Hour, are critical to the long-term patient outcome, the ability to remotely monitor the patient, thus allowing experts in the coordination center to guide the paramedical staff in managing the patient, facilitates access to care and, most importantly, access to care by a specialist. In addition, the protocol-based (triage) classification of emergency cases contributes in dispatching the most appropriate resources for each type of emergency. Based on objective data acquired at the scene of the emergency episode upon arrival of the dispatched resources, the initial decision made by the dispatcher with the assistance of appropriate protocols, has been shown correct in 82% of all cases recorded during 2002 (~40,000). This percentage represents a substantial improvement compared to the accuracy of decisions made prior to the introduction of HYGEIAnet systems and services.

The impact of ICT on the overall quality of care delivered has been greatly enhanced with novel methods of continuous education. Pre-hospital health emergency interventions involve both professional and non-professional health operators necessitating the provision of proper training for everyone. Training should be geared towards rendering the trainees capable of recognizing an emergency situation at hand, and especially enabling them to deal with the situation in a correct manner. However, in most European countries, proper training of the emergency operators is still a critical issue. In general, training of non-professionals mainly addresses three issues concerned with (a) the content, 'what to do' in the case of an emergency situation, (b) the methodology, 'what steps to take' when faced with such an emergency, and finally (c) the improvement of one's attitude, 'the lowering of the psychological barriers' in the presence of an emergency. In traditional emergency operator training, the trainee acquires the third aspect mentioned above, mainly after the end of the training course and during a real-life emergency situation. In most cases, the psychological impact of accident scenarios on operators, such as the distress of the victim, the presence of blood and the behavior of the patient's relatives, is not tested in advance. Also, traditional training methods do not adequately address the issue of 'knowledge retention.' According to Braslow et al. (1997), two months after the end of a traditional classroom instruction only 36% of trainees were still rated competent in Computerized Patient Record (CPR).

Being aware of the limitations of traditional emergency care training has led to the participation in a dedicated project (Project JUST, www.just-web.org), co-funded by the European Commission, with the objective to design and develop a complementary training course for non-professional health emergency operators. One of its objectives was to support the traditional learning phase and improve the retention capability of the trainees. This was achieved with the use of advanced IT techniques, which provide adequate support and can help to overcome the present weaknesses of the existing training mechanisms.

The main features of the resulting training course were based on three aspects, those concerned with the capability of the individual for self-learning, the benefits of interactivity between the system and the user and the extensive use of multimedia. These considerations resulted in the employment of a hybrid technological solution, the web/CD, which presents the optimal integration between the two media, even though there was an expected overhead for system and information design. Extensive usability testing and clinical trials were carried out in order to assess the effect of continuous training through the use of technology. One important finding from the analysis of the user satisfaction responses related to the question whether the web/CD suited their style and pace of learning. The resulting response showed that 'novice' users agreed more with the statement, when compared to the 'expert' users. Other evidence indicates that there was a drastic improvement for all trainees after attending the course. The above evidence supports the argument that significant benefits and performance improvements can be achieved through the innovative use of modern ICT for the effective re-engineering of organizational processes and the continuous improvement of knowledge and skills.

Home Tele-Management of Patients

A technological platform has been designed to support the tele-monitoring and tele-management of patients with asthma by health care providers at a distance. Children suffering from asthma did not visit the University Hospital. Instead, tele-medicine sessions were scheduled with the medical expert located at the University Hospital.

Dedicated software components allowed the acquisition of clinical data from the various medical devices connected to the platform and their transmission displayed in real time to the expert. The medical devices incorporated in the platform include an *Electronic Stethoscope*, an *ECG*, an

Electronic Scale, a *Peak Flow Meter* and a *Spirometer*. In respiratory diseases, pathological changes occur predominantly in the smaller airways necessitating the use of a spirometer for measuring the lung volumes.

The home care platform has been deployed in the context of HYGEIAnet as a modular platform able to support home care services in different clinical and social domains. An initial technical evaluation study was conducted to assess the platform's operational characteristics under real-life conditions. Issues such as required bandwidth for optimal performance, robustness, ease of use and real-time performance were evaluated. The results obtained reveal that the platform exhibits characteristics that prove its usefulness and effectiveness for the follow up monitoring of patients with chronic diseases from a distance (Traganitis et al., 2001).

In addition, extended clinical trials were conducted for evaluating the clinical effectiveness of the platform for the tele-management of patients with pediatric asthma (ATTRACT, 2000). The evaluation of clinical results suggest a relatively high rate of health improvement, and can therefore be considered as strong evidence for the effectiveness and efficiency of the homecare services in supporting the delivery of tele-services to citizen's with chronic diseases. Medical staff provided brief information on what they liked about the system, which was categorized as follows:

1. Avoidance of patient transportation to hospital; increased accessibility towards patient
2. Quality, precision and personalization of doctor–patient communication because of one-to-one conversation and personal attention
3. Provision of comfort, physical as well as psychological reassurance and feeling of security, and overall friendliness of process
4. Ease of use
5. Quality of image and possibility of visual contact with the patient
6. Insight into patient's daily life, possibility of using the system to optimize material and medical staff resources, possibility of educating patients on topics such as medical complications and technological advances

Quantitative evaluation of the eHealth trial (home tele-management of childhood asthma) based on the analysis of doctors' reports on 45 individual patients. Table 2 presents summary information judged as most useful for anyone interested in gaining insight on whether use of the system improved patients' health or their health care habits.

An interesting finding also emerged from this data: there were 19 instances (48% of patients) where a medical staff member reported some regimen change decision (i.e., treatment or medication change) through tele-consul-

Table 2. Health-Related Changes for Patients Through Use of the System, as Reported by Medical Staff in HYGEIAnet (Qualitative Data).

Patient-Related Health and Health Care Changes	Proportion (%) in Sample	Patients ($N = 45$)
1. ACTUAL HEALTH IMPROVEMENT – total cases	67	30
Symptom improvement	49	22
Dramatic improvement or patient free of symptoms	18	8
2. REGIMEN ADJUSTMENT BY DOCTOR – total cases	60	27
Treatment adjustment	49	22
Medication adjustment	11	5
Additional diagnosis/treatment	11	5
3. PATIENTS CHANGING THEIR HABITS – total cases	16	7
Increased medication compliance	2	1
Better utilization of medication devices	9	4
Increased patient's understanding of treatment goals/compliance	4	2
4. CRISIS AVOIDANCE – total cases	7	3
Saved hospital visit	4	2
Saved urgent care visit	2	1

tation, in combination with some type of health improvement or crisis avoidance for the corresponding patient. If one considers the nature of chronic asthma, this result suggests a relatively high rate of health improvement, and can be interpreted as strong evidence for the effectiveness of medical tele-services, in terms of significant patients' health improvement through the possibility of closer and more precise follow-up treatment of patients.

eHealth Services

Modern technology opens up for entirely new ways of working in collaborative work environments across distributed organizations by offering mobile, ad hoc trusted services over heterogeneous universal communication lines. It supports working-out-of-workspace by providing seamless delivery-on-demand of content and establishes multimodal exchange of knowledge among people, machines and devices. In implementing this vision of innovative eHealth services, a technological infrastructure has been developed based on shared workspaces. Its deployment in HYGEIAnet has demonstrated that eHealth services offer tangible clinical, social and economic benefits to all concerned.

The backbone of the collaboration platform is Jabber, a scalable open-source server implementing the IMPP XML protocol for instant messaging and presence notification. To support medical collaboration, Jabber was extended with a shared workspace component that supports subscription and notification on content updates. The messenger of the portal, now the centerpiece in medical collaboration, facilitates a smooth transition from asynchronous to synchronous interaction. Each shared workspace corresponds to a 'chat room,' where users interact sharing multimedia clinical data relevant to a particular episode of care. Various medical device components have been developed and integrated with the eHealth platform, in compliance with relevant interoperability standards. These include a spirometer, ECG devices of different manufacturers, real-time vital signs monitor, real-time 12-lead ECG and a digital stethoscope. Integration with the clinical systems managing the electronic health record segments in primary health care provides access to local clinical data of the patient.

Based on the suspected medical problem and the current clinical context, predefined document templates following the HL7/CDA ANSI standard are automatically filled out with relevant clinical data. These electronic documents are reviewed and digitally signed by the responsible physician. Smartcards and a regional Public Key Infrastructure are used to ensure authorization, confidentiality, integrity and non-repudiation. Digital signatures of clinical items follow the W3C/ IETF standard for signatures in XML.

Deployment of the platform in the domain of Cardiology and initial clinical evaluation revealed significant economic and clinical benefits. Available results indicate that 10% of the cardiac patients of the test population were involved in a tele-consultation session during a period of 6 months, thus making medical expertise instantly available to remote and isolated populations, as reported in detail in (Chronaki et al., 2001). The eHealth service enables instant availability of medical expertise to remote and isolated populations and allow for the remote management of cardiac episodes, thus increasing access to care. A rather strong diagnostic impact was also noticed: only in 9 out of 21 cases was the patient immediately transferred to the hospital. Since the health care centers are in remote locations and all the patients seen would normally have been referred and transported to the Regional hospital for evaluation, this represents a clear saving of both time and cost.

Integrated Electronic Health Record

Within the modern health care environment, the creation and efficient access by all authorized users to a single I-EHR for every citizen is the cornerstone for supporting continuity of care and the emerging, novel eHealth services, by ensuring prompt and secure access to relevant information resources. Developing an I-EHR service requires the resolution of complex technical issues. The most critical one is the specification and development of a set of generic and domain specific middleware common services and their integration for the creation of the required HII, enabling the required semantic information integration and data security and confidentiality.

The arguments for deploying an I-EHR service are so compelling that a number of countries are striving to develop workable models (Siman, 2000). An I-EHR is a collection of all of an individual's lifetime health data, generated during relevant interactions with the health care system (NCVHS, 2001). A scalable I-EHR would provide the means to access all available clinical information, at an organizational, regional, national or even international level, and to meet the challenges posed by patient mobility and the fact that an individual's health data usually resides at many specialized and geographically dispersed clinical information systems (Fig. 2).

The real and specific problem that underlies the I-EHR concept is co-ordinated resource sharing and problem-solving in dynamic, multi-institutional virtual organizations. This sharing is, necessarily, highly controlled, with resource providers and consumers defining clearly and carefully just what is shared, who is allowed to share and the conditions under which sharing occurs.

The task, therefore, from the technological viewpoint is to make data and information securely available in this inter-enterprise environment where needed, when needed and in the format needed. In defining the R&D issues to be resolved for the creation of an I-EHR for every citizen, we start from the perspective that effective creation of a Virtual Health care Organization requires that we are able to establish efficient and dynamic sharing relationships among any potential participants.

Today, the most promising approach towards achieving these objectives is based on a federation of autonomous clinical information systems and a modular underlying HII, with services facilitating the seamless integration of and unified access to the distributed clinical data of a citizen (Tsiknakis et al., 2002).

The I-EHR service, as it has been developed and used, provides a de-centralized view of the life-long, multimedia patient medical record by

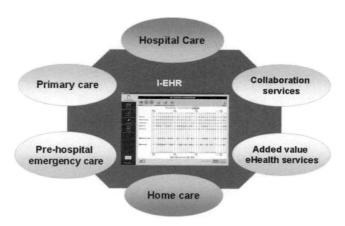

Fig. 2.   Health Care Domain Application Areas: Clusters of Telematic Services and
the I-EHR Continuum of Care.

dynamically integrating clinical information residing in a variety of heterogeneous, self-consistent clinical information systems. The I-EHR interface,
presented in Fig. 3, allows end-users to navigate in the I-EHR information
space at various levels of abstraction and supports the viewing of patient
demographic data, the time and location of a citizen's encounters with the
health system and actual medical data presented according to the Subjec-
tive-Objective-Assessment-Plan (SOAP) model.

Deployment of an I-EHR service in the context of HYGEIAnet, as well as
in the South and East Belfast Trust (SBT) in Northern Ireland, has revealed
a number of clinical and operational benefits, which are discussed in a following section. At the same time, a formal risk analysis of the I-EHR service
revealed that user confidence, in relation to the trust and security infrastructure of the RHIN, is an important factor influencing user adoption.

Nevertheless, the findings to date are extremely encouraging and suggest
that the I-EHR service can benefit not only the patients, but also health
professionals by fostering their collaboration and serving as a tool for continuing education. Available evidence also indicates that, in addition to
providing support for continuity of care, the I-EHR is a valuable tool for
basic and clinical research, medical decision-making, epidemiology, evidence-based medicine and in formulating public health policy. The adoption
of an I-EHR service is dependent on a number of factors, including I-EHR

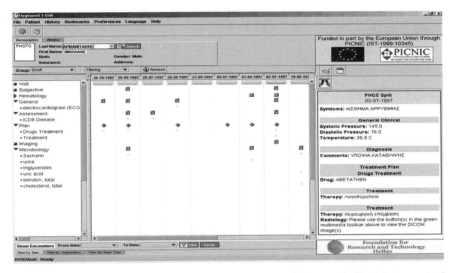

Fig. 3. The Graphical User Interface of the Integrated Electronic Health Record of a Citizen.

accessibility, interface usability and security, as well as legal and other non-technical considerations.

IMPACT ON HEALTH CARE PERFORMANCE

A gradual introduction, over the last three years, of a number of innovative services has taken place in the context of the HYGEIAnet RHIN with the objective of enhancing traditional care and improving performance through the use of ICT. However, the introduction of ICT completely transformed the processes at hand. In the pre-hospital health emergency sector, no traditional approach was able to provide the type and quality of services enabled through the eHealth services described earlier. In addition, prior to the deployment of the eHealth cardiology services (tele-cardiology) the majority of patients were referred and transported to the Regional or University Hospital, creating an excessive flow of patients to tertiary care and significant bottlenecks. Similarly, prior to the deployment of the tele-monitoring of children with asthma, all children had to be transported to a specialist, at least once a month, for follow-up. Visits to specialists resulted in significant cost for the family as they entailed losing work and school days and expensive traveling costs.

There is no apparent competing alternative for these services. One could argue that remote primary health care facilities could be staffed with the necessary specialists to provide the required level of expertise locally. The cost of such an approach would be significant, even if the required specialists were willing to be located in remote and isolated areas. Alternative technological solutions may exist, but we are not aware of any that are as scalable and conform to the requirements for interoperability of systems and services based on an open architecture and the use of adopted or de facto standards.

Initial and ongoing evaluation of HYGEIAnet services indicates that patients and health professionals have both benefited from the deployment and use of the services. The acceptance of HYGEIAnet services from medical staff and patients have resulted in a relatively high rate of health improvement, cost containment, improved quality of care and easier access to health services. Collaborations among providers and consumers of health care have improved and continuing education has become a possibility. HYGEIAnet has facilitated the accessibility of medical expertise towards patients, has allowed the optimization of material and medical staff resources and rendered possible the education of patients on topics such as medical complications and technological advances. HYGEIAnet services have enhanced a sense of well-being by providing physical comfort in one's own home, by avoiding transportation to a hospital and waiting for medical attention and by providing security and reassurance through friendly and timely service. More specifically, the observed benefits can be categorized as follows.

Economic Benefits

Expert opinion is available through RHIN services reducing the rate of patient referrals to the specialists. As a result, there has been a significant reduction in hospitalization days, loss of workdays of family members and relatives and duplication of unnecessary examinations.

Access to Care Benefits

Access to care has greatly improved in all categories where eHealth services have been employed. The tele-cardiology services allow instant access to medical expertise from remote and isolated populations. Pre-hospital health emergency episodes are remotely managed allowing experts of the coordination center to guide the paramedical staff in their management of the patient facilitating access to care and, most importantly, access to care by a specialist. Patients using the home care services mention how tele-monitoring has helped them substitute the need to physically visit the doctor or the hospital, thus counteracting limited mobility due to patient's age, health condition or lack of time. In addition, it has substituted the need to physically visit friends and social contacts, helping towards combating loneliness and isolation of people with limited mobility.

Quality of Care Benefits

The evaluation of the pre-hospital emergency services revealed a substantial improvement in the accuracy of classifications of emergency cases and therefore an increase in the number of appropriate decisions. Also, personnel training had a significant impact on the quality of care delivered. Regarding eHealth services for the remote management of chronic diseases, the quality and precision of doctor–patient communication has improved. The process is friendly and provides physical as well as psychological reassurance, feeling of security and insight into patient's daily life. Other advantages include increase in patient's autonomy, better quality of life and better environment.

BARRIERS TO IMPLEMENTATION

The impediments to creating viable, integrated delivery systems that rely on computerized information revolve around the fragmentation problem: many pieces of information, in many formats, on many platforms, in many stakeholder environments, to many geographic locations. The technical issues in creating such an environment have not been a significant problem for HYGEIAnet. Rather, most of the issues blocking information system (IS) implementation revolve around the organizational changes associated with the move towards integrated RHIN. The Ministry of Health in Greece has recognized the importance of patient-centered care and information systems in the organization of the health care sector (see the appendix for a brief presentation of the Greek health care system). However, policy does not explicitly address the development of the health care sector and information systems in parallel. Implementation efforts remain local based on personal initiative. Despite the ability of ICT to improve the efficiency and effectiveness of health care services, there are several technical, economic, organizational and behavioral barriers to the diffusion of information technologies.

The deployment and use of HYGEIAnet was inhibited by conservative attitudes, questionable self-sustainability, unclear reimbursement systems, computer illiteracy among medical personnel, organizational structures not supporting ICT and legal and social barriers to the exchange of patient information. Financial limitations were also an issue. Implementation of ICT requires large capital investment, while the rate of return is often perceived as more uncertain than that on other investment alternatives. Other issues include the inability of management to adequately support the implementation initiative, failure to understand the range of services associated with continuum-of-care delivery systems, inability to overcome individual stakeholder resistance to allowing information to flow among all entities within the RHIN and inability to convince major organizations such as Regional Hospitals to accept a role as team player in the integrated care delivery environment of a RHIN.

Legal and standards-related barriers were also encountered, relating to privacy, confidentiality and security, as well as to the lack of standards for health care information systems. Several stakeholders were concerned with individual and organizational behavior that might result in improper use and access of personal health data by unauthorized parties. The lack of comprehensive and broadly accepted, by all health care industrial stakeholders, standards for the definition, collection, communication and storage of health data, is retarding system integration and the creation of truly integrated RHIN. As long as public policy regarding the confidentiality and privacy of health-related information continues to be lacking, the growth of RHIN and eHealth services will be inhibited, while technical capabilities to ensure security are no longer an issue.

Other barriers were centered on the problems encountered during transition to integrated service delivery systems within an RHIN. In the past, information had been considered proprietary. The development of an integrated RHIN and eHealth services raised a key question: should access to information determine competitive advantage or should information be made available among stakeholders so that market advantage is based on creative use of information rather than access to information? Ownership of patient information has been the subject of much debate. However, governing the stewardship of and access to medical information is the more urgent and practical issue. Legislation is required, which should identify the rules by which information can be shared, and provide guidelines allowing access based on the 'need-to-know' principle.

These barriers are not unique to the implementation initiative of HYGEIAnet. Several authors (Kaplan, 1987, 1994; Tanriverdi & Iacono, 1999; Tonnesen, LeMaistre, & Tucker, 1999) deal with the difficult issue of encouraging physicians to become hands-on users of clinical information systems at the point of health care delivery. Since the mid-1990s, an increasing number of articles (Ash, 1997; Ash, Gorman, Lavelle, Lyman, & Fournier, 2001; Lorenzi, Riley, Blyth, Southon, & Dixon, 1997) have been published, offering lists of recommendations and strategies for practitioners to be aware of when implementing ICT. Despite these recommendations, following an ideal recipe has not proven particularly useful (Pare & Elam, 1998). There is no cookbook for success and failure in IS implementation (Poulymenakou & Holmes, 1996). Success and failure should be studied as a situation-specific event for the particular ICT. Only then could implementation strategies be developed and implemented. The following section discusses change processes in HYGEIAnet implementation and presents the key factors involved in the initial deployment and subsequent rollout of systems and services.

CHANGE MANAGEMENT IN HYGEIANET IMPLEMENTATION

Several times, it has been acknowledged that the isolated implementation of ICT, however appropriate, will not succeed unless attention is given to the management of social issues relating to the organization and its environment (Hackney, Dhillon, & McBride, 1997). However, the efficient and effective management of change to overcome organizational and cultural issues has not been adequately addressed. To encourage change, a major part of implementation initiatives concentrates on removing resistance through educational programs, establishment of new priorities and patterns of behavior. Alas, this essentially linear view of governance that assumes the possibility of identifying logical links between cause and effect has resulted in comprehensive prescriptions that do not work (Beer, Eisenstat, & Spector, 1990; Smith & Stacey, 1997).

An alternative view of change emerges when treating health care systems as complex adaptive systems (Plsek & Greenhalgh, 2001; Plsek & Kilo,

1999). Instead of change being coupled with resistance, change is treated as an inherent capacity of organizations, as a process of self-organization. During a process of self-organization, events take place and structures emerge that can neither be anticipated nor predicted.

The introduction of HYGEIAnet in the regional health care system of Crete required interconnected changes. However, contrary to implementation initiatives elsewhere, HYGEIAnet did not involve a central body to force change against employees in a tight time schedule or to plan an explicit implementation strategy. HYGEIAnet was a pilot and a model initiative based on collaboration between the Foundation for Research and Technology and interested health organizations. Technologies were disseminated with the goodwill and interest of health care employees. The implementation was essentially organic while use of the available technologies relied solely on the decision of the end-users. For this reason, HYGEIAnet is a particularly useful case to study change 'springing from within.'

Instead of developing exact implementation plans to cultivate the necessary conditions for generating change, HYGEIAnet implementation methods focused on loose control, encouragement of innovation and direction-setting. These methods produced faster results than the traditional plan and control mentality (Kouroubali, 2003). In contrast, plans often take too long and are usually not accurate or not followed.

Cumulative international experience (Iakovidis, Wilson, & Healy, 2004) has shown that within the enormous complexity of implementation efforts, there are three fundamental factors that are essential and required for an implementation effort to succeed over time. These factors are (a) a champion that persists with the deployment and diffusion of systems, (b) a length of time of a minimum 5–6 years and (c) significant financial grants to support and maintain the effort. HYGEIAnet experience supports these findings. The Foundation of Research and Technology (FORTH) has been a major champion in advancing and promoting health care systems and innovative services to the region of Crete. Since the early 1990s, FORTH has developed HYGEIAnet technologies and has coordinated their regional implementation. During these years, FORTH has persistently educated and motivated the health care community of Crete towards its vision of region-wide integrated health care services. The process of change is an ongoing event that needs to be followed longitudinally throughout the years. Implementation of HYGEIAnet has been an ongoing process since 1997, a significant amount of time to witness the gradual transformation of services and mentalities. Change has been incremental but steady. However, despite the strong leadership skills and vision of FORTH and the experience of gradual but constant change in the health care sector, financial support, the third major component of successful implementations, has been mainly from R&D funds brought in by FORTH but National funding has been largely lacking in Crete. It is only today, after long periods of evaluating benefits, that there are signs of managerial commitment to guarantee funding for the next phases of development and related operational costs. It is our experience that ongoing funding of development, maintenance and support of new technologies is fundamental in assisting the continuous process of change. Education and support of end-users and maintenance of systems and services do not seize to be of major importance even after the initial implementation has taken place. These three major factors have been present to different degrees throughout the history of HYGEIAnet implementation, with the presence of FORTH as a champion as the major driving force.

The implementation strategy focused on creating a critical mass of stake-holders who engaged personally with the available technologies and disseminated them within their health care organizations. Several of the barriers mentioned above, were overcome at a local level by the goodwill and interest of the people involved in the implementation effort. Goodwill and interest coupled with a sense of responsibility is described by the Greek word *philotimo*. *Philotimo* means literally 'friend of honour.' Several end-users involved in the implementation of HYGEIAnet possessed this valuable attribute that drove them to incorporating ICT in their daily activities with the objective of improving health care outcomes.

As Lyytinen and Hirschheim (1987) have pointed out, implementation is rarely solely a success or a failure. Similarly, while HYGEIAnet implementation was well received by most health care employees and patients, several of the barriers mentioned above still remain due to lack of appropriate public policies, legislation and funding. However, use of new technologies was wide spread and change from traditional practices did occur in many instances. The organic nature of HYGEIAnet implementation allowed the study of change springing spontaneously from within the health organizations as a process of 'self-organization.' Several factors were identified to play an important role in enhancing self-organization. Some of these factors include incentives, education, leadership, communications and culture.

Incentives

Since the beginning of the implementation effort, it became evident that incentives would play a critical role towards creating the initial critical mass of users required for successful deployment and diffusion of HYGEIAnet systems and services. Early in the process, a political and strategic decision was taken not to offer financial incentives for using innovative technologies. This decision was taken knowingly that the project had to rely on incentives that could last throughout the years and not just while money lasted. As a result, HYGEIAnet implementation gave incentives that were aligned with its vision of improving health care practices and patient outcomes. The critical mass of end-users was created with the benefits of the use of the technologies and services as its major incentive. The innovative technologies focused on improving the daily practice of health care workers, providing strong research tools to enhance scientific collaborations, assisting in research publications, clinical trials and epidemiological studies. The implementation effort offered computer training for free to all interested health care employees within Crete and introduced computers and Internet where none was available before.

Education

One of the major components involved in successful implementation of ICT is education. Having coordinated a huge, region-wide effort to train and educate over 1,100 end-users prior to the introduction of system and services in their organizations, our experience showed that education in both a holistic approach to health care and information systems is important. Information systems education introduces medical students and health care providers to the applications of technology in medical practice and provides them with the basic computer skills. Hands-on practice and on-the-job training during the first days of operation was necessary to facilitate integration of the computer into the actual workday. High priority was placed on demonstrating the usefulness of the technology and the way it supports individual services and work performance. As Anderson (1997) notes "response to implementation is shaped by physician perceptions of the usefulness of the system as well as of the changes it will bring to the performance of everyday jobs in the organization." Similarly, in Crete, employees decided to use the technologies and services to improve their daily practice. As mentioned previously, many of the technologies revolutionized practice, offering possibilities unavailable through traditional health care.

Continuing education also played an important role in the transition towards holistic care, community awareness and management of chronic disease. The shift from acute care to chronic illness care calls for providers, managers and patients with knowledge that goes beyond illness, care and provider specialty. In Crete, education increased the information flow in health organizations where HYGEIAnet was deployed, and provided opportunities for self-organization. Exposure to information benefited health care organizations and allowed change in proactive ways to improve performance as demonstrated in the various eHealth services of HYGEIAnet.

Education initiatives addressed all interested health care employees. Many skeptical health care employees attended training sessions. Some of them did change their negative attitudes but did not choose to use the systems available. The creation of a critical mass of users, however, resulted in a momentum that in many cases did not exempt skeptical users. As the technology is used daily and established routines gradually depend on ICT services, skeptical health care workers are obliged to follow the new trends. Mentality change is often the first step towards self-organization.

Leadership

In Crete, the natural tendency of agents to change had been greatly influenced through leadership. Individuals as leaders, mentors, change agents and consolidators made a huge difference to the deployment and use of HYGEIAnet (Kouroubali, 2003). Successful leaders created the conditions to effectively support self-organization through availability of information, relationship and identity. Dependency is deeply rooted in most organizations. Employees often had to be encouraged to exercise initiative and explore new areas of competence. Encouragement and cultivation of innovative activities have helped accelerate progress towards the vision for quality of care.

In Greece, doctors often see quality as being mainly an individual responsibility rather than a collective effort encompassing other people, processes and especially systems. Although care teams can significantly contribute to improvements of care, most health care professionals do not engage in teamwork to improve health care services. Formal and informal leaders in Crete health care organizations have recognized the usefulness of HYGEIAnet technologies and services in improved communications among health care providers and have taken active steps in establishing health care teams (Kouroubali, 2003). Similarly, to any changes in the public health care sector, good communication and leadership skills were essential towards creating a spirit of collaboration and teamwork.

Despite the major influence that local leadership can have on reorganizing health care with innovative technologies, governmental policy is particularly important in recognizing, encouraging and developing initiatives that are already taking place. Considering existing components could help build on already available technology and alleviate part of the budgetary load of such efforts.

Health care leadership could be a process of unlocking the capacity of transformation within the health care team in facing global health care challenges (Anderson, 1999). The complex adaptive systems approach to leadership introduces the notion of facilitation rather than hard control and planning (Anderson & McDaniel, 2000), in addition to treating health care system as a whole rather than split into individual parts. A complex adaptive systems view of health care leadership helps alleviate the anxiety introduced when strategies and planning encounter uncertainty.

Communications

Growing world evidence suggests that organized systems of care, and not just competent health care providers, are imperative to address the new demands of health care. Several authors acknowledge a required change in the way health care is viewed (Anderson & McDaniel, 2000; Plsek & Greenhalgh, 2001; Zimmerman, Lindberg, & Plsek, 1998). Health and 'health' care rather than 'illness' care require a view of the human condition that transcends disease. To change and improve practice, it is essential to shift the focus towards improving care as a whole, offering relationship-centered care and developing skills of reflective practice (Miller, McDaniel Jr., Crabtree, & Stange, 2001). Peckham (1999) points out the importance of good communications within the organization to achieve such an interconnected change in health services. Currently, vertical and horizontal communication in the Greek Health Care System is imperfect. In Crete, the exchange of information among health care workers played a vital role in the publicity and promotion of HYGEIAnet services and technologies. Crete, being an island, is contained within specific boundaries and information spreads through word-of-mouth and movement of health care workers within the region. Subsequently, the regional implementation of health care information systems allowed for better communication across sites.

Organized systems of care include all levels of health care, the patient interaction level, the health care organization and community level and the policy level. All these levels interact and influence each other. Health care information systems are "a prerequisite for coordinated, integrated, and evidence-informed health care" (WHO, 2002, p. 37). As HYGEIAnet has demonstrated, health information networks can facilitate sharing of health care-related information among the various actors in the field. Sharing of information resources is generally accepted as the key to substantial improvements in productivity and better quality of care, while horizontal and vertical channels of communication are required to address the new approach to health care.

Culture

Consumer demands for information and participation in decision-making will eventually transform the nature of clinical management and the respective roles of providers and patients in ways that could not be anticipated (Coye & Detmer, 1998, p. 766). Physicians will have to comply with these new trends to accommodate changing consumer demands. These realizations became important for Crete as more and more people were familiar with IT and access the Internet. Patients were better informed about their illnesses, treatment options, prognosis and relevant best practices. Providers needed the support of appropriate databases and communication technologies to stay up-to-date with the vast amount of information that is gradually becoming available to all audiences through the Internet. Working towards a vision of integrated health care and encouraging personal responsibility has succeeded in creating a critical mass of individuals that use information technologies out of their personal goodwill and interest.

Processes of change and key factors discussed in this section have been important in most implementation efforts throughout the world. However, these factors must be explored within their context, as they will play out in different ways in different environments. Even within Crete, similar health care organizations differed in their organization, staff constitution and work practices making each one of these factors unique in its detail in different settings. Taking this implementation effort as a model and through close examination of change processes and innovative practices could facilitate similar implementation efforts in other regions.

CONCLUSION

The health care industry is undergoing a massive restructuring in response to concerns about rising costs and access to services. Health care organizations are transforming themselves from standalone operations and businesses into health care systems supporting a continuum of care. Thus integrated RHINs evolve.

Once stakeholders are linked into real or virtual RHINs, they must strategically align their IT with their new business objectives, often adding additional functionality. Not only must information technologies be integrated within each individual organization (intra organizational), they must also work cohesively and seamlessly across the multiple organizations that have linked together into an RHIN (enterprise wide) and, ultimately across multiple RHIN (inter enterprise). The extent to which they can achieve this usually determines their ability to deliver higher quality, more cost-effective, patient-centered care and, hence, their long-term competitiveness.

So compelling are the arguments for an integrated lifelong EHR within the context of RHINs that a number of countries around the world – including the U.S., Canada, several EU countries and Australia – are striving to develop workable models along with their vision for their national HII (U.S. Department of Health and Human Service, 2001; Canada Health Infoway, 2003; UK Department of Health, 2002; NHIG, 2004).

At the end of 2003, the Medicare Prescription Drug Improvement and Modernization Act (MMA) of 2003 was signed in the U.S. including, among other new initiatives, important provisions for Health Information Technology (HIT). MMA requires the Centers for Medicare and Medicaid Services (CMS) to develop standards for electronic prescribing, expected to be a first step towards the widespread use of EHRs (Thompson & Brailer, 2004). In addition, the MMA requires the establishment of a Commission on Systemic Interoperability to provide a road map for interoperability standards in order for the majority of the U.S. citizens to have interoperable electronic health records within 10 years.

In Canada, the Canadian Infoway (Canada Health Infoway, 2004), an independent, nonprofit corporation initiated, as the result of the Canadian federal government's announcement in September 2000, to accelerate the development and adoption of modern systems of IT in health care, aims to foster the development of secure and interoperable EHR systems across Canada. Its objectives are to develop mechanisms to enable consumers to access health information that they can use, to facilitate the work of health care providers through technology and to create a unified network of electronic health records across the continuum of care.

In Europe, the UK National Health Service (NHS) information strategy for health (NHS, 2001) identified six levels of EHR ranging from simply providing support for clinical administrative data at level one (1), through remote order entry and results reporting at level three (3), to comprehensive tele-medicine and multimedia services at level six (6). This particular classification represents an evolutionary approach to the development of an I-EHR service. Already, the NHS Information Authority Electronic Record Development and Implementation Programme (ERDIP) has now formally closed (ERDIP, 2004), having delivered quite a large number of lessons learned.

In Germany, the central associations of self-administration committed themselves in 2002 "to develop a new infrastructure for telematics on the basis of a general framework architecture, to improve and/or introduce the electronic communication (electronic prescription, electronic discharge letter by the physician) and to introduce the former health insurance card as an electronic health card in the future" (Dietzel & Riepe, 2004). The target set is to have 80 million electronic health cards distributed in 2006 that will be capable of giving access to medical data, and therefore lead-in to the Electronic Patient Record.

Our experiences in developing HYGEIAnet indicate that the successful and efficient development and deployment of state of the art ICT requires the coordinated actions of many stakeholders, including public authorities, industry, technology providers and research teams. Authorities must support the necessary infrastructures and provide the academic and organizational conditions required for this support.

The incorporation of innovative ICT solutions in daily routines often changes the relationship between patients and health professionals. The shareable, ubiquitous and I-EHR is a fundamental requirement for integrated care. Communication within and across all levels of care is a prerequisite for the harmonious development of this new medical practice. Novel eHealth services change traditional and established organizational structures and enable new models of service provision. There is documented evidence from a number of trials that such novel service delivery models provide significant economic and quality of care cost benefits. Nevertheless, specific challenges, such as legal, inter-operability and funding, need to be effectively addressed in order to ensure the widespread adoption of systems and services supporting integrated and continuous care.

REFERENCES

Anderson, J. G. (1997). Clearing the way for physicians' use of clinical information systems. *Communications of the ACM, 40*(8), 83–90.

Anderson, P. (1999). Complexity theory and organization science. *Organization Science, 10*(3), 216–232.

Anderson, R. A., & McDaniel, R. R. (2000). Managing health care organizations: Where professionalism meets complexity science. *Health Care Management Review, 25*(1), 83–92.

Ash, J. (1997). Organizational factors that influence information technology diffusion in academic health sciences centers. *Journal of the American Medical Informatics Association, 4*(2), 102–111.

Ash, J., Gorman, P., Lavelle, M., Lyman, J., & Fournier, L. (2001). Investigating physician order entry in the field: Lessons learned in a multi-center study. Paper presented at the MedInfo 2001, London, UK.

ATTRACT. (2000). *Deliverable 6.2: Results from Demonstration Phase.*

Bates, D. W. (2000). Using information technology to reduce rates of medication errors in hospitals. *British Medical Journal, 320*, 788–791.

Beer, M., Eisenstat, R. A., & Spector, B. (1990). *The critical path to corporate renewal.* Boston, MA: Harvard Business School Press.

Braslow, A., Brennan, R. T., Newman, M. M., Bircher, N. G., Batcheller, A. M., & Kaye, W. (1997). CPR training without an instructor: Development and evaluation of a video self-instructional system for effective performance of cardiopulmonary resuscitation. *Resuscitation, 34*, 207–220.

Canada Health Infoway (2003). *EHRS blueprint – An interoperable EHR framework*, Version 1.0, July. http://knowledge.infoway-inforoute.ca/CHIPortal/EHRSearch/EHRS + Blueprint/

Canada Health Infoway (2004). http://www.infoway.ca/

Chronaki, C., Lees, P. J., Antonakis, N., Chiarugi, F., Vrouchos, G., Nikolaidis, G., Tsiknakis, M., & Orphanoudakis, S. C. (2001). Preliminary results from the deployment of integrated teleconsultation services in rural crete. *In: Proceedings of the 28th annual computers in cardiology congress, Rotterdam, The Netherlands* (pp. 671–674), 21–25 September.

Contandriopoulos, A. P., Lauristin, M., & Leibovich, E. (1999). Values norms and the reform of health care systems. In: R. B. Saltman, J. Figueras & C. Sakellarides (Eds), *Critical challenges for health care reform in Europe* (pp. 339–361). Buckingham: Open University Press.

Corrigan, J., Kohn, L., & Donaldson, M. (Eds) (1999). *To err is human: Building a safer health system.* Washington: Committee on Quality of Healthcare in America, Institute of Medicine.

Coye, M. J., & Detmer, D. E. (1998). Quality at a Crossroads. *The Milbank Quarterly, 76*(4), 759–769.

Dawson, S. (1999). Managing, organising, and performing in health care: What do we know and how can we learn? In: A. L. Mark & S. Dopson (Eds), *Organisational behaviour in health care: The research agenda* (pp. 7–24). Basingstoke: Macmillan.

Deloitte & Touche. (2000). *The Emerging European Health Telematics Industry; Market Analysis.* Prepared for the European Commission-Directorate General Information Society.

Dietzel, T.W., & Riepe, C. (2004). *Modernizing healthcare in Germany by introducing the eHealthcard.* Swiss Medical Informatics, No 52.

ERDIP (2004). *HS Information Authority's Electronic Record Development and Implementation Programme (ERDIP).* http://www.nhsia.nhs.uk/erdip/

Grimson, J. (2001). Delivering the electronic healthcare record for the 21st century. *International Journal of Medical Informatics, 64*, 111–127.

Hackney, R., Dhillon, G., & McBride, N. (1997). Primary care information technology within the NHS: The concept of markets and hierarchies on systems exploitation. *International Journal of Public Sector Management, 10*(5), 388–395.

Iakovidis, I., Wilson, P., & Healy, J. C. (Eds) (2004). *E-health: Current situation and examples of implemented and beneficial e-health applications* (Vol. 100). Amsterdam: IOS Press.

Institute of Medicine. (2001). *Crossing the quality chasm: A new health system for the 21st Century*. Washington, DC: National Academy Press.

Kaplan, B. (1987). The medical computing 'lag': Perceptions and barriers to the application of computers to medicine. *International Journal of Technology Assessment in Health Care, 3*(1), 123–136.

Kaplan, B. (1994). Reducing barriers to physician data entry for computer-based patient records. *Topics in Health Information Management, 15*(1), 24–34.

Katehakis, D., Tsiknakis, M., & Orphanoudakis, S. C. (2002). A healthcare information infrastructure to support integrated services over regional health telematics networks. *Health IT Journal, Medical Records Institute, 4*(1), 15–18.

Kouroubali, A. (2003). *Implementation of health care information systems: Key factors and the dynamics of change*. Cambridge: University of Cambridge.

Lorenzi, N. M., Riley, R. T., Blyth, A. J. C., Southon, G., & Dixon, B. J. (1997). Antecedents of the people and organizational aspects of medical informatics: Review of the literature. *Journal of the American Medical Informatics Association, 4*(2), 79–93.

Lyytinen, K., & Hirschheim, R. (1987). Information systems failures – a survey and classification of the empirical literature. In: P. I. Zorkoczy (Ed.), *Oxford surveys in information technology*, (Vol. 4, pp. 257–309). Oxford: Oxford University Press.

Miller, W. L., McDaniel, R. R., Jr., Crabtree, B. F., & Stange, K. C. (2001). Practice jazz: Understanding variation in family practices using complexity science. *The Journal of Family Practice, 50*(10), 872–878.

Ministry of Health. (2000). *Healthcare in Greece*. Ministry of Health and Welfare. http://www.mohaw.gr/gr/theministry/nomothesia/

NCH. (2000). *Reducing medical errors and improving patient safety; success stories from the front lines of medicine*. The National Coalition of Healthcare and The Institute for Health care Improvement. http://www.ihi.org/IHI/Topics/PatientSafety/MedicationSystems/Literature/ReducingmedicalerrorsandimprovingpatientsafetySuccessstoriesfromthefront linesofmedicine.htm

NCVHS. (2001). *Information for health: A strategy for building the National Health Information Infrastructure*. Washington, D.C.: National Committee on Vital and Health Statistics.

NHIG (2004). *National Health Information Group and Australian Health Information Council (AHIC)*. National Health Information Management Information & Communications Technology Strategy. http://www.ahic.org.au/publications/index.html

Pare, G., & Elam, J. J. (1998). Introducing information technology in the clinical setting. *International Journal of Technology Assessment in Health Care, 14*(2), 331–343.

Peckham, M. (1999). Developing the national health service: A model for public services. *The Lancet, 354*, 1539–1545.

Pellegrino, E. (2001). *Physician philosopher: The philosophical foundation of medicine*. Charlottesville, VA: Carden Jennings Publishing Co.

Plsek, P. E., & Greenhalgh, T. (2001). Complexity science: The challenge of complexity in health care. *British Medical Journal, 323*, 625–628.

Plsek, P. E., & Kilo, C. M. (1999). From resistance to attraction: A different approach to change. *The Physician Executive*, November–December, *25*(6), 40–42.

Poulymenakou, A., & Holmes, A. (1996). A contingency framework for the investigation of information systems failure. *European Journal of Information Systems, 5*(1), 34–47.

PriceWaterhouseCoopers. (1999). *HealthCast 2010; smaller world, bigger expectations.* http://www.pwchealth.com/cgi-local/hcregister.cgi?link = pdf/hc2010.pdf

Siman, A. J. (2000). An agenda for the future: A national electronic health record system. *HCIM&C, XIV*(1), 33–34.

Sissouras, A., Karokis, A., & Mossialos, E. (1994). Greece. In: *The reform of health care systems: A review of seventeen OECD countries.* Paris: OECD.

Smith, M. Y., & Stacey, R. (1997). Governance and cooperative networks: An adaptive systems perspective. *Technological Forecasting and Social Change, 54*, 79–94.

Tanriverdi, H., & Iacono, C. S. (1999). Diffusion of telemedicine: A knowledge barrier perspective. *Telemedicine Journal, 5*(3), 223–244.

Thompson, T. G., & Brailer, D. J. (2004). *The decade of health information technology: Delivering consumer-centric and information-rich health care. Framework for strategic action.* Washington, DC: Department of Health and Human Services, National Coordinator for Health Information Technology. Available from: http://www.hhs.gov/healthit/strategicfrmwk.html.

Tonnesen, A. S., LeMaistre, A., & Tucker, D. (1999). Electronic medical record implementation barriers encountered during implementation. Paper presented at the AMIA Annual Symposium.

Traganitis, A., Trypakis, D., Spanakis, M., Condos, S., Stamkopoulos, T., Tsiknakis, M., & Orphanoudakis, S. C. (2001, 25–28 October). Home monitoring and personal health management services in a regional health telematics network. Paper presented at the 23rd Annual International Conference of the IEEE Engineering in Medicine and Biology Society, Istanbul.

Tsiknakis, M., Katehakis, D., & Orphanoudakis, S. C. (2002). An open, component-based information infrastructure for integrated health information networks. *International Journal of Medical Informatics, 68*(1–3), 3–26.

UK Department of Health (2002). *Delivering 21st century IT support for the NHS*, National Strategic Programme, June. http://www.dh.gov.uk/assetRoot/04/06/71/12/04067112.pdf.

UK NHS Information Authority (2001). *An information strategy for the modern NHS 1998–2005.* A national strategy for local implementation, July . http://www.nhsia.nhs.uk/def/pages/info4health/contents.asp.

U.S. Department of Health and Human Services (2001). *Report and recommendations from the National Committee on vital and health statistics: Information for health, report and recommendations from the National Committee on vital and health statistics.* Washington, DC, November 15. http://www.ncvhs.hhs.gov/nhiilayo.pdf.

WHO. (2002). *Innovative care for chronic conditions: Building blocks for action* (No. WHO/NMC/CCH/02.01). France: World Health Organization.

Zimmerman, B. J., Lindberg, C., & Plsek, P. E. (1998). *Edgeware: Insights from complexity science for health care leaders.* Irving, TX: VHA Publishing.

APPENDIX. GREEK HEALTH CARE SYSTEM

The Greek National Health Service (NHS) was founded in 1983. Around that time, National Health Systems were established in most Southern European countries (Sissouras, Karokis, & Mossialos, 1994). The Greek NHS is based on the following principles:

- State responsibility for the provision of health care services
- Equity in the delivery of health care services
- Decentralisation of planning
- Development of primary health care services
- Prohibition of private practice for public doctors.

The Ministry of Health and Welfare is the principal authority in the provision and financing of the NHS (Ministry of Health, 2000). The NHS structure is based upon the regional and district divisions of the country. There are 13 regions and 53 districts in Greece. Each of the regions has at least one regional hospital, usually a university teaching hospital. In each district, there is at least one hospital designated as the district hospital. The NHS provides health care services to all citizens from its national treasury.

The Greek NHS is highly centralized and regulated. Its strong legal framework is determined centrally and politics play an important role. The Ministry of Health regulates and controls the organization and management of hospitals as well as their finances. The Ministry determines the number and type of employed personnel, their terms of employment and salary levels. Hospital administrations cannot employ or reduce the number of personnel without the approval of the Ministry. Also, financial management is so strictly regulated that hospital managers cannot reallocate expenditures according to their sense of need. Health centers are administratively and financially under the auspices of their district hospital, and therefore, follow the same restrictions.

In 2001, the government began to implement a plan to reform the Greek NHS. The core principle of reform was the decentralization of services to a series of regional health systems. According to recent legislation, regions are responsible for planning and co-ordinating regional development and local health activities. The new governing Regional Councils attempt to strengthen primary care services and promote preventive care programs. The Regional Councils aim to modernize health care and address the particular problems of health care institutions in their areas. Regional Councils are recent and one can only speculate about their future effectiveness.

THE RELEVANCE OF HEALTH CARE ACCESS SYSTEMS: AN EXPLORATORY STUDY OF SEVEN INDUSTRIALIZED COUNTRIES

Petri Parvinen and Grant T. Savage

ABSTRACT

A common observation is that both single- and multi-payer health care systems will achieve lower overall costs if they use primary care gatekeeping. Questioning this common wisdom, we focus on the health care access system, that is, the way in which patients gain access to health care. Gatekeeping, the use of primary care providers to control access to more specialized physician and hospital services, has come under intense scrutiny in the United States and in Europe. The few international comparative studies that have focused on the issues of quality of care, cost containment, and patient satisfaction find weak or no support for common assumptions about gatekeeping. Hence, we examine the institutional environments in seven countries in order to: (a) define and categorize health care access systems; (b) identify the components of a health care access system; (c) explore the notion of a strategic fit between health care financing systems and access system configurations; and (d) propose that the health care access system is a key determinant of process-level cost efficiency. Drawing upon institutional and governance theories, we posit

International Health Care Management
Advances in Health Care Management, Volume 5, 331–373
ISSN: 1474-8231/doi:10.1016/S1474-8231(05)05012-3

that the structure and organization of an access system is determined by how it addresses six essential questions: Who is covered? Which services are included? What are the points of access? How much time elapses before access? What are the ways of selecting among points of access? and Are services and their quality the same for everyone? This analytical framework reveals that national health care access systems vary the most in their points of access, access times, and selection mechanisms. These findings and our explanations imply that access systems are one of the only tools for demand management, that any lasting change to an access system typically is implemented over an extended time period, and that managers of health care organizations often have limited freedom to define governance structures and shape health care service production systems.

THE RELEVANCE OF HEALTH CARE ACCESS SYSTEMS: AN EXPLORATORY STUDY OF SEVEN INDUSTRIALIZED COUNTRIES

International comparative research on the institutional environment of health care has concentrated on studying the influence of financing systems on health care organizations. For example, recent studies of Organization for Economic Cooperation and Development (OECD) data by Anderson and Reinhardt and their colleagues demonstrate that both single- and multi-payer health systems that provide universal coverage are able to spend considerably less than the United States, in large part, because of the monopsonistic power of the payers of health care (Anderson, Reinhardt, Hussey, & Petrosyn, 2003; Reinhardt, Hussey, & Anderson, 2004). A common observation is that both single- and multi-payer health care systems will achieve lower overall costs if they use primary care gatekeeping.

Questioning this common wisdom, we focus on the health care access system, that is, the way in which patients gain access to health care. The dominant configurations internationally for health care access systems include primary care *gatekeeping* and *open access* to specialist care. There is also an emergent access system, *organized integration*, which coordinates the care of patients across service delivery organizations (e.g., clinics, hospitals, nursing homes). In the United States, organized integration occurs when a primary care physician coordinates patient care with specialists within an organizational framework – such as a staff model health maintenance organization (HMO) – which allows providers to share incentives, goals, and culture (Lawrence, 2001).

Gatekeeping, the use of primary care providers (e.g., general practice physicians and/or nurse practitioners and physician assistants) to control access to more specialized physician and hospital services, has come under intense scrutiny in the United States and in Europe (Ferris, Chang, Blumenthal, & Pearson, 2001; Lawrence, 2001). In a head-to-head comparison, Feachem and his colleagues examined the cost efficiency and performance associated with organized integration within Kaiser Permanente's HMOs in the United States versus gatekeeping in the United Kingdom's national health service (NHS). Their findings showed that the costs within the two systems of care were similar, but organized integration led to superior performance in prompt and appropriate diagnosis and treatment (Feachem et al., 2002). Additional studies confirm and add to these findings, showing that the postponement of medical measures leads to complications, which require more costly and less reliable measures than would have been the case if care had been delivered in a prompt and appropriate manner (Ham, York, Sutch, & Shaw, 2003; Light & Dixon, 2004).

In counterpoint, advocates argue that gatekeeping has emerged in countries with scarce medical resources, ensuring equity by judiciously matching health care services, including specialty referrals, to health care needs. Moreover, gatekeeping increases the levels of first contact care with primary care physicians, thereby reducing patients' self referrals. However, there is little evidence that gatekeeping has had much effect on patients' referral rates in the United States, a health care environment rich in specialists (Forrest, 2003; Forrest, Majeed, Weiner, Carroll, & Bindman, 2003).

Similarly, the few multi-national comparative studies that have focused on the issues of cost containment and patient satisfaction find weak or no support for common assumptions about gatekeeping. Delnoij and her colleagues (Delnoij, Van Merode, Paulus, & Groenewegen, 2000) conducted an 18-country comparative study to investigate whether gatekeeping controlled health care costs. She and her colleagues found that gatekeeping lowered the growth of ambulatory care costs, but did not significantly impact the overall level of health care costs. Congruent with other studies, Delnoij et al. found that the level of health care costs was most strongly correlated with gross domestic product (GDP). In a separate study, Wensing and his colleagues hypothesized that primary care physicians who were gatekeepers would be less favorably viewed by patients than their counterparts in nations without gatekeeping mechanisms. Their 17-country comparison found no support for this hypothesis, and they concluded that patients were highly satisfied with primary care physicians across various national health care systems (Wensing, Baker, Szecsenyi, & Grol, 2004). Nonetheless, their data show wide variation in patient satisfaction across different gatekeeping systems.

Indeed, Delnoij and her colleagues call for further research to understand micro level mechanisms and to distinguish the effects of gatekeeping from other structural aspects of health care systems (Delnoij et al., 2000). Heeding this call, we examine the institutional environments in seven countries in order to: (a) define and categorize health care access systems; (b) identify the components of a health care access system; (c) explore the notion of a strategic fit between health care financing systems and access system configurations; and (d) propose that the health care access system is a key determinant of process-level cost efficiency.

As a necessary first step, we provide an overview of some institutional characteristics of the health systems in the seven countries examined. National health system access and financing systems are of particular interest since these structures may either encourage or hinder different types of primary care practices. Significantly, at the national level, systems of financing and organizing health care impact how the delivery of care is configured by physician participation.

WHAT IS A HEALTH CARE ACCESS SYSTEM?

Definitions, Components, and Categorizations

A health care access system is the set of processes that leads a patient to enter a health care system. The key issues include who is empowered to make decisions and how alternatives are perceived by these decision makers, as well as the implications of their decisions on costs, quality, and efficiency in production. Our analysis of health care access systems incorporates a distinction between the patient's initial access to the health care system and the handoff access opportunities that the patient and/or the health care professionals have in sending the patient to further care. Specifically, we posit that the structure and organization of an access system is determined by how it addresses six essential questions: (1) Who is covered? [Eligibility]; (2) Which services are included? [Coverage]; (3) What are the points of access? [Accessibility]; (4) How much time elapses before access? [Timeliness]; (5) What are the ways of selecting among points of access? [Choice]; and (6) Are services and their quality the same for everyone? [Equity].

The determinants of an access system can be used to analyze both initial access (the patient's entry into the health care system) and handoff access between points of care. Given the components that are put forward for analyzing access systems, there is a danger that categorizing access systems as either gatekeeping, open access or organized integration is an oversimplification. Within any one type of an access system, there may be a great amount of variability. For example, there are a number of different access logics underlying organized integration (Shortell, Gillies, & Anderson, 1994; Shortell, Gillies, Anderson, Erickson, & Mitchell, 1996). Moreover, there are different versions of open access (Murray & Tantau, 1999; Oldham, 2001). We propose, therefore, the novel idea that it is a gross oversimplification to look at primary care gatekeeping as a uniform access system.

Any new access system categorization can be interpreted and expanded, and new categorizations made, by analyzing them in terms of the six determinants of an access system. Distinguishing among open access, advanced access, and carve out (Grandinetti, 2000; Murray & Berwick, 2003) is an example of how the same determinants can be applied to analyze different conceptualizations. While we need a typology of access systems, the definitions for different types need to be refined. In this study, access systems in seven countries are analyzed with this need in mind.

Theoretical Stance

We adopt an institutional perspective to organization and management. Access systems are a vital element in the determination of the institutional structure of production in the health care industry (Coase, 1937). Institutional theory discusses regulative, normative, cultural, and cognitive pillars of institutional structure (Scott, 2000), all of which are highly influenced by the access system in health care. The access system is embedded in a set of societal institutional constraints that vary from country to country. Legislation is a good example. The extent to which access is guaranteed by law varies from country to country. This has an immediate effect on how the access system operates. For example, primary care gatekeeping works very differently depending on whether access is determined and planned at the organizational level (e.g., United Kingdom) or whether it is guaranteed by law (e.g., Sweden, Finland). Moreover, cultural norms and values determine whether the access system can differentiate between patients. Patient cognitions of themselves and the qualities of the health care system also determine how access systems work (Stewart et al., 1997). As the interplay between the financing system and the access system can be analyzed as question of the institutional and contextual environment (Tolbert, 1985), institutional theory is clearly useful for the study of access systems.

When institutional theory is brought to the level of organizations, governance theory becomes useful (Williamson, 1999). Governance theories of the firm (e.g., agency theory, transaction cost economics, property rights theory, complete and incomplete contracting theory) produce tools for analyzing actor behavior and economic outcomes in access systems. The key governance concepts from the perspective of access systems are risk, information, and incentives.

The propensity to use health care services is naturally dependent on the perception of risk by key decision makers (e.g., patients or providers). On one hand, initial access is dependent on patient risk preferences, as they influence the likelihood and way in which services are entered (Stewart et al., 1997; Zivin & Bridges, 2002). In the United States, as in many other countries, third-party payers impose user charges and other mechanisms to shape patients' risk preferences. On the other hand, handover access is crucially the question of physicians' risk preferences, as they decide whether patients are hospitalized or referred to physician specialists (Franks, Williams, Zwanziger, Mooney, & Sorbero, 2000). Again, third-party payers attempt to shape physician preferences through various incentives and oversight mechanisms, such as utilization review.

The operation of access systems is also highly dependent on information. Governance theory provides useful concepts such as information asymmetries, imperfect information, and bounded rationality for the study of health care access. Information asymmetries concerning access generally emerge between patients and professionals, as treating professionals are unable to deliver information concerning the right points of access to patients. Imperfect information about access is present in all healthcare systems and grows more severe whenever the access system is changed. Bounded rationality has an impact whenever the access system is too complex for some patients to understand.

As noted in our discussion of risk preferences, incentive structures are a natural tool for analyzing the choices of actors in the access system. From a theoretical economics perspective, patients view a healthcare access system as a menu of options. Depending on the patients' utility functions and their incentive structures, patients will 'shop' for the right access type based on preferences shaped by urgency, satisfaction, perceived quality, waiting time, preferred method of contact, and the probability of attaining care. Abusing the access system, e.g., using emergency services for obtaining non-urgent treatments or skipping gatekeeping are typical examples of behaviors that combine incentive and information-related explanations (Grumbach, Keane, & Bindman, 1993; Burnett & Grover, 1996; Boushy & Dubinsky, 1999).

INSTITUTIONS, ORGANIZATIONS, FINANCING, AND ACCESS SYSTEMS

In what follows, we compare the health care institutional environments, organizations, financing systems, and access systems in seven industrial countries: Canada, the United States, the Netherlands, the United Kingdom, Finland, Sweden and Germany. These countries have similar per capita GDP and health care technology, but varied means of financing and organizing health care services. Drawing upon data from OECD (2004) and the World Health Organization (WHO, 2004), we make rudimentary comparisons among the seven countries (see Appendices A–G). Other sources include national and ministry databases, the European Union's European observatory on health care systems, and research published in refereed journals.

We systematically evaluate the health care financing systems, the organization of the delivery of health care services, the methods for controlling costs, and the management of quality in the seven countries. Included in the comparisons are statistics about health care costs, sources and modes of financing, hospital stays, performance indicators, and health insurance.

Financing Systems

National health care systems display three distinct means of financing care: (1) national health services (e.g., the United Kingdom and Sweden) funded through general taxation; (2) national compulsory insurance (e.g., Canada); or (3) a mixture of compulsory social and private insurance (e.g., Germany, Netherlands, and the United States). Of the countries compared, the United States (see Appendix G) is unique in its reliance primarily on voluntary rather than compulsory employer-based private health insurance, and secondarily on social health insurance (i.e., Medicare) and other publicly funded health insurance (e.g., Medicaid). Financing can be broken out into two aspects: the direct versus indirect provision of health services by various national governments (Abel-Smith, 1992). Direct financing of health services occurs if the main health insurer or government – whether national, regional, or local – owns health care facilities and employs health care professionals, as in Sweden (see Appendix E) and the United Kingdom (see Appendix F). Indirect financing, in contrast, occurs if the main insurer or government contracts for the provision of various health services. For example, the provincial and regional governments in Canada (see Appendix A) and the sickness funds (insurance companies) in Germany (see Appendix C) and the Netherlands (see Appendix D) contract with providers for health services.

Fig. 1 compares the sources of revenue for health expenditures in each of the seven national health systems. In contrast to the United States, universal access is offered by the four countries at the top (the U.K., Sweden, Canada, and Finland) and the two countries at the bottom (Germany and the Netherlands) of Fig. 1. These countries rely primarily on either taxation (single-payer) or compulsory social and private insurance (multi-payer). Universal access to health care within any of these national health systems does not come without some rationing and limiting access to secondary and tertiary health care (McKee & Figueras, 1996). Generally speaking, single-payer national health systems are more efficient than multi-payer systems, while gatekeeping systems of care are better able to control costs. This point

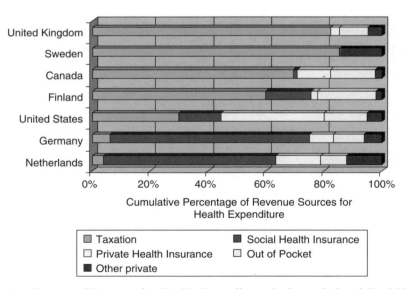

Fig. 1. Sources of Revenue for Health Expenditures in Seven Industrialized Nations. *Source*: WHO (2004).

is underscored by the percentage of GDP that the United Kingdom (7.6%), Finland (7.3%), Sweden (8.9%), and Canada (9.7%) devoted to health care versus that expended by the Netherlands (8.9%), Germany (10.7%), and the United States (13.9%) in 2001 (OECD, 2003). The non-universal, but multi-payer form of financing within the United States leads not only to high costs, but also to limited access for the uninsured and uneven quality (Keeler & Brodie, 1993; Schneck, 2000; Malin, Keeler, Wang, & Brook, 2002; Schackman et al., 2001; Reinhardt et al., 2004).

However, even countries with stable forms of financing are facing problems sustaining their health systems. In the Netherlands, physician-practice restrictions have been imposed because of excessive growth in costs. Because of these restrictions, a good number of physicians have taken early retirement. Co-payments have been introduced, and various procedures have been eliminated from the care package (Busse, 2002b). Major controls have been exerted on the pharmaceutical industry in these same countries. Agreements to lower prices of certain medications as much as 40% have been introduced. Additionally, in some instances, a limited list of approved medications have been implemented (Dixon & Mossialos, 2002). In most places of Scandinavia (e.g., Denmark, Norway, Sweden, and Finland), extensive financing of medical services has been curtailed in part through shifting the burden of payment of physicians from the public to the private sector (Koivusalo, 1999; Hjortsberg & Chatnekar, 2001; León & Rico, 2002; Vallgårda, Thomson, Krasnik, & Vrangbæk, 2002; Lian, 2003).

Despite the extensive research about the differences and characteristics of different financing systems, establishing a direct link between financing systems and the efficiency of the health care system has proven difficult (Magnussen & Solstad, 1994; Aas, 1995; Kroneman & Siegers, 2004). Prior explanations for differences and increases in health care costs and spending based on financing systems have been merited, but offer only partial explanations for the variance among national health systems.

A more nuanced understanding of the impact of financing systems occurs if the mediating influence of health care access systems is recognized. For example, there are major differences in the access systems of different forms of, basically technically similar, private health insurances. A private, personal health insurance can operate with a number of different access systems depending on who finances the private insurance and on the national institutional health care context. Both in Canada and the United States, private health insurance that is entirely paid for by the individual basically gives open access to any form of treatment (this is reflected in the insurance premiums). However, in the United States, private health insurance policies partially paid for by the employer, even if the employer's share is small, allow this third-party payer to shape the individual's preferences for initial access.

Moreover, access systems often explain important processes that financing systems cannot explain. For example, there are major differences in the utilization of specialized care between Finland (see Appendix B) and Sweden (see Appendix E), where the financing systems are virtually the same but the access systems are different. In Sweden, there is open access to a wide range of specialized health care services under the public system; in contrast, access to virtually all specialized care is governed through gatekeeping in Finland. As a result, during 2003, Swedes had 1.5 encounters per inhabitant per year with specialists, resulting in over 13.4 million total encounters (Socialstyrelsen, 2004), while Finns only had 1.2 encounters per inhabitant per year with specialists, for a total of 6.1 million encounters (STAKES, 2004). Interestingly, Swedish–Finnish ratios of total health expenditure per capita (8.9% : 7.3%) and total costs of specialized care per inhabitant (1009 EUR : 670 EUR) follow a very similar pattern (Socialstyrelsen, 2004; STAKES, 2004).

Access Systems

Clearly, how health care is financed at the national level does not determine the structure of its access system. For example, the NHS in the United Kingdom (see Appendix F) and the NHS in Sweden (see Appendix E) as single-payer, socialized health systems rely on general taxation and provide direct services to their citizens via NHSs. Yet they have remarkably different ways of structuring their systems of care for physicians and patients. Sweden provides its citizens with open access to physician specialists; in contrast, the United Kingdom and Finland limit access to specialists through a well-developed gatekeeping system of primary care. Similarly, both Germany (see Appendix C) and the Netherlands (see Appendix D) rely on multi-payer, mixed market systems of social and private health insurance to fund indirectly the services provided by physicians, hospitals, and other providers. On the one hand, Germany allows its citizens open access to physician specialists in ambulatory settings; on the other hand, the Netherlands imposes primary care gatekeeping. Canada, which has a single-payer health system with indirect services, also imposes gatekeeping (see Appendix A). The United States, with its multi-payer system of public and private funding, uses mostly open access, with some gatekeeping and relatively little organized integration (see Appendix F).

The variation in health care access systems is not directly linked to the overall supply of physicians in each of these national health systems, but is related to the ratio of general practitioners (GPs) to specialists. Fig. 2 contrasts the ratio of GPs to the ratio of all physicians (number per thousand) for each of the seven countries. Note that Germany and the Netherlands have the highest ratio of total physicians (3.2 and 3.3 per thousand) to population, but the Netherlands has the higher proportion of GPs (1.9 versus 1.29 per thousand). This relationship is also found in Canada which has approximately a fifty-fifty split between GPs and specialists (CIHI, 2002). The anomaly in this relationship seems to be the United Kingdom, which has low ratios for both GPs (0.60) and total physicians (2.0 per thousand). The apparently low number of GPs is also something that the NHS has attempted to address in the past few years, both through a program for retaining GPs (Hastie, 2001) and through a public–private partnership program for upgrading GP clinical facilities (Kmietowicz, 2001; Royal College of General Practitioners, 2003).

A Six Component Analysis of Access Systems

Viewing access systems in terms of the six components (who is covered, access time, services, points of access, selection mechanism, and service quality) provides a fine-grained analysis, which may better explain the

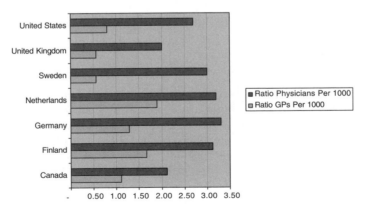

Fig. 2. General Practitioner and Total Physician Ratio to Population for Seven Countries. *Source*: CIHI (2002); Dixon and Mossialos (Eds) (2002); OECD (2003); and Royal College of General Practitioners (2003).

efficiencies and deficiencies of different systems. All six components can be applied to analyze both initial access and handoff access. Conceptually, we classify quality differences, population coverage, and service coverage as general access system issues in Table 1. However, we examine points of access, access times, and the selection mechanisms between access points separately for both initial access and for handoff access. The six components' analysis reveals that what differs between various national health care access systems are the points of access, access times, and the selection mechanisms. For national health systems with universal coverage, population and service coverage, as well as quality assurance, work in different ways but in a similar extent and with a similar logic. Also, there are significant variations among national systems that use gatekeeping systems to control handoff access. The same variation applies to national systems that allow open access for specialist care. Thus, gatekeeping and open access as key distinctions between health care access systems seems oversimplified.

ACCESS SYSTEMS, FINANCING SYSTEMS, AND COST: A QUESTION OF FIT

Most countries use a mixture of price controls and limits on capacity, rather than explicit rationing, to manage costs (Reinhardt et al., 2004). Based on our discussion of the financing systems and analysis of the access systems in these seven countries, it seems relevant to try to establish a more fine-grained linkage between different access systems and costs.

Health Care Costs and Access Systems

Conceptually, the different attributes of a health care access system should have a direct link to costs. Who is covered, with which services, and with what level of quality are a matter of customer segmentation and organization differentiation and involve the explicit rationing of health services. In other words, segmenting patients and attempting to provide the proper and sufficient care, but not more, has an explicit link to costs. In turn, points of access and their selection mechanism relate to allocative efficiency (Palmer & Torgerson, 1999). That is, these mechanisms attempt to maximize net benefit by allocating demand accurately to existing resources. Access time, both for initial access and for the handover access, has a correlation to cost; as waiting times increase, care costs increase (Johannesson, Johansson, &

Table 1. Analyzing Initial and Handoff Access Systems on Six Components.

	General Access			Initial Access			Handoff Access		
	Who is Covered?	Which Services are Included*?	Are Services and their Quality the Same for Everyone?	Access Time	Points of Access (in Addition to ERs)	Selection Mechanism between Access Points	Access Time	Points of Access	Selection Mechanism between Access Points
Canada	National system covering all residents	AM, IP, PH PRMED, CH, PRV, PRT, HOM	Regional and hospital-specific differences	Dependent on regional queue status	GPs	Urgency (otherwise designated)	Dependent on regional queue status	Mostly autonomous non-profit hospitals	Gatekeeping
Germany	All sickness fund members (99.8% of population)	NPH, AM, PH, IP, HC, DC, RH, screening	Regional and hospital-specific differences	Dependent on sickness fund	GPs, private practices, hospitals	Patient discretion	Dependent on sickness fund-hospital relationship	Designated hospitals for each sickness fund	Open access or organized integration
Finland	All through national system	PRV, PH, PRMED, IP, AM, DC, LTC, RH, HOM, MEN	Regional differences, attempts to unify	Guaranteed access within three days	GPs in health centers	Urgency (otherwise designated)	Consultation guaranteed in 3 weeks, treatment in 3 months	Region-specific hospital defined in referral	Gatekeeping
Netherlands	All obliged to obtain insurance (3 systems)	PRV, IP, AM, PH, MEN, LTC, PRV, PRMED, RH, sick leaves	Yes (strict quality control)	Dependent on insurance system	GPs	Urgency (otherwise designated)	Dependent on hospital	Mostly autonomous non-profit hospitals	Gatekeeping
Sweden	All through national system	PRV, PH, PRMED, IP, AM, DC, LTC, RH, MEN	Yes (widespread quality systems and monitoring)	Guaranteed access within one week (?)	Health centers (multi-profession)	Limited patient discretion	Guaranteed access within one month	Three hospital categories dependent on need	Open access
United Kingdom	All through NHS	PRV, OP, AM, PH, MED, DC, MH, RH	Highly variable depending on hospital and specialism	Highly variable	GPs and mid-level nurses	Patient chooses GP within locale	Dependent on district queue status	3 hospital types, depending on needed specialist	Gatekeeping

Table 1. (*Continued*)

	General Access		Initial Access			Handoff Access		
	Who is Covered?	Which Services are Included*?	Are Services and their Quality the Same for Everyone?	Access Time	Points of Access (in Addition to ERs)	Selection Mechanism between Access Points	Access Time	Points of Access	Selection Mechanism between Access Points
United States	85% of population covered	Usually at least IP, AM, PH. Private also PRV, DC, PRMED	Quality control widespread and extensive despite other differences	Dependent on insurance system – generally one day	GPs, family practices, clinics, hospitals	Variable patient discretion	Some private plans guarantee access time	For-profit, non-profit, and public hospitals; multi- and single-specialty clinics	Gatekeeping, open access, or organized integration

Soderqvist, 1998; Propper, Croxson, & Shearer, 2002). The impact of the access system on spending and cost requires an elaborate understanding of how an access system drives patient and professional behavior. Looking at the differences between usage, costs, and patient behavior, it seems that the linkage is strong but complex. Hence, we posit the following proposition:

Proposition 1. The attributes of the health care access system are a significant driver of health care spending and costs. As the effect is mediated through the perceptions and behavior of individual patients and professionals, this link is desperately multifaceted.

Health Care Access and Financing Systems

However, similar access systems may yield different cost results. Comparing out-of-pocket spending versus private insurance yields an interesting insight. The share between out-of-pocket spending and private insurance differs from one access system to another. Out-of-pocket payments are relatively more common in Finland and the U.K., whereas private insurance is common in the Netherlands and Canada. All four countries have a gatekeeping system. Where out-of-pocket and private spending together constitutes a large share of total spending, health care costs per capita tend to be higher (U.S.A., Canada). Furthermore, health spending in gatekeeping countries (the U.K., Finland, the Netherlands, and Canada) tends to have a lower share of GDP. These relationships are, however, more indicative than apparent (Delnoij et al., 2000).

Thus, there is reason to believe that there is a more complex relationship beyond the immediate relationship between access systems and cost. Our discussion of out-of-pocket costs suggests that principle-agent decision-making affects cost efficiency. The access system and the financing system together define who makes the decisions concerning what health services are wanted, what services are needed, and what services will be provided. This decision-making process is the basic premise of health care demand management. Hence, we suggest in the following proposition that a strategic fit between an access system and a financing system leads to a more knowledgeable, actionable, and ultimately, efficient decision-making process.

Proposition 2. Attaining a fit between the health care access and financing systems correlates with achieving efficiency in health care at the level of the system.

Health Care Access Systems and Process-Level Efficiency

How can the degree of fit be assessed? This is where basic governance theory becomes useful. Applied governance theory examines process problems in health care (Gaynor, Rebitzer, & Taylor, 2004; Parvinen, Reijonsaari, & Kämäräinen, 2004). It distinguishes between problems emerging from the governance modes in which decision-making is organized and the governance practices that determine action outcomes. Governance analysis reveals that situations are harmful where information asymmetries and/or incentive asymmetries in the presence of weak or non-existing monitoring prevail. Opportunistic behavior, partial optimization of individual tasks in a care chain, or property rights violations all lead to sub-optimal efficiency outcomes in an entire care process.

For example, the degree of fit could be assessed by the relative share of care decisions made by decision-makers other than those who legitimately should be making them. Outcomes of such misappropriated decisions could also be studied. These might include the number of visits that are unnecessary or provided in an inappropriate setting, useless treatments, pointless ancillary services, etc. This approach, however, begs the question: Are there configurations of access and financing systems that obtain better economic efficiencies than others? Our examination of the seven countries unveils some issues that give reason to doubt so. Comparing the otherwise relatively similar Swedish and Finnish systems reveal that the costs for diagnostic specialized care are much higher in Sweden. Patients can enter specialized clinics without the triage imposed by primary care gatekeeping in Finland. This Swedish access system does not necessarily lead to more treatments, but it does increase diagnostic costs significantly. For example, practically all radiological examinations in Sweden are performed in hospitals (Lantto, 2000). On the other hand, hospitalization from emergency departments in Finland is very high due to the fact that many primary care physicians work at regional emergency departments and tend to place patients in the hospital overnight for monitoring.

A good access-financing system configuration organizes not only clinical and medical knowledge, but also knowledge about patient processes to the relevant decision-making nexuses within the access system. Physicians making allocation decisions often lack the incentives to rationalize process costs related to the entire patient process, or even have an incentive against rationalizing them, as is the case when a 'fee per service' system is used in private sector operations. The degree of finance-access fit in a health care system could thus also be judged on how often the cost burden, process cost information, and decision-making power is conjoined. This is also why interest groups are designing gatekeeping systems for services typically paid out-of-pocket, e.g., plastic and ophthalmic surgery.

In order to be able to study process-level efficiency in health care, a total quality management perspective to patient processes and care processes arguably is the most useful. The patient-oriented approach is a relevant starting point for process analysis, because patient processes are often cross-functional and span organizational borders (Tarte & Bogiages, 1992; Vissers, Hasman, & Stapert, 1998). They provide a challenge for the traditional production-oriented approach, which is often designed to optimize the performance of single organizations or functions inside an organization, leading to sub-optimization of the whole service production process from the patients' point of view (Rummler & Brache, 1995; Lillrank, Kujala, Kämäräinen, & Kronström, 2003). In a patient-oriented approach, process-level data, both case-based and aggregate, are collected. Measures such as activity-based service costs, throughput times, resource utilization, turnover rates, order penetration points, care form options, and system output can then be employed (see Table 2). Clearly, there is an urgent need for research linking access systems, financing systems, and process level efficiency. Any attempt to verify access system–financing system fit would need to permeate patient process efficiency measures.

Proposition 3. Health care access systems have a direct relationship to efficiency at the level of discrete patient processes.

IMPLICATIONS FOR POLICY AND RESEARCH

The different attributes and processes within a health care access system provide a basis for analyzing how institutional configurations impact and how care is organized and delivered to patients. However, access system categorizations need to be refined through further research. For example, the different varieties of gatekeeping systems and their key attributes should be researched. Moreover, we should be aware that besides access to care and a system of financing, there are other institutional issues that influence how health care services are organized. From the viewpoint of health care managers and policy-makers, the question is how access systems should be prioritized vis-à-vis other issues in health care management.

The first implication from this exploratory study is that managing access systems is essentially the management of an evolutionary mechanism. The

Table 2.   Patient Process Attributes within Different Health Care Access
Systems.

Process Attribute	Examples of Issues for Study
Process goals	Process goals and objectives (medical and non-medical)
	Management of patient and other stakeholder expectations
Process input	Patients knowledge of particular health care service
	Factors determining who has access to care
	Variation in patients "quality" (medical and non-medical)
	Patient expectations and behavior
	Patient volume
Care form options	Alternative care forms that are available
	Latest medical technology utilization
	The geographical location of services
	Use of subcontracted medical services
Decision making process	Decision-making process to select care form
	Factors upon process performance optimization is based on
	Decision making at each phase of the process
	Authority of medical professional
Competence of personnel	Level of medical competence of personnel
	Service orientation of medical and non-medical personnel
Resource utilization	Health care system shared resources
	Process dedicated resources
	Use of other resources (e.g., physiotherapist)
	Total cost of patient episode (including e.g., employers)
Temporal dimension	Waiting times and patient episode time categories
	Resource availability and allocation
	Non-medical factors used to determine patient order of priority
Process output	Quality of care, outpatient status, patient satisfaction
	Process efficiency and effectiveness
	Meeting other stakeholder expectations

institutional environment and organization-level governance are both key
determinants of the prevailing access system. Access systems have evolved
alongside changes in the modes and resources of the various financing systems. The management of evolution, be it in an industry business model
logic, network structure, or health care access systems, is a question of
systematic action and the management of inertia and cognitions in the long
term (Porac, Ventresca, & Mishina, 2002). Abrupt moves change little.
Plans to change access systems should operate on a 20-year horizon rather
than a quarterly basis. Iteration and incremental continuous improvement is
necessary. Access system management is not improved through environmental jolts imposed through either abrupt market or policy changes.

The second implication is that health care access systems should be managed more actively. This exploratory study shows that access systems are one of the only tools for demand management in publicly financed national health care systems. Despite the evident linkages to the financing system and especially its historical evolution, there are opportunities to manage access systems creatively under any given institutional setting.

Nevertheless, and thirdly, physicians, administrators, and managers of health care organizations have limited freedom within institutionalized environments to define governance structures that shape health care service production systems. Policy-makers are the primary shapers of access systems. The degrees of freedom for managers seem to be more dependent on access system policy than on the financing system. Policy-makers should engage in active dialogue with health care stakeholders about the access system in order to craft good access-financing system fits. Moreover, our study suggests that traditional financing system-centered policy is perhaps not the easiest or the most direct way for achieving process efficiency.

As with any exploratory inquiry, we are left with additional questions. Should the access system be developed first and the financing system next? The United States and the United Kingdom are not the only nations wrestling with access systems and attempts to provide integrated care. The Netherlands, Canada, and Sweden also are looking at ways to provide coordinated care across different forms of health service delivery organizations, especially for patients with chronic conditions (Dixon & Mossialos, 2002; Smith, 2002). Each of these countries is faced with rising costs within predominately publicly financed national health systems. Should attention be first and foremost directed to access system management? Lastly, which parts of the health care system other than financing should be analyzed in the context of access systems? We hope this chapter provides a starting point for conceptualizing access systems, and thus, facilitates inquiry into research dealing with other access system-related issues.

REFERENCES

Aas, I. H. M. (1995). Incentives and financing methods. *Health Policy, 34*(3), 205–220.

Abel-Smith, B. (1992). Cost containment and new priorities in the European community. *The Milbank Quarterly, 70*(3), 393–416.

Anderson, G. F., Reinhardt, U. E., Hussey, P. S., & Petrosyan, V. (2003). It's the prices, stupid: Why the United States is so different from other countries. *Health Affairs, 22*(3), 89–105.

Birkner, B. R. (1998). National quality of care activities in Germany. *International Journal of Quality Health Care, 10*(5), 451–454.

Boushy, D., & Dubinsky, I. (1999). Primary care physician and patient factors that result in patients seeking emergency care in a hospital setting: The patient's perspective. *Journal of Emergency Medicine, 17*(3), 405–412.

Brown, L. D., & Amelung, V. (1999). Manacled competition: Introducing market reforms in the German health care system. *Health Affairs, 18*(3), 76–91.

Burnett, M. G., & Grover, S. A. (1996). Use of the emergency department for nonurgent care during regular business hours. *Canadian Medical Association Journal, 154*(9), 1345–1351.

Busse, R. (2002a). Germany. In: E. Mossialos (Ed.), *Health care systems in eight countries: Trends and challenges* (pp. 47–60). Copenhagen: European Observatory on Health Care Systems.

Busse, R. (2002b). Netherlands. In: A. Dixon & E. Mossialos (Eds), *Health care systems in eight countries: Trends and challenges* (pp. 61–73). Copenhagen: European Observatory on Health Care Systems.

Busse, R., & Riesberg, A. (2000). *Health care systems in transition: Germany.* Copenhagen: European Observatory on Health Care Systems.

CCOHTA. (2002). *FAQ.* Retrieved October 26, 2002, from http://www.ccohta.ca/entry_e.html

CIHI. (2002). *Canada's Health Care Providers.* Ottawa: Canadian Institute for Health Information.

CIHI. (2002). *Health care in Canada 2002.* Ottawa: Canadian Institute for Health Information.

CMS. (2002). *National health care source of funds.* Retrieved November 15, 2002, from http://cms.hhs.gov/researchers/pubs/datacompendium/2002/02pg15.pdf

Coase, R. H. (1937). The nature of the firm. *Economica, 4*, 386–405.

Cosca, T. (1999). Physicians. In: *1998–1999 Occupational Outlook Handbook.* Retrieved January 30, 2000, from http://stats.bls.gov:80/oco/ocos074.htm#employment

Crebolder, H. F., & van der Horst, F. G. (1996). Anticipatory care and the role of Dutch general practice in health promotion – A critical reflection. *Patient Education and Counseling, 28*(1), 51–55.

Delnoij, D., Van Merode, G., Paulus, A., & Groenewegen, P. (2000). Does general practitioner gatekeeping curb health care expenditure? *Journal of Health Services Research & Policy, 5*(1), 22–26.

Department of Finance. (2002). *Equalization Program.* Retrieved October 26, 2002, from http://www.fin.gc.ca/FEDPROV/eqpe.html

Diderichsen, F. (1999). Devolution in Swedish health care: Local government isn't powerful enough to control costs or stop privatisation. *British Medical Journal, 318*(May 1), 1157–1158.

Dixon, A., & Mossialos, E. (Eds) (2002). *Health care systems in eight countries: Trends and challenges.* Copenhagen: European Observatory on Health Care Systems.

Dixon, A., & Robinson, R. (2002). The United Kingdom. In: A. Dixon & E. Mossialos (Eds), *Health care systems in eight countries:Trends and challenges* (pp. 103–114). Copenhagen: European Observatory on Health Care Systems.

Feachem, R. G. A., Sekhri, N. K., White, K. L., Dixon, J., Berwick, D. M., & Enthoven, A. C. (2002). Getting more for their dollar: A comparison of the NHS with California's Kaiser permanente commentary: Funding is not the only factor commentary: Same price, better care commentary: Competition made them do it. *British Medical Journal, 324*(7330), 135–143.

Ferris, T. G., Chang, Y., Blumenthal, D., & Pearson, S. D. (2001). Leaving gatekeeping behind – Effects of opening access to specialists for adults in a health maintenance organization. *New England Journal of Medicine, 345*(18), 1312–1317.

Forrest, C. B. (2003). Primary care in the United States: Primary care gatekeeping and referrals: Effective filter or failed experiment? *British Medical Journal, 326*(7391), 692–695.

Forrest, C. B., Majeed, A., Weiner, J. P., Carroll, K., & Bindman, A. B. (2003). Referral of children to specialists in the United States and the United Kingdom. *Archives of Pediatrics & Adolescent Medicine, 157*(3), 279–285.

Frankish, C. J., Kwan, B., Ratner, P. A., Higgins, J. W., & Larsen, C. (2002). Social and political factors influencing the functioning of regional health boards in British Columbia (Canada). *Health Policy, 61*(2), 125–151.

Franks, P., Williams, G. C., Zwanziger, J., Mooney, K., & Sorbero, M. (2000). Why do physicians vary so widely in their referral rates? *Journal of General Internal Medicine, 15*(3), 163–188.

Gabel, J. R., Hunt, K. A., & Hurst, K. (1998). *When employers choose health plans do NCQA accreditation and HEDIS data count? (No Report 293).* New York: The Commonwealth Fund.

Gaynor, M., Rebitzer, J. B., & Taylor, L. J. (2004). Physician incentives in health maintenance organizations. *Journal of Political Economy, 112*(4), 915–931.

Grandinetti, D. A. (2000). Doctors and the Web. Help your patients surf the Net safely. *Medical Economics, 77*(5), 186–188, 194–196, 201.

Grumbach, K., Keane, D., & Bindman, A. B. (1993). Primary care and public emergency department overcrowding. *American Journal of Public Health, 83*(3), 372–378.

Ham, C., York, N., Sutch, S., & Shaw, R. (2003). Hospital bed utilisation in the NHS, Kaiser Permanente, and the US Medicare programme: Analysis of routine data. *British Medical Journal, 327*(7426), 1257–1261.

Hastie, A. (2001). The general practitioner retainer scheme. *BMJ Career Focus, 323*(7305), S2-7305–27305.

Hjortsberg, C., & Chatnekar, O. (2001). *Health care systems in transition: Sweden 2001* (Vol. 3). Copenhagen: European Observatory on Health Care Systems.

Hurst, J., & Jee-Hughes, M. (2001). *Performance measurement and performance management in OECD health systems* (Labour Market and Social Policy-Occasional Papers No. N° 47). Paris: Organization for Economic Cooperation and Development.

Johannesson, M., Johansson, P. O., & Soderqvist, T. (1998). Time spent on waiting lists for medical care: An insurance approach. *Journal of Health Economics, 17*(5), 627–644.

Jönsson, B. (1997). Economic evaluation of medical technologies in Sweden. *Social Science and Medicine, 45*(4), 597–604.

Keeler, E. B., & Brodie, M. (1993). Economic incentives in the choice between vaginal delivery and cesarean section. *Milbank Quarterly, 71*(3), 365–404.

Klazinga, N., Lombarts, K., & van Everdingen, J. (1998). Quality management in medical specialties: The use of channels and dikes in improving health care in the Netherlands. *Joint Commission Journal on Quality Improvement, 24*(5), 240–250.

Kmietowicz, Z. (2001). Evidence that public-private partnerships can increase funding is "paltry". *British Medical Journal, 323*(7319), 954b.

Koivusalo, M. (1999). Decentralisation and equity of healthcare provision in Finland. *British Medical Journal, 318*(May 1), 1198–1200.

Kroneman, M., & Siegers, J. J. (2004). The effect of hospital bed reduction on the use of beds: A comparative study of 10 European countries. *Social Science & Medicine, 59*(8), 1731–1740.

Lantto, E. (2000). *Radiologia Keski-Suomessa: Alueellinen toimintamalli 2000-luvulle [Radiology in Central Finland: Regional standards of activity]* (No.14). Helsinki: National Research and Development Centre for Welfare and Health (STAKES).

D. Lawrence (Ed.). (2001). Editorial: Gatekeeping reconsidered. *The New England Journal of Medicine, 345*(18), 1342–1344.

Le Grand, J. (2002). Further tales from the British National Health Service. *Health Affairs, 21*(3), 116–128.

Le Grand, J., Mays, N., & Mulligan, J.-A. (1999). *Learning from the NHS internal market: A review of the evidence.* London: King's Fund.

León, S., & Rico, A. (2002). Sweden. In: A. Dixon & E. Mossialos (Eds), *Health care systems in eight countries: Trends and challenges* (pp. 91–102). Copenhagen: European Observatory on Health Care Systems.

Levit, K., Cowan, C., Lazenby, H., Sensenig, A., McDonnell, P., Stiller, J., & Martin, A. (2000). Health spending in 1998: Signals of change. The health Accounts Team. *Health Affairs, 19*(1), 124–132.

Lian, O. S. (2003). Convergence or divergence? Reforming primary care in Norway and Britain. *Milbank Quarterly, 81*(2), 173, 305–330.

Light, D., & Dixon, M. (2004). Making the NHS more like Kaiser Permanente. *British Medical Journal, 328*(7442), 763–765.

Lillrank, P., Kujala, J., Kämäräinen, V., & Kronström, V. (2003). Patient in process - A new approach to managing patient processes in healthcare. Paper presented at the hospital of the future: 3rd international conference on the management of healthcare & medical technology, Warwick, Great Britain.

Magnussen, J., & Solstad, K. (1994). Case-based hospital financing: The case of Norway. *Health Policy, 28*(1), 23–36.

Malin, J. L., Keeler, E., Wang, C., & Brook, R. (2002). Using cost-effectiveness analysis to define a breast cancer benefits package for the uninsured. *Breast Cancer Research and Treatment, 74*(2), 143–153.

McKee, M., & Figueras, J. (1996). For Debate: Setting priorities: Can Britain learn from Sweden? *British Medical Journal, 312*(7032), 691–694.

Mills, R. J. (2002). *Health Insurance Coverage: 2001* (Internet No. P60-220). Washington DC: U.S. Census Bureau.

Ministry of Health, W. a. S. (2002). *Diagnosis and Treatment Combination (DBC 2003).* Retrieved November 1, 2002, from http://www.dbc2003.nl/new2/getpage.php?page=97

Ministry of Social Affairs and Health. (2004). *Health Care in Finland* (Brochure No. 11). Helsinki: Ministry of Social Affairs and Health.

Murray, M., & Berwick, D. M. (2003). Advanced access: Reducing waiting and delays in primary care. *Journal of the American Medical Association, 289*(8), 1035–1040.

Murray, M., & Tantau, C. (1999). Redefining open access to primary care. *Managed Care Quarterly, 7*(3), 45–55.

OECD. (2001). *OECD Health at a glance – how Canada compares* (PolicyBrief). Paris: Organisation for Economic Co-operation and Development.

OECD. (2003). *Health at a glance: OECD indicators 2003.* Paris: Organisation for Economic Co-operation and Development.

OECD. (2004). *OECD health data 2004: A comparative analysis of 30 countries.* Paris: Organisation for Economic Co-operation and Development.

Oldham, M. (2001). Opportunity knocked. *Health Services Journal, 111*(5780), 24.

PAHO. (2001). *Regional Core Health Data System – Country Health Profile 2001: Canada.* Retrieved October 26, 2002, from http://www.paho.org/English/SHA/prflCAN.htm.

Palmberg, M. (1997). Quality improvement in Swedish health care. *Joint Commission Journal on Quality Improvement, 23*(1), 47–54.

Palmer, S., & Torgerson, D. J. (1999). Economics notes: Definitions of efficiency. *British Medical Journal, 318*(7191), 1136.

Parvinen, P., Reijonsaari, K., & Kämäräinen, V. (2004). *A governance-process framework for healthcare research: Some exploratory evidence.* Paper presented at the British academy of management, University of Saint Andrews, UK.

Porac, J. F., Ventresca, M. J., & Mishina, Y. (2002). Interorganizational cognition and interpretation. In: J. A. C. Bauman (Ed.), *The Blackwell companion to organizations* (pp. 579–598). Malden, MA: Blackwell Publishing.

Propper, C., Croxson, B., & Shearer, A. (2002). Waiting times for hospital admissions: The impact of GP fundholding. *Journal of Health Economics, 21*(2), 227–252.

Reinhardt, U. E., Hussey, P. S., & Anderson, G. F. (2004). U.S. health care spending in an international context. *Health Affairs (Millwood), 23*(3), 10–25.

Robinson, R., & Dixon, A. (1999). *Health care systems in transition: United Kingdom.* Copenhagen: European Observatory on Health Care Systems.

Royal College of General Practitioners. (2003). *Profile of UK practices.* Retrieved May 14, 2004, from http://www.rcgp.org.uk/information/publications/information/PDF/02_OCT_03.pdf.

Rummler, G. A., & Brache, A. P. (1995). *Improving performance: How to manage the white space on the organization chart.* San Francisco: Jossey-Bass.

Sauerland, D. (2001). The German strategy for quality improvement in health care: Still to improve. *Health Policy, 56*(2), 127–147.

Schackman, B. R., Goldie, S. J., Weinstein, M. C., Losina, E., Zhang, H., & Freedberg, K. A. (2001). Cost-effectiveness of earlier initiation of antiretroviral therapy for uninsured HIV-infected adults. *American Journal of Public Health, 91*(9), 1456–1463.

Schneck, L. H. (2000). Health insurance for the "uninsurable". *Medical Group Management Journal, 47*(6), 48–52, 54, 56–57.

Scott, W. R. (2000). *Institutions and organizations* (2nd ed). Thousand Oaks, CA: Sage Publications.

Shortell, S. M., Gillies, R. R., & Anderson, D. A. (1994). The new world of managed care: Creating organized delivery systems. *Health Affairs, 13*(1), 46–64.

Shortell, S. M., Gillies, R. R., Anderson, D. A., Erickson, K. M., & Mitchell, J. B. (1996). *Remaking Health Care in America: Building Organized Delivery Systems.* San Francisco: Jossey-Bass.

Smith, P. C. (Ed.) (2002). *Measuring up: Improving health system performance in OECD countries.* Paris: Organisation for Economic Co-operation and Development.

Socialstyrelsen. (2004). *Hälso- och sjukvårdsverksamhet 2003 [Yearbook of health and medical care 2003].* Stockholm: National Board of Health and Welfare (Socialstyrelsen).

SPRI. (1998). *Health care 98 the facts* (No. Statistical Report 330). Stockholm: Swedish Institute for Health Services Development.

STAKES. (2004). *Statistical yearbook on social welfare and health care 2004.* Helsinki: National Research and Development Centre for Welfare and Health (STAKES).

Stewart, A. L., Grumbach, K., Osmond, D. H., Vranizan, K., Komaromy, M., & Bindman, A. B. (1997). Primary care and patient perceptions of access to care. *Journal of Family Practice, 44*, 77–185.

Swedish Institute. (1999). *The health care system in Sweden* (No. Fact Sheet FS 76 x Vpb). Stockholm: Swedish Institute.

Tarte, J. P., & Bogiages, C. C. (1992). Patient-centered care delivery and the role of information systems. *Computers in Healthcare, 13*(2), 44–46.

Tolbert, P. S. (1985). Institutional environments and resource dependence: Sources of administrative structure in institutions for higher education. *Administrative Science Quarterly, 30*(1), 1–13.

Tolkki, O., Ahovuo, J., Kauppinen, T., Fyhr, N., Kujala, J., & Parvinen, P. (2004). *Patient in process, benefits of reduced throughput time – case HUSpacs*. Paper presented at the EuroPACS-MIR 2004 in the Enlarged Europe, Trieste, Italy.

Vallgårda, S., Thomson, S., Krasnik, A., & Vrangbæk, K. (2002). Denmark. In: A. Dixon & E. Mossialos (Eds), *Health care systems in eight countries: Trends and challenges* (pp. 17–29). Copenhagen: European Observatory on Health Care Systems.

Vissers, M. C., Hasman, A., & Stapert, J. W. (1998). Presenting treatment protocols with Web technology. *Medinfo, 9*(Part 1), 521–524.

Wensing, M., Baker, R., Szecsenyi, J., & Grol, R. (2004). Impact of national health care systems on patient evaluations of general practice in Europe. *Health Policy, 68*(3), 353–357.

WHO. (1996). *Health care systems in transition: Sweden*. Copenhagen: World Health Organization.

WHO. (2002a). *Selected health indicators for Canada*. Retrieved October 26, 2002, from http://www3.who.int/whosis/country/indicators.cfm?country = CAN&language = english#economic.

WHO. (2002b). *Selected health indicators for Germany*. Retrieved October 26, 2002, from http://www3.who.int/whosis/country/indicators.cfm?country = DEU&language = english#economic.

WHO. (2002c). *Selected health indicators for Sweden*. Retrieved October 26, 2002, from http://www3.who.int/whosis/country/indicators.cfm?country = SWE&language = english#economic.

WHO. (2002d). *Selected health indicators for the Netherlands*. Retrieved October 26, 2002, from http://www3.who.int/whosis/country/indicators.cfm?country = NLD&language = english#economic.

WHO. (2002e). *Selected health indicators for the United Kingdom*. Retrieved October 26, 2002, from http://www3.who.int/whosis/country/indicators.cfm?country = GBR&language = english#economic.

WHO. (2004). *The world health report: 2004: Changing history*. Geneva, Switzerland: World Health Organization.

Williamson, O. E. (1999). Strategy research: Governance and competence perspectives. *Strategic Management Journal, 20*, 1087–1108.

Zivin, J. G., & Bridges, J. F. P. (2002). Addressing risk preferences in cost-effectiveness analyses. *Applied Health Economics and Health Policy, 1*(3), 135–139.

APPENDIX A. THE CANADIAN HEALTH CARE SYSTEM

Health Care Financing, Organization, and Delivery in Canada

Who is Covered?
The public system provides access to all Canadians (OECD, 2001).

What is Covered?
Services. Citizens receive coverage for ambulatory services, inpatient services, prescription medications, physician services, community health services, disease prevention programs, and health protection programs. Home care is covered at varying levels, with the national and provincial governments spending almost $3 billion on home care in 1999 (CIHI, 2002).

Cost-Sharing. Federal, territorial, provincial, and municipal governments share the cost of health care; social security paid only 1.9% of public expenditures on health in 2000.

How are Revenues Generated?
About 72% of total health care expenditures were paid with public funds in 2000. Supplementary private insurance accounted for 19.8% and out-of-pocket payments for 15.5% of total health expenditures; these sources were used primarily for drugs and dental care (WHO, 2002a).

How is the Delivery System Organized?
Physicians. Physicians organize and provide a variety of health care services, and they are compensated primarily via fee-for-service payments. Alternative plans (e.g., salary, and per diem or per capita payments) accounted for 11% of all clinical payments in 2000 (PAHO, 2001). Approximately 50% of physicians were GPs in 1998, and acted as gatekeepers for secondary and tertiary health services (CIHI, 2002).

Hospitals. Most hospitals are non-profit, autonomous entities that provide inpatient and ambulatory services, diagnostic testing, as well as other services. Hospitals are staffed with physicians, registered nurses, licensed practical nurses, registered psychiatric nurses, aides, and various other health care professionals. In many hospitals, the staff works to provide patient care through a primary care team.

Government. The Canada Health Act, passed in 1984, consolidates hospital and medical insurance into 12 inter-linked provincial/territorial health plans that are the sole payer for hospital and physician care. Additions made to the Act in 1996 and 1997 made provisions for federal contributions to health and social services. The 1996 and 1997 revisions consolidated contributions into the Canada Health and Social Transfer (CHST). The CHST transfer of taxes and cash payments equalizes funding (Department of Finance, 2002) and allows territories and provinces to control their systems of health care and social programs in accord with their own priorities. Nonetheless, the provincial and territorial health systems must meet the dictates of the Canada Health Act and provide social assistance with no minimum residency. Hence, the federal government is directly in charge of the health care services for the following groups: Royal Canadian Mounted Police, veterans, members of the armed forces, inmates in federal jails, Inuit, and status Indians.

How are Costs Controlled?

In addition to federal and provincial oversight of health care budgets, a variety of methods are used to control costs, including primary care gate-keeping, technology evaluations and rationalization (CCOHTA, 2002), and hospital budgets administered by local or regional health authorities (Frankish, Kwan, Ratner, Higgins, & Larsen, 2002).

How is Quality Measured and Improved?

On the hospital, provincial, and national levels, Canada is working to monitor levels of health performance and quality. The greater part of work to develop health indicators is taking place on the provincial level, while national efforts are still in the early stages. Significantly, in 1999, all first ministers (except the Premier of Quebec) signed a Social Union Framework, which provided a collaborative structure for social policy, including assurances for collecting and sharing health care data. In addition, two other entities have contributed to this national effort: the Canadian Institute for Health Information and the Canadian Council on Health Services Accreditation. Since 2000, the Canadian Institute for Health Information has produced annual reports on health indicators. It has worked cooperatively with the Canadian Council on Health Services Accreditation (CCHSA), which accredits hospitals. CCHSA introduced Client-Centered Accreditation in 1995 ensuring principles of quality improvement were incorporated into accreditation standards. In 2000, CCHSA's Achieving Improved Measurement (AIM) Project updated the accreditation process with standardized performance indicators based on four quality dimensions: responsiveness, system competency, client/community focus, and work life (Hurst & Jee-Hughes, 2001).

APPENDIX B. THE FINNISH HEALTH CARE SYSTEM

Health Care Financing, Organization, and Delivery in Finland

Who is Covered?
All citizens, immigrants, and residents are covered by the national health-care system.

What is Covered?
Services. Preventive care, public health care, prescription drugs, inpatient and outpatient care, dental care, long-term care and rehabilitation, and mental health care are covered.

Cost-Sharing. Patients pay for private care; user charges are imposed for some publicly provided health services.

How are Revenues Generated?
General Taxation. All residents pay income tax, which comprises two elements: a set-rate city-of-residence-specific municipal tax (15–20%) and a highly progressive national income tax. The government allocates municipalities a so-called state share every year depending on the financial condition and demographic profile of the municipality. Municipalities provide primary care services and buy hospitalized and specialized care from hospital districts. In 2002, health care expenses accounted for 7.3% of the GDP; on average, health care accounted for 25% of the municipal budgets. An extensive system of reimbursement for services, medication, and equipment that are not provided without charge by the public system, but belong to the national health care system exists. The national pension and reimbursement authority (Kela) coordinates mandatory health care and social insurance payments (on average 1.6% of gross salary) and offers partial or complete reimbursement for a variety of services, including rehabilitation, medication, the use of private sector physicians, dental care, and medical equipment.

Private and Occupational Health Plans. Private health plans are new and uncommon, as private insurance accounts for 2% of total health expenditures (WHO, 2002e). Out-of-pocket payments include payment for non-prescription medications, non-covered surgical, ophthalmic, dental, rehabilitation and elderly care services, as well as other private health care (although the latter may be entirely or partially covered through private, occupational or public health insurance). In 2000, out-of-pocket expenditures accounted for approximately 20.2% of total health care expenditures (WHO, 2004). The public system also collects minor fees for GP visits and hospital hotel services as a patient incentive for rational use of these services.

How is the Delivery System Organized?

Physicians. Municipalities in Finland organize primary care in 279 primary care centers, with smaller municipalities or group of municipalities usually having a larger health care center and larger cities running a network of health stations. A system of population responsibility, with assigned GPs for every citizen, is widely used. The usage of private primary care services is also increasing (14% in 2003) (Ministry of Social Affairs and Health, 2004). Primary care physicians make referrals to specialists. In municipal primary care organizations, most (over 90%) of the physicians are GPs, and specialists work under the hospital districts. It is not uncommon for GPs to do part-time work in the private sector, hospitals, or elsewhere. Some health centers and stations also provide minor-scale acute care services.

Hospitals. Public specialized and hospitalized care is organized into 21 hospital districts that are owned by the municipalities surrounding them (6–58 municipalities per district) (Ministry of Social Affairs and Health, 2004). The hospital district organizations run many administrative functions, attempting to provide and coordinate as many overhead services to the hospitals as possible. The public hospital system comprises (1) area-specific district general hospitals, (2) large university hospitals, and (3) specialized clinics that often work in conjunction or at least in the immediate vicinity of hospitals. A significant share of specialist work is run in private practices, whose services can also be used by the public sector through referral. The share between private and public specialist care varies tremendously from specialty to specialty, with the private sector strongly represented, e.g., eye surgery, orthopedic surgery, bypass surgery, allergy care, gyneacology, and urology services.

Government. The government has handed out much of the organizing tasks to the municipalities, but retains a strong role as a financier, legislator, and policy-maker. The Ministry of Social Affairs and Health coordinates the system (e.g., physician training, financing, employment policies, current care guidelines, norms, and rules) and works closely together with the national pension and reimbursement authority that essentially runs a public health insurance and compensation plan for the entire population.

How are Costs Controlled?
General practitioners act as gatekeepers to all government run and much of privately run specialized health care. Health care expenditure planning takes place during the government's general public expenditure planning process during the annual budget rounds. Government funding for primary and hospitalized is allocated to municipalities, whose task is to decide how spending is divided between the two. Municipalities run their own primary health care stations and are responsible for controlling their costs. The municipalities attain representation in the boards of hospital districts in return for their ownership. The costs of the hospital districts are controlled through complex and varying mechanisms ranging from hospital district management accounting practices and quarterly reporting to municipalities to benchmarking across districts and reporting to political decision-making organs. Demand management takes place through waiting lists for non-emergency care. In general, cost control is exercised in Finland extensively by all involved parties (most importantly the government, reimbursement authorities, hospital districts, and municipalities), to the extent that doubts of adverse effects emerging from partial optimization of the system have been identified (Tolkki et al., 2004). Most frequently employed cost-control mechanisms include benchmarking, budgeting, indexing, and building cost profiles for municipalities.

How is Quality Measured and Improved?
Quality management is generally common and advanced in Finnish health care organizations. The Ministry of Social Affairs and Health publishes specific quality guidelines for certain health care activities, and the League of Municipalities publishes statistics that monitor health care quality. As of 2000, 16% of Finnish health care organizations had either received or were applying for the National Quality Award, with 15% of these health care organizations applying for the ISO 9000 certificate. The first Finnish ISO 9000 quality system was adopted in 1995, and the first ISO 9002 quality certification took place in 1999. As of 1999, over 50% of Finnish hospitals had started building a quality system.

APPENDIX C. THE GERMAN HEALTH
CARE SYSTEM

Health Care Financing, Organization, and Delivery in Germany

Who is Covered?
Everyone is eligible to participate in the public system. Individuals above a determined income level have the right to obtain private coverage. Statutory health insurance covers 88% of the population. Of this 88%, mandatory members and their dependents account for 74%, while 14% of members are voluntary. Private health insurance covers 9% of the population (the affluent, self-employed, and civil servants). Free government health care for those on social welfare, police officers, and those in the military (or civil alternative) covers 2% of the population. The uninsured represent less than 0.2% of Germany's citizens (Busse, 2002a).

What is Covered?
Services. The benefits covered include health screening and prevention, non-physician care, ambulatory medical services, inpatient care, home nursing care, dental care, and some types of rehabilitation (Busse & Riesberg, 2000).

Cost-Sharing. While there have traditionally been few cost-sharing provisions, recent reforms shift costs to patients via user charges (Brown & Amelung, 1999). Co-payments exist for pharmaceuticals, non-physician care, dental treatments, ambulance transportation, and initial hospitalization or rehabilitation. Nonetheless, these charges are limited or exempted for those with low incomes, chronic illnesses, or who are under 18 years.

How are Revenues Generated?
Sickness Insurance Funds (SIFs). The chief system for financing health care is through contributions toward statutory health insurance, which had 420 sickness funds in 2000. In 2002, the average contribution rate was 14%, with that cost being shared between employee and employer. The unemployed, the homeless, and immigrants are covered through a special sickness fund financed through general revenues. In 2000, sickness funds accounted for 68.8% of total health expenditures (WHO, 2002b).

Other Sources. In 2000, the three other major sources of finance within the statutory insurance-based system included private health insurance (12.5%

of health expenditures), out-of-pocket payments (10.6% of health expenditures), and taxes (6.2% of health expenditures).

How is the Delivery System Organized?
Physicians. Only physician association members may treat members of the sickness fund on an ambulatory basis. General practitioners have no formal gatekeeper function, accounting for less than 40% of ambulatory physicians. Private-practice physicians are paid on a fee-for-service basis. Regional and national representatives of the sickness funds negotiate with the regional and national associations of physicians to determine aggregate payments.

Hospitals. There are 2030 general hospitals, of which fewer than 40% (790) are publicly owned. Private for-profit hospitals account for around 20% of the total, with non-profit private hospitals accounting for more than 40%. However, almost all of these general hospitals contract with the social insurance funds. They are staffed with salaried junior and senior doctors. However, physician medical department heads may charge private patients fee-for-service charges. The 1992 Health Care Structure Act and subsequent pieces of legislation introduced an inpatient prospective payment system. Representatives of the sickness funds negotiate with individual hospitals over prospective payment rates.

Government. The Federal Ministry for Health and the parliament are in charge of the health care at the national level. Decision-making authority is shared between the federal government and the 16 Lander (states). One of their most significant roles is to oversee the sickness funds and voluntary insurance companies, assuring a level playing field for competition. Because sickness funds vary in their income and expenditures depending upon their pools of insured people, a compensation scheme operates to equalize these differences, requiring transfers of income from low cost sickness funds to sickness funds with high expenditures.

How are Costs Controlled?
Sickness funds are the purchasers of health care for statutory health insurance. Due to competition among funds, selective purchasing has recently become an issue. Physicians' associations are given a global budget by the sickness funds. The associations use a Uniform Value Scale to pay their members. Control measures are in place for physician reimbursement in order to prevent false claims or overutilization. Sources for hospital funding

include operating costs from the sickness funds and investment costs from the Lander. The 1992 Health Care Structure Act and subsequent pieces of legislation introduced an inpatient prospective payment system. Representatives of the sickness funds negotiate with individual hospitals over prospective payment rates. A referral from an ambulatory doctor is necessary for admission to hospitals except in cases of emergency.

How is Quality Measured and Improved?
Traditionally, physician specialty societies have monitored and attempted to improve the quality of medical care through structural means. However, after passage of a revised Social Security Act on quality assurance, physicians' associations have started quality management projects. The Social Code Book V introduced the Federal Coordination Committee and the Federal Committee Hospital, as well as determining the duties of the Federal Committee for Improvement of Quality Assurance. The responsibility of these committees is to insure use of quality assurance measures (Sauerland, 2001). Many institutions and commissions also are trying to develop quality assurance activities focusing on formulating practice guidelines (Birkner, 1998).

APPENDIX D. THE DUTCH HEALTH CARE SYSTEM

Health Care Financing, Organization, and Delivery in the Netherlands

Who is Covered?
All citizens are covered under the Algemene Wet Bijzondere Ziektekosten (Exceptional Medical Expenses Act, or AWBZ) that provides funding for long-term, disability, and chronic psychiatric care. All citizens with an annual income below a set level must enroll under the Ziekenfondswet (Medical Insurance Access Act, or ZFW) into a public social insurance fund for acute and short-term health care (64% of the population in 2002). Those with an annual income above the determined level must purchase private social health insurance for medical care (Busse, 2002b). Public servants (5% of population) enroll in one of three separate insurance plans that cover medical expenses.

What is Covered?
Services. A compulsory benefit package includes preventive services, inpatient and outpatient hospital care, physician services, mental health care,

long-term care, preventive dental care, prescription drugs, rehabilitation, and sick leave compensation. Citizens may choose among providers who have contracts with their sickness or private insurance fund.

Cost-Sharing. Patients pay 20% of specialists' and pharmaceutical charges, with a maximum of about US $100 per year. Private insurers also assess apportionment charges to cover the difference between the claims and the premiums of those insured under ZFW. These losses are apportioned among private insurance policyholders under the age of 65. In 2000, out-of-pocket payments accounted for 8.6% of total health expenditures (WHO, 2002d).

How are Revenues Generated?
ZFW. Citizens with an annual income below a certain level (below €31,750 in 2003) must enroll in a sickness fund. The ZFW is funded by compulsory payroll contributions and by a flat fee set in a risk-adjusted fashion by each insurer. Retirees over 65 paid 6.8% of their pension income, and 4.8% of other earned income in 1998, plus the flat fee. Additionally, government grants (general revenue) are used to equalize funding. Sickness funds may offer supplemental policies to extend coverage; about 90% of those enrolled purchase supplemental coverage.

AWBZ. Long-term care and exceptional medical expenses are funded through fixed percentage contributions (9.6% of taxable income in 1998) from each employee (paid by employers) and from the self-employed, as well from government grants (general revenue) and through limited cost sharing.

Private Insurance. In 2000, private insurance accounted for 24.9% of total health expenditures (WHO, 2002d). However, private insurers cover about 30% of the population for acute care. As of January 1, 2002, the premium for private insurance increased an average 12%. Private insurers are required to contribute a portion of their revenues to equalize funding for the sickness insurance funds (under ZWF) that serve a disproportionate share of the elderly.

General Taxation. The central government subsidizes funding under both AZWB and ZWF; these two social insurance funds accounted for 63.5% of total health expenditures in 2000, with general revenues accounting for slightly less than 4% of total health expenditures (WHO, 2002d).

How is the Delivery System Organized?
Physicians. General practitioners have a formal gatekeeper function. For primary care patients, GPs are paid on a capitation basis under ZWF, but fee-for-service under private insurance. Specialists are paid on a scheduled fee-for-service basis.

Hospitals. For-profit and not-for-profit hospitals, may be either private or public. Physician-specialists enter into exclusive contracts with hospitals. The contracts customarily include exclusive rights to practice, along with shared income agreements that may include fee for service components. Academic hospitals increasingly have turned to straight salary compensation for physicians. However, as indicated below, these forms of physician compensation began undergoing reforms in January 2004. Most other health care professionals receive union or association negotiated salaries.

Government. The Dutch government regulates the sickness insurance funds and private insurers by mandating services to be covered and setting income-related maximums on premiums. Major reform efforts during the early 1990s to reduce government interventions in favor of a self-regulating – managed competition – system largely have been thwarted. Recently enacted reforms are noted below.

How are Costs Controlled?
Payroll and income tax premiums for AWBZ and ZFW are paid into a central regulatory body, the Sickness Fund Council. The Sickness Fund Council decides on a prospective global budget for each sickness insurance fund; it also decides on a fixed cost budget for hospital capital and maintenance expenses, paid largely through government grants. The sickness funds use both their own flat-fee premiums plus the global budget to pay for hospital and physician services. The Central Office on Health Care Tariffs (COTG) sets out guidelines for the composition and calculation of tariffs, including both fees-for-service and capitated payments to physicians and hospitals. Rather than directly setting prices, the COTG relies on setting the parameters for a bargaining process between regional providers – hospitals, physicians, and other medical professionals – and regional buyers, including both sickness funds and private insurers, for determining fees, capitation, and other prices. The COTG then reviews these prices to ensure that they are within the guidelines for each income group.

Health care reforms to increase competition among sickness funds and among providers have included (a) allowing sickness funds to selectively contract with GPs and pharmacists; (b) transforming premium setting for sickness fund and private insurers, with 90% of the premium being income-related and set by the government and 10% being a flat fee set in a risk-adjusted fashion by each insurer; and (c) relaxing regulations on negotiating fees for service and capitation rates. Beginning in January 2003, a new system based on diagnosis and treatment combination (DBC) was implemented for reimbursing hospitals and medical specialists. This prospective payment system takes into account the degree to which the demand for care falls to the hospital and the medical specialists, how demand for care should be handled, and the costs associated with this service. It differs from diagnostic-related groups (DRGs) in that the entire episode of care, including out-patient treatment, is included (Ministry of Health, 2002).

How is Quality Measured and Improved?
Based on 1989 legislation, quality management is the responsibility of both health care professionals and management, with input from insurers and patients. Three different approaches have been undertaken to manage health care quality (Klazinga, Lombarts, & van Everdingen, 1998). The National Organization for Quality Assurance in Hospitals not only conducts peer review activities of physician practices, but also supports efforts aimed at quality assurance in hospitals. In addition, 28 scientific societies accredit various medical specialties, conducting site visits that assess quality process management, use of guidelines, and the evaluation of patient satisfaction and treatment outcomes. More than 60 consensus guidelines have been developed for and by medical professionals, with input from patient organizations and third-party payers. Medical specialty and general practice associations also have created practice guidelines (Crebolder & van der Horst, 1996).

APPENDIX E. THE SWEDISH HEALTH CARE SYSTEM

Health Care Financing, Organization, and Delivery in Sweden

Who is Covered?
All citizens are covered by the system, as well as immigrants and residents (Hjortsberg & Chatnekar, 2001).

What is Covered?
Services. Preventive care, public health care, prescription drugs, inpatient and outpatient care, dental care, long-term care and rehabilitation, and mental health care are covered. Patients are able to choose the principal health care provider. Choices may also be made concerning outpatient facilities and health centers in the county council. A referral may be necessary for care outside the individual's county council.

Cost-Sharing. Voluntary health insurance that supplements the national health system coverage accounts for less than 1% of the total health care revenue. Direct user charges accounted for about 2% of total health expenditures in 2000 (León & Rico, 2002).

How are Revenues Generated?
Income and Payroll Taxes. Income taxes are levied on residents with rates determined by county councils and municipalities. The average collective rate of taxation of local income is around 30%. Health care accounts for 85% of total county expenditures and is managed and overseen at the county level. Total taxation, through county taxes (66%) and national taxes (7–11%), accounted for 77.3% of total expenditures on health care in 2000 (WHO, 2002c). National payroll taxes (8.5% of the employees' salary) are paid by the employer for social insurance, and accounted for about 25% of public health expenditures in 2000 (León & Rico, 2002).

Private Health Payments. According to WHO data, out-of-pocket expenditures accounted for 22.7% of total health expenditures in 2000 (WHO, 2002c). Dental and pharmaceutical co-payments, as well as private physician supplemental charges, are the major costs associated with out-of-pocket expenses (Hjortsberg & Chatnekar, 2001).

How is the Delivery System Organized?
Basic Care and Public Health Centers. Basic care – preventive, primary, and public health – is provided at 900 public health centers (SPRI, 1998; Swedish Institute, 1999). In addition to physicians, patients may receive care from district nurses and other mid-level providers.

Physicians. General practitioners serve as family doctors, but not as gatekeepers. Most physicians (80%) are specialists. Physicians employed by the government typically are paid a salary if they are specialists; GPs may be remunerated prospectively via capitation. Private providers may set their own fee-for-service rates, but must adhere to county and national guidelines if they are to be reimbursed by the public system. In order to be reimbursed by social insurance, private health care providers must have an agreement with the county council. Other physicians must use the regulated fee schedule or receive payment directly from the patient. Public general practitioners are employed by county councils and receive a monthly salary in relation to their qualifications and work schedule.

Hospitals. Sweden has 79 hospitals, which are divided into regional, central country, or district county hospitals according to their degree of specialization and size. The majority of hospitals are publicly funded.

Government. The National Board of Health and Welfare supervises the county councils. It also acts as the supervisory and advisory agency for health and social services, as well as licensing agency for all health care personnel. County councils have authority over primary and inpatient care, including public health and preventive care. After 1992, the role of financing changed for county councils. With the Ädel reform, local municipalities were held responsible for social welfare services to elderly individuals, as well as the disabled. They also became responsible for long-term inpatient care.

How are Costs Controlled?
To control utilization and costs, Sweden's central government has controlled physician training, capital expenditures, and equalization and incentive grants to the county councils. County councils and municipalities have imposed tight fiscal controls on the number of health care personnel and on their salaries. During the 1990s, overall employment in health care was reduced by 25% (Diderichsen, 1999). Since 1995, each county council has rationed care using the principles of human rights, individual need, solidarity, and cost-effectiveness. Many elective procedures (e.g., *in vitro* fertilization) are not performed unless the patient directly pays for the service. The 1992 Guarantee of Care Act balances these fiscal restrictions with consumer responsiveness: patients placed on a waiting list for non-acute, low priority problems should have services provided within three months (WHO, 1996). Other cost-control mechanisms include a drive for evidence-based care, as well as economic evaluations of medical technologies (Jönsson, 1997).

How is Quality Measured and Improved?
The National Board of Health and Welfare produced a set of guidelines concerning quality in 1994. These guidelines were updated in 1997 by a law

requiring the health services to implement a system of continuous quality improvement (CQI). Several national organizations are involved in this effort to diffuse CQI methods and tools throughout Swedish health care, with most of the actual CQI work performed at the local level (Palmberg, 1997). The Federation of Swedish County Councils has developed 50 health care quality registers to implement and benchmark CQI systems in health care. The Federation also promotes a competition for the Swedish Health Services Quality Award (Swedish Institute, 1999).

APPENDIX F. THE BRITISH HEALTH CARE SYSTEM

Health Care Financing, Organization, and Delivery in the United Kingdom

Who is Covered?
All residents of the United Kingdom (England, Wales, Scotland, and Northern Ireland) are covered under the National Health Service (NHS).

What is Covered?
Services. Although health services are not specified, they generally include preventive services, inpatient and outpatient hospital care, physician services, inpatient and outpatient drugs, dental care, mental health care, and rehabilitation. Citizens may choose a general practitioner within their locale.

Cost-Sharing. All hospital and specialist services are supplied without charge to the patient; however, user charges occur for outpatient drugs, dentistry, and ophthalmology. Approximately 2% of income for NHS is derived from user charges (Dixon & Robinson, 2002).

How are Revenues Generated?
General Taxation. In 2000, taxes raised by the national government accounted for 81% of total expenditures on health care, with social security contributions making up 11.2% of NHS funding (WHO, 2002e).

Private Insurance. About 11.5% of the population has private health insurance (Dixon & Robinson, 2002), which can be divided into two major forms: individual insurance (31% of all private insurance) and employment-based insurance funded by employers (59%). The remainder of private insurance is funded by premiums paid by employees. Both for-profit and non-profit companies provide private health insurance (Robinson & Dixon,

1999). Private insurance accounted for approximately 3.2% of total health expenditures in 2000 (WHO, 2002e).

Out-of-pocket payments include payment for non-prescription medications, ophthalmic and dental services, as well as private health care (although the latter may be covered through private health insurance). In 2000, out-of-pocket expenditures accounted for approximately 10.6% of total health care expenditures (WHO, 2002e).

How is the Delivery System Organized?

Physicians. The NHS has a well-developed primary care system made up of GPs and other mid-level providers (e.g., midwives and practice nurses) and other health care professionals. General practitioners make referrals to specialists. On the one hand, NHS pays GPs as independent, self-employed professionals using a mix of fixed allowances, capitation fees, and some specific fees for services. On the other hand, the NHS employs consultants (hospital-based physician specialists) directly and pays them a set salary. Consultants may supplement their salary by treating private patients. However, full-time consultants are limited to earning only 10% of their gross salary from private service. Part-time consultants face no restrictions (Dixon & Robinson, 2002).

Hospitals. Most hospitals provide general acute care services, along with some outpatient services. The NHS hospital system comprises three tiers: (1) small community hospitals (size: 50–200 beds) offering secondary care and outpatient surgery (number: 400); (2) district general hospitals offering secondary and tertiary care (number: 200); and (3) regional, typically teaching, hospitals offering specialized tertiary care. For the most part, these NHS hospitals are publicly owned with independent trust status. As of 1998, independent medical/surgical hospitals totaled 230 (Robinson & Dixon, 1999; Dixon & Robinson, 2002).

Government. As a purchaser and provider of health care, the national government retains responsibility for health legislation and general policy. However, under the Labour Party, the administration of NHS has been devolved to the Departments of Health under the leadership of the Secretaries of State in each country of the U.K. Moreover, the responsibility for purchasing health services also is being devolved, and is the responsibility of Primary Care Trusts in England, Health Boards in Scotland, local health groups in Wales, and Primary Care Partnerships in Northern Ireland (Robinson & Dixon, 1999).

How are Costs Controlled?
General practitioners act as gatekeepers to specialized care in NHS. Health care expenditure planning takes place during the government's general public expenditure planning process. The NHS funding for the following year is established during this process. To control utilization and costs, the U.K. has controlled physician training, capital expenditure, pay, and purchaser budgets. There are also waiting lists for non-emergency care. In addition, a centralized administrative system results in lower overhead costs. Other cost-control mechanisms include a drive for clinically cost-effective care, formal efficiency targets, and benchmarking.

How is Quality Measured and Improved?
Since coming to power in 1997, the Labour government has increased the funding for the NHS to improve its infrastructure. The government has also promoted quality goals by establishing measures to put people and patients at the center of the health service. The central government set up a Performance Assessment Framework to monitor how well NHS organizations are performing (Le Grand, 2002). The National Institute for Clinical Excellence (NICE) was established within the NHS in 1999 to provide patients, health professionals and the public with authoritative, robust, and reliable guidance on current "best practice" for both individual health (including medicines, medical devices, diagnostic techniques, and procedures) and the clinical management of specific conditions (Le Grand, Mays, & Mulligan, 1999).

APPENDIX G. THE UNITED STATES HEALTH CARE SYSTEM

Health Care Financing, Organization, and Delivery in the U.S.

Who is Covered?
About 85.4% of the population in 2001 was covered by either public (25.3%) or private (70.9%) health insurance. However, 10.8% of the population was covered both by public and private insurance (Mills, 2002).

What is Covered?
Services. Benefit packages vary with the type of insurance, but typically include inpatient and outpatient hospital care and physician services. Many

private plans also include preventive services, dental care, and prescription drug coverage.

Cost-Sharing. User charges vary by type of insurance, but typically include outpatient and prescription drug co-payments, as well as deductibles for hospitalization. Out-of-pocket payments accounted for 15% of health expenditures in 2000 (Mills, 2002).

How are Revenues Generated?
Medicare. This national social health insurance program covers health services for the elderly, the disabled, and those with end-stage renal disease. Administered by the Centers for Medicare and Medicaid Services (CMS), Medicare covered 13.5% of the population in 2001 (Mills, 2002). The program is financed through a combination of payroll taxes, general federal revenues, and premiums. It accounted for 17.3% of total health expenditures in 2000 (CMS, 2002).

Medicaid. A joint federal-state health benefit program covering targeted groups of the poor, e.g., pregnant women, families with children, and the disabled, Medicaid is administered by the states, which operate within broad federal guidelines overseen by CMS. It covered 11.2% of the population in 2001 (Mills, 2002) and accounted for 15.6% of total health expenditures in 2000 (CMS, 2002). The program is financed by general federal tax revenues (9.1% of total health expenditures in 2000), which match tax revenues raised by each state (6.5% of total health expenditures in 2000). The ratio of matching federal funds varies for each state depending upon its per capita income.

State Children's Health Insurance Program (SCHIP). A state-federal health benefit program targeting poor children, SCHIP is jointly administered by CMS and the states and covers about 1.6% of the population. It is funded by federal (5.3% of total) and state taxes (7.0% of total) (CMS, 2002).

Private Insurance. Provided by not-for-profit and for-profit health insurance companies regulated by state insurance commissioners, private health insurance can be purchased by individuals, although most people receive employer-based insurance. Many large employers self-fund health benefits for their employees, using insurance companies as third party administrators. Private insurance covered 70.9% of the total population, with 62.6% of the population receiving employment-based insurance in 2000 (Mills,

2002). It accounted for 32.6% of total health expenditures in 2000 (CMS, 2002).

How is the Delivery System Organized?

Physicians. General practitioners usually have no formal gatekeeper function, except within some managed care plans. While the majority of physicians are in private practice, increasingly physicians are being employed by medical group practices, health maintenance organizations, or organized delivery systems (Cosca, 1999). They are paid through a combination of methods: charges, discounted fees paid by private health plans, capitation contracts with private plans, public programs, and direct patient fees.

Hospitals. For-profit, non-profit, and public hospitals are paid through a combination of methods: charges, per admission rates, and capitation. Prospective payment based on DRGs is the norm for reimbursement in Medicare.

Government. The federal government is the single largest health care insurer and purchaser.

How are Costs Controlled?

Third-party payers and private insurers have attempted to control cost growth through a combination of selective provider contracting, discounted price negotiations, utilization control practices, risk-sharing payment methods, and other managed care techniques. Following the Balanced Budget Act of 1997, the federal government has reduced reimbursements for hospitals, physicians, and others providing services to Medicare and Medicaid recipients (Levit et al., 2000).

How is Quality Measured and Improved?

Hospitals. Almost all hospitals have established continuous quality improvement programs in order to comply with voluntary standards imposed by accrediting bodies such as the Joint Commission on Accreditation of Healthcare Organizations (http://www.jcaho.org/index.html).

Managed Care Organizations. A voluntary private–public endeavor, The National Committee for Quality Assurance (NCQA) accredits private health plans and has been instrumental in developing the Health Plan Employer Data and Information Set (HEDIS). The NCQA has had growing but limited impact on improving the quality of patient care provided through managed care organizations; participating organizations voluntarily report patient satisfaction and other measures of quality as measured using HEDIS (Gabel, Hunt, & Hurst, 1998).

Government. The federal government through the Agency for Healthcare Quality and Research funds numerous efforts to improve clinical and overall quality, including evidence-based medicine guidelines and protocols.

AUTHOR INDEX

SUBJECT INDEX

COUNTRY INDEX

393

SET UP A CONTINUATION ORDER TODAY!

Did you know that you can set up a continuation order on all Elsevier-JAI series and have each new volume sent directly to you upon publication? For details on how to set up a **continuation order**, contact your nearest regional sales office listed below.

To view related series in Business & Management, please visit:

www.elsevier.com/businessandmanagement

The Americas
Customer Service Department
11830 Westline Industrial Drive
St. Louis, MO 63146
USA
US customers:
Tel: +1 800 545 2522 (Toll-free number)
Fax: +1 800 535 9935
For Customers outside US:
Tel: +1 800 460 3110 (Toll-free number).
Fax: +1 314 453 7095
usbkinfo@elsevier.com

Europe, Middle East & Africa
Customer Service Department
Linacre House
Jordan Hill
Oxford OX2 8DP
UK
Tel: +44 (0) 1865 474140
Fax: +44 (0) 1865 474141
eurobkinfo@elsevier.com

Japan
Customer Service Department
2F Higashi Azabu, 1 Chome Bldg
1-9-15 Higashi Azabu, Minato-ku
Tokyo 106-0044
Japan
Tel: +81 3 3589 6370
Fax: +81 3 3589 6371
books@elsevierjapan.com

APAC
Customer Service Department
3 Killiney Road #08-01
Winsland House I
Singapore 239519
Tel: +65 6349 0222
Fax: +65 6733 1510
asiainfo@elsevier.com

Australia & New Zealand
Customer Service Department
30-52 Smidmore Street
Marrickville, New South Wales 2204
Australia
Tel: +61 (02) 9517 8999
Fax: +61 (02) 9517 2249
service@elsevier.com.au

30% Discount for Authors on All Books!

A 30% discount is available to Elsevier book and journal contributors on all books *(except multi-volume reference works)*.

To claim your discount, full payment is required with your order, which must be sent directly to the publisher at the nearest regional sales office above.